Platform Trial Designs in Drug Development

Chapman & Hall/CRC Biostatistics Series

Shein-Chung Chow, Duke University of Medicine
Byron Jones, Novartis Pharma AG
Jen-pei Liu, National Taiwan University
Karl E. Peace, Georgia Southern University
Bruce W. Turnbull, Cornell University

Recently Published Titles

Medical Biostatistics, Fourth Edition
Abhaya Indrayan, Rajeev Kumar Malhotra

Self-Controlled Case Series Studies: A Modelling Guide with R
Paddy Farrington, Heather Whitaker, Yonas Ghebremichael Weldeselassie

Bayesian Methods for Repeated Measures
Lyle D. Broemeling

Modern Adaptive Randomized Clinical Trials: Statistical and Practical Aspects
Oleksandr Sverdlov

Medical Product Safety Evaluation: Biological Models and Statistical Methods
Jie Chen, Joseph Heyse, Tze Leung Lai

Statistical Methods for Survival Trial Design With Applications to Cancer Clinical Trials Using R
Jianrong Wu

Bayesian Applications in Pharmaceutical Development
Satrajit Roychoudhury, Soumi Lahiri

Platform Trials in Drug Development: Umbrella Trials and Basket Trials
Zoran Antonijevic and Robert A. Beckman

For more information about this series, please visit: https://www.crcpress.com/go/biostats

Platform Trial Designs in Drug Development

Umbrella Trials and Basket Trials

Edited by
Zoran Antonijevic and
Robert A. Beckman

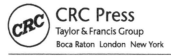

CRC Press is an imprint of the
Taylor & Francis Group, an **informa** business

A CHAPMAN & HALL BOOK

CRC Press
Taylor & Francis Group
6000 Broken Sound Parkway NW, Suite 300
Boca Raton, FL 33487-2742

© 2019 by Taylor & Francis Group, LLC
CRC Press is an imprint of Taylor & Francis Group, an Informa business

No claim to original U.S. Government works

Printed on acid-free paper

International Standard Book Number-13: 978-1-138-05245-1 (Hardback)

Visit the Taylor & Francis Web site at
http://www.taylorandfrancis.com

and the CRC Press Web site at
http://www.crcpress.com

Contents

Preface ix
Acknowledgments xiii
List of Contributors xv

Part I   Overview of Platform Clinical Trials 1

1   I-SPY2: Unlocking the Potential of the Platform Trial 3
    Laura Esserman, Nola Hylton, Smita Asare, Christina Yau,
    Doug Yee, Angie DeMichele, Jane Perlmutter, Fraser Symmans,
    Laura van't Veer, Jeff Matthews, Donald A. Berry, and Anna Barker

2   The Challenges with Multi-Arm Targeted Therapy Trials 23
    Ryan J. Sullivan and Keith T. Flaherty

3   Basket Trials at the Confirmatory Stage 37
    Robert A. Beckman and Cong Chen

4   Harnessing Real-World Data to Inform Platform
    Trial Design 55
    Daphne Guinn, Subha Madhavan, and Robert A. Beckman

5   Impact of Platform Trials on Pharmaceutical Frameworks 73
    Zoran Antonijevic, Ed Mills, Jonas Häggström, and
    Kristian Thorlund

Part II   Stakeholders 83

6   Friends of Cancer Research Perspective on Platform Trials 85
    Jeffrey D. Allen, Madison Wempe, Ryan Hohman, and Ellen V. Sigal

7   Regulatory and Policy Aspects of Platform Trials 97
    Rasika Kalamegham, Ramzi Dagher, and Peter Honig

8   Multi-Arm, Multi-Drug Trials from a Reimbursement
    Perspective 119
    Anja Schiel and Olivier Collignon

9 Highly Efficient Clinical Trials: A Resource-Saving Solution
   for Global Health 125
   Edward J. Mills, Jonas Häggström, and Kristian Thorlund

10 Decision Analysis from the Perspectives of Single and
   Multiple Stakeholders.....................................141
   *Robert A. Beckman, Carl-Fredrik Burman, Cong Chen,
   Sebastian Jobjörnsson, Franz König, Nigel Stallard, and
   Martin Posch*

11 Optimal Approach for Addressing Multiple Stakeholders'
   Requirements in Drug Development 153
   Zoran Antonijevic and Zhongshen Wang

Part III Statistical Methodology.....................165

12 Primary Site Independent Clinical Trials in Oncology..........167
   Richard M. Simon

13 Platform Trials 181
   Ben Saville and Scott Berry

14 Efficiencies of Platform Trials 197
   Satrajit Roychoudhury and Ohad Amit

15 Control of Type I Error for Confirmatory Basket Trials 211
   Cong Chen and Robert A. Beckman

16 Benefit-Risk Assessment for Platform Trials...................231
   Chunlei Ke and Qi Jiang

17 Effect of Randomization Schemes in Umbrella Trials
   When There Are Unknown Interactions between
   Biomarkers..253
   Janet J. Li, Shuai Sammy Yuan, and Robert A. Beckman

18 Combinatorial and Model-Based Methods in Structuring
   and Optimizing Cluster Trials...............................265
   Valerii V. Fedorov and Sergei L. Leonov

Part IV Conclusions 287

19 An Executive's View of Value of Platform Trials 289
David Reese and Phuong Khanh Morrow

Index. 295

Preface

Platform trials, including umbrella and basket trials, test multiple therapies in one indication, one therapy for multiple indications, or both. As readers will learn in this volume, these novel clinical trial designs have the potential to dramatically increase the cost-effectiveness of drug development, leading to more life-altering medicines for people suffering from serious illnesses. Further, these medicines may be available at lower cost. Necessity is indeed the mother of invention in this instance, as the increasing cost of drug development is becoming unsustainable. Two particular problem areas are rare diseases, in which it may be quite difficult to accrue sufficient patients for traditional trial designs, and oncology, where increasing molecular understanding is creating small biomarker-defined subgroups from which it is also a challenge to accrue, and where the large number of such subgroups and the corresponding larger numbers of experimental therapies create a combinatorial explosion of reasonable testable clinical trial hypotheses.

Our intention was to recruit the key leaders and innovators in this domain, to give them free rein to discuss what they felt to be most important with minimal editorial constraints, and to cover the topic from multiple perspectives, including some that are unconventional. We have indeed been fortunate to collect thoughts from many of those who broke new ground to form and advance this field, and from a variety of creative thinkers viewing these trial designs from perspectives as diverse as quantum computing, patient's rights to information, and international health.

We begin this book with an overview of platform trials from multiple perspectives. The first two chapters following this introduction present the case for platform clinical trials by describing the benefits and associated challenges of two of the most influential, I-SPY2 and NCI-MATCH, written by their principal investigators and colleagues. In contrast to these two platform trials focusing on the exploratory stage of drug development, the next chapter proposes a new basket design potentially acceptable at the confirmatory stage. The section concludes with chapters describing the use of real world data to optimally design platform trials, and how to optimally deploy platform trials at the level of pharmaceutical portfolios.

The second part of the book describes views of and impacts on key stakeholders: patients, regulators, and payers. They are presented in the first three chapters of this section respectively, and written by expert representatives. These perspectives are followed by a discussion of potential global health benefits of perpetual platform trials. The final chapters of the second section address complexities of decision making in the presence of multiple stakeholders. The first focuses on alignment among multiple stakeholders, while the other proposes optimal development pathways in the presence of differing stakeholders' requirements.

In Part III, renowned statisticians discuss a variety of methodological issues. This section contains some chapters that go into mathematical detail. The first two chapters provide an overview of statistical designs and tools for basket trials and platform trials in general, including applications. The subsequent chapters cover a variety of topics, including estimating efficiencies of platform trials, Type I error control in the basket trial design proposed in Part I, benefit-risk assessment within platform trials, and the problem of patient allocation to strata when they are positive for multiple biomarkers. The section ends with a visionary application of quantum computing to platform trials.

An executive's view of the value of platform trials for pharmaceutical companies concludes the book.

Given the approach in creating it, this book is a snapshot of a very dynamic field poised to greatly influence the development of experimental therapies. This dynamic nature was immediately evident when we held the first teleconference with authors, and there were several competing definitions of basic terms such as "platform trial," "master protocol," and "umbrella trial." Under these circumstances, selecting the book's title was challenging and controversial. We included basket trials in the book, although for some authors this was inconsistent with the book's original title, "Platform Trials." We learned that some would not include basket trials in the definition of platform trials. Accordingly, we changed the title to "Platform Trials in Drug Development: Umbrella Trials and Basket Trials," so that it would be clear to all readers that basket trials are included. We regret that some of our authors would clearly find this title logically inconsistent. The reader should be alert to the fact that authors were permitted to write their chapter with their preferred definitions of terms, and therefore the definitions are specific to the individual chapters.

More generally, we made no attempt to harmonize disagreement and debate, and there are some opinions herein that we do not share, as well as some obvious contradictions between chapters (for example, two of the chapters on basket trials, 4 and 16, disagree with the concluding chapter's analysis of type I error in these designs). Thus, while the book provides answers to many questions about this new field, the questions may be answered in different and occasionally conflicting ways. Rather than providing facts and answers, the primary purposes of this book are to stimulate more questions and to catalyze further innovation.

Robert A. Beckman
Washington, DC

Zoran Antonijevic
Chapel Hill, North Carolina

Acknowledgments

This book is a project of the Drug Information Association Adaptive Design Scientific Working Group, and the editors would like to acknowledge the contributions of its more than 200 members from around the world to our perspective on adaptive designs. We would like to thank our accomplished and intellectually diverse author group for high quality contributions that made our jobs as editors much easier. Finally, we would like to thank our wives, Gordana Sekulic and Susan Beckman, for their patience during the process of putting the book together.

Z. A.
R. A. B.

Contributors

Jeffrey D. Allen
Friends of Cancer Research
Washington, DC

Ohad Amit
Glaxo Smith-Kline
Philadelphia, Pennsylvania

Zoran Antonijevic
Z-Adaptive Design, Chapel Hill
North Carolina; Drug Information
Association Adaptive Design
Scientific Working Group
Washington, District of Columbia

Smita Asare
I-SPY Trial Operations, Quantum
Leap Health Care Collaborative
San Francisco, California

Anna Barker
Complex Adaptive Systems Initiative
Arizona State University
Tempe, Arizona

Robert A. Beckman
Departments of Oncology and of
Biostatistics, Bioinformatics, and
Biomathematics, Lombardi
Comprehensive Cancer Center
and Innovation Center for
Biomedical Informatics,
Georgetown University
Medical Center, Washington,
District of Columbia; Drug
Information Association Adaptive
Design Scientific Working Group
Washington, District of Columbia

Donald A. Berry
Berry Consultants, LLC, Austin
Texas; Department of Biostatistics

MD Anderson Comprehensive
Cancer Center
Houston, Texas

Scott M. Berry
Berry Consultants, LLC
Austin, Texas

Carl-Fredrik Burman
Department of Mathematical
Sciences, Chalmers University of
Technology, Gothenburg, Sweden
Statistical Innovation, Advanced
Analytics Centre, AstraZeneca R&D
Molndal, Sweden

Cong Chen
Merck & Co., Inc.
Kenilworth, New Jersey

Olivier Collignon
European Medicines Agency
London, UK

Ramzi Dagher
Pfizer, Inc., New London/Norwich
Connecticut

Angie DeMichele
Department of Medicine
University of Minnesota
Minneapolis, Minnesota

Laura Esserman
Departments of Surgery and
Radiotherapy, Breast Care Center
and Breast Oncology Program
University of California San Francisco
San Francisco, California

Valerii V. Fedorov
ICON Clinical Research
North Wales, Pennsylvania

Keith T. Flaherty
Henri and Belinda Termeer
Center for Targeted Therapy,
Massachusetts General
Hospital Cancer Center
Boston, Massachusetts

Daphne Guinn
Program in Regulatory Science
Department of Pharmacology
Georgetown University
Medical Center
Washington, District of Columbia

Jonas Häggström
MTEK Sciences, Vancouver, British
Columbia, Canada; Knowledge
Integration and Trial Services
The Bill & Melinda Gates
Foundation
Seattle, Washington

Ryan Hohman
Friends of Cancer Research
Washington, District of Columbia

Peter Honig
Pfizer Inc.
Philadelphia, Pennsylvania

Nola Hylton
Department of Radiology
University of California San Francisco
San Francisco, California

Qi Jiang
Seattle Genetics Inc.
Bothell, Washington

Sebastian Jobjörnsson
Department of Mathematical
Sciences, Chalmers
University of Technology
Gothenburg, Sweden

Rasika Kalamegham
Genentech, Inc.
Washington, District of Columbia

Chunlei Ke
Biogen, Inc.
Cambridge, Massachusetts

Franz König
Center for Medical Statistics
Informatics, and Intelligent
Systems, Medical
University of Vienna
Vienna, Austria

Sergei L. Leonov
ICON Clinical Research
North Wales, Pennsylvania

Janet J. Li
Pfizer, Inc.
San Francisco, California

Subha Madhavan
Department of Oncology
Innovation Center for Biomedical
Informatics and Lombardi
Comprehensive Cancer Center
Georgetown University
Medical Center
Washington, District of Columbia

Jeff Matthews
Department of Surgery, University
of California San Francisco
San Francisco, California

Edward Mills
MTEK Sciences, Vancouver, British
Columbia, Canada; Knowledge
Integration and Trial Services
The Bill & Melinda
Gates Foundation
Seattle, Washington

Phuong Khanh Morrow
Amgen, Inc.
Thousand Oaks, California

Jane Perlmutter
Gemini Group
Ann Arbor, Michigan

Martin Posch
Center for Medical Statistics,
Informatics, and Intelligent Systems
Medical University of Vienna
Vienna, Austria

David Reese
Amgen, Inc.
Thousand Oaks, California

Satrajit Roychoudhury
Pfizer, Inc.
New York, New York

Benjamin R. Saville
Berry Consultants, LLC
Austin, Texas

Anja Schiel
Norwegian Medicines Agency
Oslo Norway

Ellen V. Sigal
Friends of Cancer Research
Washington, District of Columbia

Richard M. Simon
Biometrics Research Program and
Computational and Systems
Biology Branch, National
Cancer Institute, Bethesda
Maryland; Current address
Rich Simon Consulting
Potomac, Maryland

Nigel Stallard
Warwick Medical School, The
University of Warwick
Coventry, UK

Ryan J. Sullivan
Department of Hematology/
Oncology, Massachusetts General
Hospital Cancer Center
Boston, Massachusetts

Fraser Symmans
Department of Pathology, MD
Anderson Comprehensive
Cancer Center
Houston, Texas

Kristian Thorlund
MTEK Sciences, Vancouver, British
Columbia, Canada; Knowledge
Integration and Trial Services, The
Bill & Melinda Gates Foundation
Seattle, Washington

Laura van't Veer
Helen Diller Family Comprehensive
Cancer Center, University of
California San Francisco
San Francisco, California

Zhongshen Wang
Incyte Corporation
Wilmington, Delaware

Madison Wempe
Friends of Cancer Research
Washington, District of Columbia

Christina Yau
Department of Surgery
University of California
San Francisco
San Francisco, California

Doug Yee
Department of Pharmacology
Microbiology, Immunology
and Cancer Biology
University of Minnesota
Minneapolis, Minnesota

Shuai Sammy Yuan
Merck & Co., Inc.
Kenilworth, New Jersey

Part I

Overview of Platform Clinical Trials

1

I-SPY2

Unlocking the Potential of the Platform Trial

Laura Esserman, Nola Hylton, Smita Asare, Christina Yau, Doug Yee,
Angie DeMichele, Jane Perlmutter, Fraser Symmans, Laura van't Veer,
Jeff Matthews, Donald A. Berry, and Anna Barker

Modern drug discovery, fueled by high throughput technologies, combinatorial chemistry, rational drug design, and increasingly powerful information processing, has become progressively efficient and productive. So much so, that the number of new cancer therapeutics in development doubled over the span of a decade.[1] As of 2015, there were 836 individual cancer drugs at various stages in the pipelines of America's biopharmaceutical companies, including 83 for breast cancer and 132 for lung.[2] An estimated 80% of these are first-in-class therapies and 73% are potential "personalized" medicines.[3] On paper at least, we have an embarrassment of riches. But it is a different story in practice.

On average, it takes 10–15 years for a new therapeutic to successfully navigate preclinical and clinical testing and gain marketing approval. Rising costs, particularly for late stage clinical trials, put the average investment required for a new agent past the US$2 billion mark.[4]

Not only is new drug development a high stakes game, it is also high risk, particularly in oncology: fewer than 1 in 20 agents entering clinical trials ultimately gain approval.[5] Two-thirds of agents evaluated in large, expensive phase 3 trials fail to receive approval. The requirement for large patient numbers to achieve statistical certainty in our current trial model compounds our problems. As we prepare for the age of personalized medicine, we must also prepare for the inevitable subdividing of diseases, particularly cancers, into smaller and smaller subsets, making it harder and harder to achieve target enrollment.

Few would argue that our current approach of using successively larger, single agent randomized controlled trials (RCTs) is efficient, in terms of time, money, and resources; it has resulted in inordinately large investments with low yields. Perhaps more importantly, it continues to struggle to meet the needs of patients, who are increasingly demanding better, more personalized treatments.

Faster "Knowledge Turns"

This need for "something better" is what has fueled the principal mission of the I-SPY program: to accelerate the development of improved treatments for early breast cancers at high risk of recurrence. In practice, this has meant nothing less than developing a platform trial model that was smaller, more targeted, faster, more efficient, cheaper, and demonstrating that it could be successfully put into practice. However, from the beginning, I-SPY was designed to be much more.

The overarching goal has been not simply to demonstrate a new trial model in a single indication, but to re-engineer the clinical trial in a manner broadly applicable in oncology and beyond. Conceptually, the goal is to move away from discrete, single agent trials, towards a continuously updated "learning" platform that employs biological information (biomarkers) to progressively optimize the targeting of agents to the patients or subtypes in which they are most effective.

This accelerated learning approach is rooted in the concepts described by former CEO and co-founder of Intel, Andy Grove, PhD who, in a 2005 article in JAMA, compared development cycles between healthcare and the semiconductor industry.[6] The rate of progress in the latter is often represented by "Moore's Law," which states that the number of components per integrated circuit (and therefore the processor power) doubles every two years.[7] This rapid rate of progress, Grove argues, relies on rapid "knowledge turns" and early indicators of success or failure during the development process for a new or improved product. In his industry, knowledge turns are measured in *months*.

By the same measure, a knowledge turn in healthcare (including oncology), is essentially the transit time to move from a proposed treatment to the analysis of trial results. In drug development, knowledge turns are measured in *years*—in many indications, even *decades*. One can point to any number of factors contributing to the extended development times in clinical drug development.

Protocol Approvals

Most investigators are all too aware of the complex processes and multiple approvals required to initiate a single trial—that is, each and every trial.

This redundancy is one of the most significant sources of inefficiency in our system—every principal investigator, company, or cooperative group needs to run their own trial, and for every agent evaluated, a brand-new protocol is written, requiring multiple repetitions of the reviews and regulatory approvals, contracting, and start up time. Then, to make matters worse, at the end of the trial, all the contracts, documentation, and approvals are essentially voided, forcing us to start over on the next (often very similar) trial. This kind of waste of human and intellectual capital would be unacceptable in any other industry, but for clinical trials, it has been the norm for decades. Only recently, with the introduction of the master protocol, have we begun to explore more expedient means of getting to the same place.

Smarter Outcomes

All it takes is a quick glance at the typical timeline for oncology trials and it becomes clear that the most significant contributor to the long knowledge turns in drug development are in follow-up—a consequence of the distant outcome measures that are required. Take for instance, the use of disease-free survival (DFS) as an endpoint in either neoadjuvant or adjuvant therapy trials in oncology. This alone condemns this industry to progress at a snail's pace, as it establishes our baseline for obtaining results as 5–10 years—this is the lion's share of the healthcare knowledge turn. Although there is little question DFS remains the gold standard of efficacy, it is important to recognize that perfection (in terms of endpoints) clearly comes at a cost of excruciatingly slow development times. For this reason, validating an early surrogate outcome measure was one of the mission-critical objectives of I-SPY.

As we have learned in I-SPY, the neoadjuvant approach has important advantages over adjuvant therapy in this regard. By starting with systemic therapy as the first treatment (rather than surgical removal), it provides an opportunity to directly assess tumor response to therapy. It allows us to maximize what we learn about the effects of the therapy and to do so very early after treatment, rather than 5–10 years down the road. This has clear advantages not only for the purposes of the trial, but for optimizing care and redirecting treatment to clinical trials or other interventions in the event of a poor response.

Smarter Approach

Another key contributor to the extended development times is that all agents are first tested in the metastatic stage, not only for phase 1 (safety), but for phase 2 and 3, prior to being tested in the early disease phase. Testing novel agents earlier in the disease course (early stage) in the setting of high risk for early recurrence can cut years off the development time. As well, this means testing agents when the disease is more curable, before patients have had multiple treatments and the possibility of developing resistance, and while the immune system is more intact; all contribute to an increased likelihood to improve the chance of a meaningful response, while improving the knowledge turns.

Of course, unlike processor chips, in which great pains are taken to ensure they are identical in both construction and operation, the nature of diseases like cancer couldn't be more different. Cancers are heterogeneous in multiple ways, they are dynamic, and they adapt to external stimuli. Because this heterogeneity cannot be ignored, I-SPY was designed to embrace it. Biomarkers can fuel adaptive designs to help determine how an agent performs among different molecular subtypes of breast cancer,[8] ultimately speeding the transition of drugs from phase 2 to phase 3 trials, and increasing the chances of success in phase 3 by using a more targeted approach.

I-SPY2: Design

The I-SPY Program goals were, from the beginning (and they remain) lofty. It was designed to integrate and link phase 1 (I-SPY Phase 1), phase 2 (I-SPY2), and, in time, Phase 3 (I-SPY3) evaluations to establish a dynamic pipeline of novel agents. We aim to accelerate the identification of the subset of high risk breast cancer patients that benefit from novel agents or combinations, rapidly validate them, and shepherd them into clinical use (Table 1.1). The centerpiece of the program is I-SPY2, our ongoing, adaptively randomized phase 2 study that features multiple simultaneous experimental arms with a common control and a master-protocol. [9,10]

I-SPY2 is focused on the evaluation of new agents for neoadjuvant treatment of breast cancers with a high risk of recurrence. It is a precompetitive collaboration among multiple academic, pharmaceutical, bio-technology, governmental, and advocate stakeholders. New agents are administered in combination with standard neoadjuvant therapy (which serves as the common control arm) consisting of 12 weekly cycles of paclitaxel, followed by 4 cycles of anthracycline-based chemotherapy (Figure 1.1).

The critical feature that enables many elements of the I-SPY2 approach is the use of a master protocol, which allows multiple drugs from multiple companies to be in the trial for evaluation simultaneously. As a biomarker-driven study, all consenting participants undergo baseline assessments for hormone receptor (HR) status, HER2 status and a 70-gene assay[11] ("Mammaprint" from Agendia, Irvine, CA") that correlates with risk of recurrence. Each patient is then classified into one of eight prospectively defined disease subtypes. The adaptive-randomization algorithm, continuously updated during the study as each patient reaches the primary endpoint, assigns patients to competing drug regimens (20% are assigned to control)

TABLE 1.1

I-SPY2 is designed to increase the success rate of phase 3 trials, understand which subset of disease has the biggest benefit for specific agents and reduce the time and cost of running phase 3 trials.

Principle	Solution
Test agents where they matter most	• Neoadjuvant setting, poor prognosis cancers • Integrate advocates into trial planning
Rapidly learn to tailor agents	• Adaptive Design • Neoadjuvant therapy • Integration of biomarkers, imaging
Optimize Phase 3 trials	• Graduate drugs with predicted probability of success in Phase 3 trials for given biomarker profile
Drive Organizational Efficiency	• Adaptive Design • Master IND & Master CTA • Test drugs by class, across many companies • Shared cost of profiling • Financial support separated from drug supply • Shared IT Infrastructure, caBIG • Protocol & ICF structure to minimize delays
Use Team Approach	• Democratize access to data • Share credit and opportunity • Collaborative process for development

on the basis of current Bayesian probabilities of each agent achieving a pathological complete response within the patient's biomarker subtype (Figure 1.2). In other words, randomization in I-SPY2 preferentially assigns women to arms that have a higher likelihood of achieving a good outcome in their tumor subtype. This approach is designed for efficiency, in terms of the time and number of patients required to reach statistical significance. The algorithm uses a longitudinal model based on pathologic complete response (pCR) assessed histologically at time of surgery (I-SPY's primary endpoint), as well as MRI functional tumor volume measures taken at various time-points during treatment (Figure 1.3). Therefore, unlike standard RCTs, the number (and baseline tumor characteristics) of patients that end up being assigned to each experimental arm/agent in I-SPY2 is influenced by the trial results.

For the purposes of assessing the efficacy of each arm/agent, ten clinically relevant "signatures" were defined prospectively. These are similar to the subtypes used in randomization, but also broader categorizations such as "all patients," "all HR+ patients," etc. As the trial progresses, each arm/agent is continually assessed against pre-defined criteria for success ("graduation") or failure (futility) within each of the ten signatures.

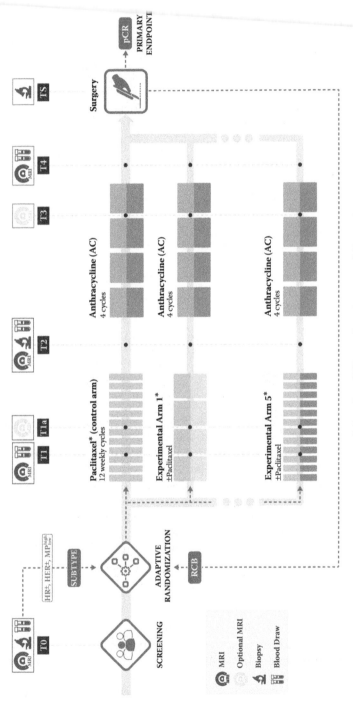

FIGURE 1.1

Study schema for the I-SPY2 platform trial for neoadjuvant treatment of early breast cancer at high risk of recurrence. The study permits efficient evaluation of multiple experimental agents within an adaptively randomized, biomarker-driven design.

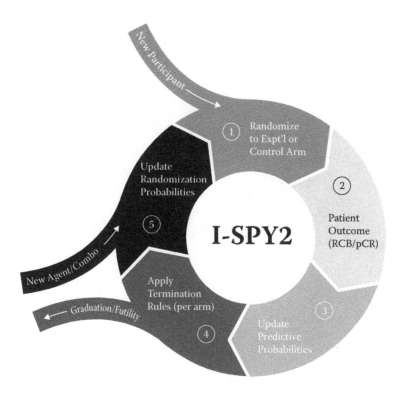

FIGURE 1.2
In I-SPY2, the randomization probabilities of incoming patients assign patients to one of up to five experimental therapies (or control) on the basis of probabilities of success within a particular biomarker subtype. These probabilities are continuously updated as patients reach the primary endpoint, assessment of pathologic complete response at time of surgery.

An agent graduates from I-SPY2 if the predictive probability of it showing statistical superiority over control in a 1:1 randomized, 300-person phase 3 trial of patients with the graduating signature(s) is >85%. Futility is declared if the predictive probability of an agent's success in the hypothetical phase 3 trial <10% for all signatures, or if the arm reaches the maximum enrollment of 120 patients without graduating in any signature. Graduation or futility results in an immediate halt to enrollment for that particular arm, which is communicated to investigators only after all enrolled patients complete surgery.

Given its Bayesian adaptive approach, results from I-SPY2 are reported differently than other RCTs. As illustrated in Figure 1.4, I-SPY results are reported in terms of probabilities for each of the 10 signatures: i) the estimated (mean of the distribution of) pCR rate in the agent/control arms for the given signature; ii) the (Bayesian) probability that the agent

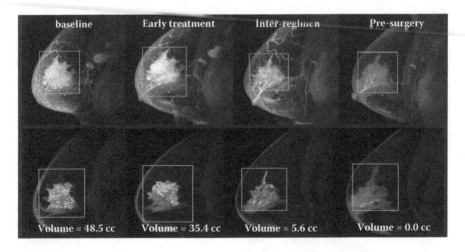

FIGURE 1.3
Serial MRI measurements of functional tumor volume are used to impute treatment response to inform the I-SPY2 adaptive randomization algorithm.

is superior to control; 3) the (Bayesian) probability of success in the hypothetical 300-patient phase 3 trial.

I-SPY2 is not only about knowledge turns, but also about knowledge generation. Serial biopsies and blood draws are taken during the course of treatment; as of April 2017, over 46,000 bio-specimens have been collected from >1000 patients, representing an uniquely rich resource for the evaluation of hypothesis-testing biomarkers (or "qualifying biomarkers," Table 1.2), typically based on mechanism of action, and hypothesis generating biomarkers, which are more exploratory in nature. All I-SPY2 biomarker work is conducted in a CLIA certified lab.

Progress

It is important to remember, that in 2008, when I-SPY was in the planning stages, there was scant experience with models other than the standard "agent vs. control" randomized clinical trial model. Prior to this point, trials were focused on agents from one company only, and did not include agents from more than one company. Also, there was some doubt that Institutional Review Boards would approve a platform trial. Although there was vigorous discussion of the potential of using adaptive approaches and Bayesian statistical models in oncology trials, there were limited examples from which to draw.[12,13] Similarly, at that time, the use of a master protocol was

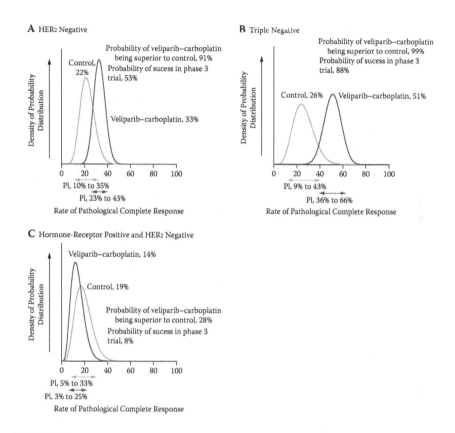

FIGURE 1.4

Example of how I-SPY2 results are reported through probability distributions of estimated pCR rates, Bayesian probabilities of superiority over control, and the Bayesian probabilities of success in a hypothetical 300-patient phase 3 trial. Results are tabulated for each of the 10 clinically relevant signatures. Reproduced from Rugo, et. al, 2016.[9]

largely untested, having been employed only in one or two cases and in limited context.[14]

I-SPY2 is therefore one of the earliest, and is currently the longest running platform trial, having been continuously enrolling and evaluating new agents since it opened in October, 2010. So, how has it performed in terms of the two primary goals of improved efficiency and efficacy?

Over its seven years of operation, I-SPY2 has entered 14 agents into the trial, with more combinations expected this coming year. A total of 11 agents have completed evaluation. The time an agent spends in the study, whether reaching graduation or stopped for futility, is between 10 and 24 months. The multiple simultaneous arms and common control use this time very efficiently, translating into the completed evaluation of about

TABLE 1.2

Categories of biomarkers in I-SPY2

Type	Standard	Qualifying	Exploratory
Definition	Routine biomarkers that are embedded within the adaptive randomization algorithm to segment the population	Biomarkers based on mechanism of action, used for hypothesis-testing related to treatment response to new agents	Hypothesis-generating biomarkers, intended to generate ideas for future studies or qualifying biomarkers
Endpoints	**ER/HER2 IHC; FISH Mammaprint** • FDA cleared 70 gene assay (used to determine randomization eligibility) • IDE (filed with FDA) for 44K array **MR Volume** • used to impute response to treatment in patients who have not yet gone to surgery • IDE (filed with FDA)	**Signatures** • DNA Repair Deficiency • AKT pathway • HER pathway • Hi-2 (Mammaprint) • Immune Signatures **Platforms** • 44k Agilent Array • Reverse Phase Protein Arrays • Vectra Multiplex Staining Environment	• RNA Seq • DNA Seq • Circulating DNA • Circulating tumor cells

two agents per year. This marks a significant departure from a decade-long trend that has seen the average duration of phase 2 single-agent oncology trials swell to 40 months.[15]

As of January 1, 2018, 2216 patients had been screened for I-SPY2 and 1265 enrolled and adaptively randomized. Because the size of patient cohorts are not fixed in I-SPY's adaptive model, the number of patients ranged from 52 to 120, with an average of 80 patients (excluding one agent halted for safety reasons), which is comparable to most phase 2 oncology studies.

I-SPY2 has been equally successful in meeting its goals in terms of improving breast cancer treatment efficacy. There have been several notable successes to date:

- validated the efficacy and safety of pertuzumab in locally advanced breast cancer, after it received accelerated approval while under investigation in I-SPY2. Only 54 patients were required in this arm;

- pembrolizumab, an immunotherapy that entered the trial in November 2015, graduated 11 months later and received breakthrough designation in triple-negative disease, partly based on I-SPY2 results;
- the efficacy of a graduated agent combination (veliparib plus carboplatin), where 90 patients were enrolled, was confirmed in a 750-patient phase 2 study (BrighTNess) to evaluate the contributions of each agent in the combination. The trial showed the same result as I-SPY, but revealed that the increase in pCR was due to carboplatin;
- neratinib, an anti-HER2 tyrosine kinase inhibitor that graduated in early 2013, moved forward as a second-line therapy in the setting of residual disease following neoadjuvant therapy.

Seven of the 11 completed agents graduated in at least one subtype with the net results that on average, a woman entering I-SPY2 today has double the chance of achieving a complete response (no tumor left at the time of surgical resection) relative to when the trial started. Furthermore, three-year follow-up results presented in late 2017, and which included ~750 patients treated with 11 different regimens (including control) showed that women who achieved a pCR—regardless of therapy or subtype—had improved 3-year event-free and distant recurrence-free survival, with a hazard ratio of 0.24.[16]

In other words, pCR is a strong and robust predictor of long-term outcome following neoadjuvant therapy in patients with a high risk of early recurrence, regardless of tumor subtype. In practical terms, this means that following neoadjuvant therapy, in which systemic therapy is administered before surgery, the complete disappearance of tumor tells us which women have had their risk of early recurrence shift from high-risk to low-risk, and which women remain in the high-risk category. This provides important opportunities for both treatment-sparing to limit toxicities in those at low risk, and treatment redirection or supplemental treatment in high risk women.

Perhaps most importantly for I-SPY2, the high degree of fidelity between pCR and long-term outcome is validation that pCR is the viable early readout of efficacy originally envisioned as driving faster knowledge turns.

Lessons from I-SPY2

The success of I-SPY2 cannot be attributed to one or two factors alone, but are the result of synergy that has been created in deconstructing and then re-engineering our approach to phase 2 clinical drug development.

Clearly, the use of a master protocol/master IND is one of the critical enabling tools that makes trials such as I-SPY possible. The master protocol model employed by I-SPY brings an abundance of operational efficiencies.

For instance, under the master protocol, when an agent leaves the trial, new agents are introduced modularly through protocol amendments. Amendments to already-approved protocols are faster and more efficient, avoiding the need for repeated review of all study procedures, creating a seamless process that avoids disruption of enrollment as drugs enter and leave the trial.

All amendments currently require local IRB review at each clinical site, and so rules have been established to ensure continuity and consistency across sites. Because I-SPY is continuously recruiting for at least one arm, when IRBs of the sites with 50% enrollment approve an amendment, the protocol is activated for the network of sites with approval, while the other sites are on put hold from randomizing to that arm. As there have been significant moves towards the use of central IRBs, (or IRBs of record), I-SPY will be moving towards central review to bring additional efficiencies.

The use of a master protocol has also facilitated the development of one of the most important approaches that makes I-SPY function—its precompetitive model for collaboration among the many stakeholders in the trial.

Precompetitive Model

In essence, it means that all stakeholders acknowledge their alignment with the goals of the study up-front and must agree that no single organization is entitled to a competitive advantage over the others, as a condition of participation.

The I-SPY2 precompetitive collaboration currently involves multiple pharmaceutical companies. Once an agent drops, leaves, or graduates from the trial, there is an aggressive timeline for results reporting which includes making information available to the research community. The collaboration is coordinated and managed by the Quantum Leap Healthcare Collaborative (QLHC), a 501(c)3 not-for-profit, which serves as the sponsor and honest broker for new knowledge generated in the course of the trial. The original sponsor of the trial was the Foundation for the National Institutes of Health (FNIH). Several non-profit and foundation sponsors provide a broad base of funding support, removing the potential for undue influence by any single organization. Having QLHC as sponsor is clearly advantageous, providing faster contracting, budgeting and hiring of central resources than normally seen in an academic environment.

In practical terms, for I-SPY2 this has meant that among the first activities in building a relationship with a new stakeholder or drug developer is to provide them with the "term sheet" that outlines the rules of participation, as well as the standard I-SPY2 contract. It is also made clear that the contract is non-negotiable—no changes to the standard contract are entertained. The standardization of contracts among all stakeholders is critical to establishing a level playing field, and is especially important in ensuring equality among partner drug developers. To date, only a handful of potential partners have found this to be a non-starter and walked away, the majority accepting the contracts as written.

As a consequence of this approach, new agents are able to enter the study much more quickly, without the need to renegotiate terms in each case. I-SPY2 expends very little personnel time or salary on contracting and subcontracting processes. In fact, the bulk of the effort mostly amounts to answering questions and clarifications, rather than negotiations.

Importantly, this equality of stakeholders and harmonized approach to contracting also extends to clinical site subcontracts. It is, of course, well known that delays in contract and budget negotiation are among the most often reported reasons for delays in site initiation[17,18] and it appears the problem is increasing: industry average site-contract cycle times have doubled in the past 5 years.[19] By precluding lengthy negotiations over details such as publication, authorship policy, data ownership, etc., I-SPY sites are able to focus efforts on other start-up activities.

Regulatory Pathway

Among the early lessons learned by I-SPY investigators was the realization that a platform that reduced both cost and time for phase 2 development was not necessarily all that the pharmaceutical and biomarker companies were looking for. Initially, the enthusiastic partners were those companies looking to I-SPY to establish proof-of-concept, or to quickly identify potential pathways, evaluate targets or sensitive subpopulations. But for most, there was a critical missing ingredient: *a clear path toward drug registration and companion diagnostic approval.*

This realization led the I-SPY executive team to organize a May 2011 workshop in which all stakeholders (including the FDA) came together to explore potential regulatory paths for biomarker-drug combinations derived from I-SPY2 and similar trials. The key question put to the attendees was "What is the most efficient way to generate evidence needed for regulatory review and approval?" The consensus view was that the early endpoint used in I-SPY2, pathologic complete response (pCR), at least in the context of a screening phase 2 trial should be an acceptable endpoint for accelerated approval in patients with high-risk biology (predicted to have early recurrence), meeting the definition of an endpoint "that is reasonably likely to predict a clinical outcome."[20,21]

The FDA concurred, and shortly afterwards issued guidance for accelerated approval of neoadjuvant agents in breast cancer based upon the endpoint of pCR.[22] Armed with a clear path to registration and a level playing field for all stakeholders, there has been an increased willingness to enter new agents into I-SPY2.

Although I-SPY clearly benefitted from a willing and collaborative FDA in this process, there were some elements that were by design. Prior to launching I-SPY2, we conducted the I-SPY1 pilot trial (CALGB 150007 and

150012/ACRIN 6657) in which one a primary goal, among others, was to assess the suitability of pCR and MRI lesion volume change as a surrogate endpoint in our target population, early breast cancer at high risk for recurrence. A key finding from the phase 2 I-SPY1 was that pCR was a better predictor of recurrence-free and event-free survival when taken in the context of tumor biology and evaluated within individual subsets based on hormone receptor (HR) and HER2 status.[23] Also, MRI volume change and MRI final volume was predictive of 3-year event free survival, and predictive of pCR.[24] As discussed, below, MRI volume change is used during the course of treatment to inform the adaptive randomization algorithm.

Engaging Investigators

While effective engagement of drug developers is an essential component of I-SPY, so too is the ability to attract and retain high quality investigators. In general, for the average investigators in a large collaborative network, there can often be a large imbalance between the effort required and the resulting academic recognition. One of the ways I-SPY attempts to distribute the professional benefits to our academic investigators is by assigning a pair of "drug chaperones" for each investigational agent (or agent combination), essentially co-principal investigators for that arm of the study. The chaperone role comes with both responsibility and reward. Chaperones help to write the agent's amendments, manage issues relating to the drug arm for which they are the chaperone, monitor safety signals, write abstracts, and analyze primary efficacy results. Chaperones are first authors on presentations and manuscripts of the primary study results. In addition, there are clearly defined rules dictating the requirements for (and order of) authorship which let all investigators know, up front, what they can expect. I-SPY also provides many opportunities for leadership within the study, with dedicated working groups for agent selection, biomarker studies, trial operations, imaging, informatics, pathology, statistics, advocacy, safety, and quality of life. Although coordinated centrally, working group activities go beyond recommendations, and directly influence the conduct of the trial, and each are encouraged to innovate and publish. These strategies are enhanced by an overall culture of collaboration and innovation that has been carefully developed and is continuously reinforced.

Standardization

While much of the emphasis in I-SPY has been to increase the rate of knowledge turns in neoadjuvant therapy for breast cancer, improving the quality of both care and the resulting data has been equally important. In much the same way that standard contracts are used among all stakeholders, I-SPY has relied upon highly standardized operational and scientific processes as a manner that improves both efficiency and quality.

Take for example the multiple MRIs performed as part of the protocol. Because the adaptive randomization algorithm relies upon longitudinal MRI measures of functional tumor volume change (ΔFTV), these analyses must be reported in real time, making consistency between clinical sites, operators and image analyses imperative. In fact, one of the key goals of the I-SPY1 trial was not only to validate MRI as a measure of tumor response to therapy, but also to evaluate and demonstrate the high degree of consistency in quantitative MRI that can be achieved across multiple clinical sites.[25–27] To date, of over 6000 MRI exams have been performed in I-SPY2, with more than 98% meeting strict quality standards and deemed analyzable for the primary imaging end point, ΔFTV.

Similarly, significant effort was extended to reduce potential variability in the overall primary endpoint, pathologic complete response. In practice and across clinical trials, the definition of pCR varies, sometimes including conditional assessment of axillary nodes, others considering only the primary tumor site. The solution for I-SPY was the use of the "Residual Cancer Burden" score (RCB), which provides a more granular assessment, in which pCR is represented by an RCB score of zero (on a scale of 0–3).[28] Importantly, for both MRI and pathology assessments, standardized protocols were accompanied by extensive site training, qualification testing, and an ongoing quality assurance program. Much of the strength of our pCR and long-term outcome data can likely attributed to the tighter definitions and high degree of fidelity of these measures.[16]

For these and other site generated data, I-SPY has well-established training for site personnel. Quality assurance measures that are an ongoing part of I-SPY2 require that all clinical sites demonstrate their ability to follow the standardized protocols and yield reproducible results. The QA program includes measures such as MRI functional volume change measures, pathology (using RCB), standards for axillary surgical management and identification of the tumor and sample processing and quality control in the CLIA-certified I-SPY lab, among others.

Unlocking the Potential of the Master Protocol

Perhaps the most significant advantage of the master protocol is that it establishes a dynamic trial environment, which permits a trial to make adjustments, improvements, and even iterative evolutions over time, through the use of protocol amendments. As of the first quarter of 2018, the I-SPY2 trial is now on its 18th protocol amendment. We have had no significant issues gaining approval across multiple local IRBs for any of them.

The flexibility this affords has allowed us to fine tune the trial operationally, validate emerging biomarkers and even MRI methodologies within the trial, seamlessly integrate supplemental studies on the fly and—most importantly—it has allowed the trial to evolve along with changes in the standard of care and in our understanding of breast cancer.

Conclusion

To address the costs, time, and inefficiencies that plague the RCT, from the outset, the I-SPY2 team embraced the concept of the "platform trial." A platform trial, performed under a single master protocol, facilitates evaluating multiple treatments simultaneously. Additionally the I-SPY2 trial also features an adaptive design which supports declaring treatments superior (graduation), dropping unsuccessful treatments for futility, and adding new therapies as the trial proceeds.

The platform trial has proven to be ideal to achieve the goals of the I-SPY2 team. Master protocols support the investigation of multiple drugs in a single disease or single/multiple drugs in multiple diseases. The FDA supports several types of master protocols including umbrella trials, basket trials, and platform trials. I-SPY2 employs a master protocol that supports studying multiple therapies in breast cancer and eliminating and adding therapies on the based on a decision algorithm. Beyond being a platform trial, I-SPY2 is a learning system that can be continued indefinitely.

With the emergence of new immunotherapies with apparent large gains in efficacy in several breast cancer subtypes, this flexibility has become increasingly important. As standards of care continue to increase in multiple cancers, all clinical trials will need a dramatically different approach. We will be faced with the ethical question of whether we can withhold, even temporarily, very effective treatments in lieu of experimental therapies with unpredictable results. Regardless, without assurance that they will receive treatment that gives them the best possible chance at a cure, why would patients want to volunteer to be part of a trial?

In the future of drug development in oncology, patient-centered trials become a necessity. As we have more and more effective treatment options at our disposal, minimizing toxicities and safeguarding patient quality of life become increasingly important endpoints. The future of I-SPY2 and other phase 2 and phase 3 platform trials is undoubtedly one in which our measures of success are radically changed, moving towards our composite or hybrid endpoints that incorporate measures of both efficacy and safety/toxicity.

I-SPY amendment 18 marks I-SPY2's first steps in this direction, by introducing a strategy for de-escalation of treatment in patients with a strong, early response to treatment. Future amendments will focus on escalation of therapy in poor responders, by providing poor responders the opportunity to change to biologically targeted treatments while remaining enrolled in I-SPY2. These advances are a reflection of the culture of innovation that began in the early days of I-SPY and continues to this day. With each step, we grow closer to our ultimate goal of establishing a next-generation adaptive, patient-focused learning system, where healthcare knowledge turns are measured in months, not years.

References

1. PhRMA. Cancer drugs in development. U.S. number 2005–2015. www.statista.com/statistics/268805/number-of-cancer-drugs-in-development-since-2005/. Published 2015. Accessed November 28, 2017.
2. PhRMA. Medicines in development for cancer. phrma-docs.phrma.org. http://phrma-docs.phrma.org/sites/default/files/pdf/oncology-report-2015.pdf. Published 2015. Accessed November 28, 2017.
3. DiMasi JA, Grabowski HG, Hansen RW. Innovation in the pharmaceutical industry: New estimates of R&D costs. *J Health Econ.* 2016;47:20–33. doi:10.1016/j.jhealeco.2016.01.012.
4. Tufts Center for the Study of Drug Development. *Personalized Medicine Gains Traction but Still Faces Multiple Challenges.* Vol. 17; 2017.
5. Thomas DW, Burns J, Audette J, Carroll A, Dow-Hygelund C, Hay M. BIO industry report: Clinical development success rates 2006–2015. bio.org. www.bio.org/sites/default/files/Clinical%20Development%20Success%20Rates%202006-2015%20-%20BIO,%20Biomedtracker,%20Amplion%202016.pdf. Accessed December 30, 2017.
6. Grove AS. Efficiency in the health care industries: A view from the outside. *JAMA.* 2005;294(4):490–492. doi:10.1001/jama.294.4.490.
7. Moore's Law. Wikipedia. https://en.wikipedia.org/wiki/Moore%27s_law. Published January 29, 2018. Accessed February 2, 2018.
8. Esserman LJ, Berry DA, DeMichele A, et al. Pathologic complete response predicts recurrence-free survival more effectively by cancer subset: Results from the I-SPY1 TRIAL–CALGB 150007/150012, ACRIN 6657. *J Clin Oncol.* 2012;30(26):3242–3249. doi:10.1200/JCO.2011.39.2779.
9. Rugo HS, Olopade OI, DeMichele A, et al. Adaptive randomization of veliparib–carboplatin treatment in breast cancer. *N Engl J Med.* 2016;375(1):23–34. doi:10.1056/NEJMoa1513749.
10. Park JW, Liu MC, Yee D, et al. Adaptive randomization of neratinib in early breast cancer. *N Engl J Med.* 2016;375(1):11–22. doi:10.1056/NEJMoa1513750.

11. Cardoso F, Van't Veer LJ, Bogaerts J, et al. 70-Gene signature as an aid to treatment decisions in early-stage breast cancer. *N Engl J Med*. 2016;375(8):717–729. doi:10.1056/NEJMoa1602253.

12. Chow S-C, Chang M. Adaptive design methods in clinical trials—A review. *Orphanet J Rare Dis*. 2008;3:11. doi:10.1186/1750-1172-3-11.

13. Ledford H. Clinical drug tests adapted for speed. *Nature*. 2010;464:1258.

14. Ledford H. "Master protocol" aims to revamp cancer trials. *Nature*. 2013;498:146–147.

15. Alsumidale M, Schiemann P. Why are cancer clinical trials increasing in duration? Applied clinical trials. www.appliedclinicaltrialsonline.com/why-are-cancer-clinical-trials-increasing-duration. Published August 31, 2015. Accessed August 30, 2017.

16. Yee D, I-SPY2 Trial Investigators. Pathological complete response predicts event-free and distant disease-free survival in the I-SPY2 trial. *Cancer Research*. 2018;78(4 Suppl). doi:10.1158/1538-7445.SABCS17-GS3-08.

17. Dilts DM, Sandler AB. Invisible barriers to clinical trials: The impact of structural, infrastructural, and procedural barriers to opening oncology clinical trials. *J Clin Oncol*. 2006;24(28):4545–4552. doi:10.1200/JCO.2005.05.0104.

18. Lamberti MJ, Zuckerman R, Howe D, Shapiro L, Getz KA. Factors influencing investigative site willingness and ability to participate in clinical trials. *Ther Innov Regul Sci*. 2011;45(3):377–390. doi:10.1177/009286151104500316.

19. KMR Group. Site contracts from weeks to months: Results from KMR Group's site contracts study. kmrgroup.com. https://kmrgroup.com/wpcontent/uploads/2016/08/2016_08_24_KMRGroup_Site_Contracts_Study_Results.pdf. Published August 24, 2016. Accessed January 5, 2018.

20. Esserman LJ, Woodcock J. Accelerating identification and regulatory approval of investigational cancer drugs. *JAMA*. 2011;306(23):2608–2609. doi:10.1001/jama.2011.1837.

21. Prowell TM, Pazdur R. Pathological complete response and accelerated drug approval in early breast cancer. *N Engl J Med*. 2012;366(26):2438–2441. doi:10.1056/NEJMp1205737.

22. Food and Drug Administration. Guidance for Industry: Pathological complete response in neoadjuvant treatment of high-risk early-stage breast cancer: Use as an endpoint to support accelerated approval. fda.gov. www.fda.gov/downloads/Drugs/GuidanceComplianceRegulatoryInformation/Guidances/UCM305501.pdf. Published October 2014. Accessed November 26, 2017.

23. Esserman LJ, Berry DA, Cheang MCU, et al. Chemotherapy response and recurrence-free survival in neoadjuvant breast cancer depends on biomarker profiles: Results from the I-SPY1 TRIAL (CALGB 150007/150012; ACRIN 6657). *Breast Cancer Res Treat*. 2012;132(3):1049–1062. doi:10.1007/s10549-011-1895-2.

24. Hylton NM, Gatsonis CA, Rosen MA, et al. Neoadjuvant chemotherapy for breast cancer: Functional tumor volume by MR imaging predicts recurrence-free survival-results from the ACRIN 6657/CALGB 150007 I-SPY 1 TRIAL. *Radiology*. 2016;279(1):44–55. doi:10.1148/radiol.2015150013.

25. Li W, Arasu V, Newitt DC, et al. Effect of MR imaging contrast thresholds on prediction of neoadjuvant chemotherapy response in breast cancer subtypes: A subgroup analysis of the ACRIN 6657/I-SPY 1 TRIAL. *Tomography*. 2016;2(4):378–387. doi:10.18383/j.tom.2016.00247.

26. Hylton NM, Blume JD, Bernreuter WK, et al. Locally advanced breast cancer: MR imaging for prediction of response to neoadjuvant chemotherapy—Results from ACRIN 6657/I-SPY TRIAL. *Radiology*. 2012;263(3):663–672. doi:10.1148/radiol.12110748.

27. Newitt DC, Aliu SO, Witcomb N, et al. Real-time measurement of functional tumor volume by MRI to assess treatment response in breast cancer neoadjuvant clinical trials: Validation of the Aegis SER software platform. *Transl Oncol*. 2014;7(1):94–100. doi:10.1038/s41523-017-0025-7.

28. Symmans WF, Peintinger F, Hatzis C, et al. Measurement of residual breast cancer burden to predict survival after neoadjuvant chemotherapy. *J Clin Oncol*. 2007;25(28):4414–4422. doi:10.1200/JCO.2007.10.6823.

2

The Challenges with Multi-Arm Targeted Therapy Trials

Ryan J. Sullivan and Keith T. Flaherty

Introduction

The concept and framework for development of drugs for oncology has changed dramatically over the past 75 years. The first era of medical oncology, The Chemotherapy Era, was based on the premise that malignant cells are more susceptible to cellular poisons targeting cell division than non-malignant cells. These so-called cytotoxic chemotherapies are a diverse set of drugs with quite specific "targets" including DNA binding elements (e.g., alkylating agents, platinum-based agents), mimics of DNA bases that intercalate into DNA (e.g., purine and pyrimidine analogs), enzymes that unwind DNA (topoisomerase I and II inhibitors), and microtubules (e.g., taxanes, vinca alkaloids), among others. The therapeutic window varies amongst agents and classes of agents, but generally, cytotoxic chemotherapy is challenging to give over a prolonged period of time due to the cumulative effects of these agents on the bone marrow. And, the concept of predictive biomarkers to prospectively guide clinical development was entirely absent.

With the identification of oncogenes that drive tumor proliferation and preserve cell survival, a new class of agents have been developed to specifically target oncogenic pathways and/or specific mutated oncogenes. There now have been remarkable examples of successful drug development that have changed the treatment landscape for several diseases including, though not exclusively, chronic myelogenous leukemia (CML), epidermal growth factor receptor (EGFR) mutated lung cancer, and BRAF mutant, malignant melanoma (1–3). In each of these cases, the presence of the drug target, whether the BCR/ABL fusion protein resulting from the 9:21 chromosomal rearrangement in CML or oncogenic mutations in a host of solid tumor and hematologic malignancies, ultimately has served as the defining biomarker to select patients most likely to benefit from target inhibition. However, in the case of CML, BCR/ABL fusions are nearly ubiquitously present (4). So clinical development of imatinib in CML could proceed without regard for prospective patient selection based on this molecular feature. With the successful development of the molecularly targeted therapies for a diverse set of diseases, the paradigm of drug development has changed from testing an agent in a specific disease (e.g., paclitaxel in breast cancer) to testing an agent (or a combination of agents) in a molecularly defined subset of a disease (vemurafenib in BRAF-mutant melanoma). More recently, the concept of developing targeted agents against specific targets that are present across a number of diseases (e.g., NTRK fusions) have led to an emergence of so-called basket trials (5). And the logical extension of these trials is multi-arm, targeted therapy trials that enroll patients with a wide variety of molecular alterations in numerous malignancies onto one of a number of cohorts offering molecular targeted therapy predicted to inhibit the identified aberration.

As clinical trials become increasingly complex, a number of key issues have been identified. First and foremost, every trial that involves the treatment of a molecularly defined cohort must utilize an accurate and reliable test to identify the specific molecular alteration. If the molecular feature is rare in certain cancer types, then it becomes critical that screening can be done in the background of a patient's treatment, as advanced cancer patients cannot put treatment decisions on hold while being screened for a biomarker that is unlikely to be present. Second, trial sponsors must determine whether or not to test the agent in only patients with the specified alteration, in one disease or across many, and as a single-agent or in combination. From a regulatory perspective, the US FDA has typically required some demonstration of specific efficacy in a biomarker positive population, by having evidence of inefficacy in biomarker negative patients. Third, the design of the larger multi-arm studies often is hampered by either limited treatment options (e.g., based on a single pharmaceutical company's approved agents and those in the pipeline) or the challenges of working with multiple companies in the same study. Fourth, statistical challenges including appropriate end-point selection are present and need to be thought through carefully. What follows is a description of how the targeted therapy clinical trial landscape evolved over a short period of time with a particular focus on how the aforementioned challenges have been overcome as numerous multi-arm, multi-drug targeted therapy trials have opened in the past two years.

Historical Targeted Therapy Model (One Test, One Treatment)

The Development of EGFR Inhibitors in Non-Small Cell Lung Cancer

The recognition that EGFR signaling was important in non small cell lung cancer (NSCLC) preceded the identification of oncogenic mutations in EGFR (6). Following suit, EGFR inhibitors, such as gefitinib and erlotinib, were initially developed in advanced NSCLC independent of EGFR mutation (7,8). Based on the data from this study of erlotinib, this agent was approved for use broadly in patients with advanced NSCLC, independent of mutation status. Of note, several lessons were learned from these early studies. First, erlotinib was associated with improved survival outcomes, compared to placebo, whereas gefitinib was not, except in prespecified subgroups of patients (never smokers, patients of Asian descent). Second, significant responses were seen, with both drugs, in approximately 8–9% of patients. Third, a subset of patients had remarkable responses that were long lasting (9).

It was this third finding that was so intriguing about the EGFR inhibitors and led to further investigation. In fact, it was clear early on these agents were more effective in the setting of an *EGFR* mutation, and that these "exceptional responders" were indeed patients with oncogenic *EGFR* mutations (3,10,11). However, in subsequent years, the development of erlotinib, gefitinib, and more recently afatinib and osimertinib, have been in mutation positive patients only (12,13). In fact, osimertinib is a remarkable agent in that it is approved for patients with *EGFR* mutations that developed in response to prior EGFR inhibitors, as it is an inhibitor of the EGFRT790M oncoprotein, which is the most common form of EGFR inhibitor resistance (12).

The Development of BRAF Inhibitors in Melanoma

The identification of oncogenic mutations at the 600 position in *BRAF* in 2002 led to a rapid clinical development plan to bring BRAF inhibitors to patients with BRAF mutant melanoma (14). The earliest preclinical data was described with the multi-targeted tyrosine kinase inhibitor (TKI) sorafenib (15). Since the discovery of *BRAF* mutations in cancer came around the same time that sorafenib was making its way into the clinic as a VEGF, PDGF, and RAF (of both B- and C-isoforms) inhibitor, it logically was tested in patients with melanoma (16). While there were a number of trials of sorafenib as a single-agent or in combination with chemotherapy and other "targeted" therapies, including two randomized phase III studies of carboplatin and paclitaxel plus or minus sorafenib, the basic conclusion from all these studies were that sorafenib was not an effective therapy for patients with melanoma (17–20). Interestingly, despite it being a purported BRAF inhibitor, a trial of sorafenib specifically in *BRAF* mutant melanoma was never performed, although post-hoc analysis of the E2603 study, *BRAFV600E* mutational status was not predictive of better outcome with sorafenib in combination with chemotherapy (carboplatin and paclitaxel; CP). Interestingly, copy number alterations of *RAF1* (*CRAF*), *KRAS*, and *CCND1* was associated with improved outcomes with triplet therapy compared to CP; presumably, according to the authors, through sorafenib effects of CRAF (21,22). Based on this data, a revised conclusion of the benefit of sorafenib in metastatic melanoma is that it is ineffective in *BRAF* mutant melanoma, but may have some benefit in other molecular subsets that upregulate CRAF. Thus, the development of sorafenib in melanoma failed precisely due to the overestimation of its effects on one molecularly defined population and underestimation of its effects on others; although in fairness, the technology was not available to routinely categorize these other subsets until more recently.

Out of the underwhelming data with sorafenib, came a new approach with more specific inhibitors of BRAF. Vemurafenib, the first of these, demonstrated high-response rates in *BRAFV600E* mutant melanoma and no responses in a limited number of patients non-*BRAF* mutated melanoma (2). Furthermore, emerging preclinical data highlighted that vemurafenib and dabrafenib, the second such inhibitor to be developed, were potent inhibitors of *BRAFV600*-mutated cancer cells and the mitogen activated protein kinase (MAPK) pathway but would paradoxically activate MAPK signaling in non-mutated cell lines, in particular those with active activating *NRAS* mutations (23,24). Based on the early clinical and preclinical data, these drugs were only developed in *BRAF* mutated malignancies (2,25). Following the early clinical success of vemurafenib and dabrafenib, two randomized controlled trials were launched (one with each agent) and demonstrated superiority of vemurafenib and dabrafenib against chemotherapy (26,27). These studies led to the FDA-approval of vemurafenib in 2011 and dabrafenib in 2013.

A key component to the development of these agents was the co-development of a clinical assay that would have adequate sensitivity and specificity to detect the *BRAFV600E* mutation. Additionally, as *BRAFV600K* mutations are present in 5–20% of *BRAFV600* mutant melanomas, consideration to detecting this mutation was also important. Both Roche (vemurafenib) and GlaxoSmithKline (GSK; dabrafenib) selected real-time polymerase chain reactions (PCR) assays and designated these as companion diagnostics (28,29). The distinguishing features of these assays, the cobas® 4800 *BRAF* (Roche) and the THXID®BRAF (bioMerieux), is that they are quite specific and adequately sensitive for tissue containing 50% or more tumor and can be implemented in most clinical/molecular pathology laboratories. Importantly, the THXID®BRAF is better at identifying *BRAFV600K*, as the cobas® 4800 *BRAF* assay is only approximately 70% sensitive for the detection of this specific mutation (29). With the FDA-approval of vemurafenib and dabrafenib, the respective companion diagnostics were also approved.

Multiplexed Assays (One Test, Many Potential Treatments)

The examples of *EGFR* mutant NSCLC and *BRAF* mutant melanoma are illustrative in that they highlight the concept that a drug development plan that emphasizes identifying the patients most likely to benefit will be rewarded. Additionally, the identification of patients with the specific mutation/aberration to be targeted is as critical as identifying an agent to target the alteration. As such, the pathway most often chosen by companies is either to develop, or partner with a company that will develop, a companion diagnostic. While this strategy is sound, the challenge in the clinical world is that tissue is often limited, and sequentially testing a formalin fixed paraffin embedded (FFPE) block is time and tissue consuming, and may impact negatively on clinical care. For example, in non-small cell lung cancer, there are two histological (squamous and adenocarcinoma), four molecular (*EGFR* mutation, BRAF mutation, ALK fusions, and *ROS1* fusion), and one immunohistochemical (IHC; programmed death 1 ligand, PDL1) tests that need to be performed to adequately decide frontline therapy. Thus, the development of multiplexed assays that can perform all the required analyses with the least amount of tissue is necessary. Furthermore, with the reduced cost of sequencing, these types of approaches are likely more cost-effective than performing sequential testing or multiple single-plexed assays in parallel.

Tissue

The original multiplexed assays were developed to identify specific point mutations using multiple labelled probes that could be distinguished from each other with a unique identifier. For example, MassARRAY (Sequenom) is a system that utilizes PCR allelic specific extension primers to point mutations designed to be different but known masses, such that individual mutations might be identified using mass spectrometry (30). Another PCR-based assay, SNaPshot also leveraged allelic specific primers and extension steps to allow for differential and known times to travel through a capillary electrophoresis apparatus (31). The initial use of these was to develop panels of targetable mutations that might be identified in a particular disease (e.g., NSCLC). Over time, these panels increased to include more loci on more genes, and were adopted by a number of academic cancer centers. Yet, one of the key limitations of these approaches is that it only allows for the detection of point mutations, which limit the comprehensive analysis of genes where mutations occur at many loci, thus this approach is excellent for assessing hot spot mutations such as *EGFR* or *BRAF*, but poor at evaluating loss of function mutations in tumor suppressor genes such as *P53* and *NF1*. Additionally, these assays are unable to detect gene amplifications or deletions, which may be as relevant as point mutations on oncogenesis and treatment selection.

With the cost of sequencing reducing and the development of computational platforms allowing for more reliable interpretation of exome sequencing data, it was only a matter of time for the development, and commercialization of multiplexed assays to be developed that utilize massively parallel (next generation) sequencing (NGS). The advantage of these approaches are several, including the ability to analyze a larger percentage of (or the entire) a gene, the ability to detect amplifications and deletions, the capacity to distinguish a genetic aberration as germ line or somatic, and more relevant to the immunotherapy world, the ability to calculate a total mutational burden (32). The major disadvantage of available NGS platforms currently is the relatively slow turnaround time, with results returned typically in 3–4 weeks. In the metastatic cancer population, this can pose significant challenges when relying on these tests to navigate the care of patients present with symptomatic or otherwise aggressive disease features. The first and, to date, most successful commercial venture has been Foundation Medicine, which currently offers a product that can analyze over 300 genes for point mutations, amplifications, deletions, some rearrangements, and can calculate tumor mutational burden and microsatellite instability that may predict immunotherapy response (33). Furthermore, this platform, in the form of the FoundationOne CDx™ assay, has been FDA-approved in 2017 as a companion diagnostic for a number of disease subsets in melanoma (*BRAFV600E/K* mutant), NSCLC (*BRAFV600E* mutant, *EGFR* mutant, *ALK* rearranged), colorectal cancer (*KRAS* mutant as exclusion for cetuximab), and breast cancer (*BRCA1/2* alterations for the use of the PARP inhibitor rucaparib). A second NGS assay, Oncomine™ Dx Target Test, that can detect point mutations or deletions in 23 genes, as well as ROS1 rearrangements, has been approved by the FDA in 2017.

Blood

Mutation detection in circulating tumor DNA (ctDNA) dates back 20 years, but with advances in PCR techniques, in particular digital droplet PCR (ddPCR), and the lowering of sequencing costs allowing for ultra-low power (ULP) whole genome sequencing (WGS), the routine and reliable detection of ctDNA in patients with metastatic solid tumors is possible (34). The obvious value of accurate blood-based genetic analysis is that hard-to-biopsy patients would not need to have tissue acquisition and analysis performed to help in treatment selection. However, to date and despite analytic sensitivity and specificity of greater than 95%, the major challenge of ctDNA analysis is that a significant minority of patients have undetectable ctDNA levels, including approximately 20% of NSCLC patients and over 30% of patients with melanoma (35,36). Furthermore, the most reliable assay for ctDNA point mutation is ddPCR, which is difficult to multiplex. More recently, NGS approaches have been implemented to analyze ctDNA for copy number variation and gene alteration identification utilizing a number of techniques including ULP-WGS, targeted exosome sequencing, and hybrid-capture based sequencing (37). To date, none of these techniques has been FDA-approved as a companion diagnostic, but as these types of assays are now offered commercially (e.g. FoundationACT®, Foundation Medicine; Guardant360, Guardant Health) this is likely to change in the near future.

Development of Multi-Arm Targeted Therapy Trials

The origins of the multi-arm targeted therapy trial can be clinical trials called "basket" trials that enroll patients with a specific mutation to a particular treatment independent of tumor type. One of the first of these trials enrolled patients with *BRAFV600* mutant malignancies to receive vemurafenib (38). The trial had eight disease-specific cohorts and one "others" cohort, which was not disease specific other than patients must not be a candidate for one of the other cohorts. This design incorporated a straightforward endpoint, response rate at first assessment (8 weeks), and offered a glimpse of the activity of BRAF inhibitors across a number of different malignant histologies. Similar studies have been carried out with a number of agents, including immunotherapies (39–41). In many ways, these trials, which largely have been replaced by phase I trials, open multiple cohorts in "dose expansion" after the identification of the maximum tolerated dose and/or recommended phase 2 dose. However, in either case, the design of these studies is quite straightforward, and the selection of an appropriate efficacy endpoint which is easy to interpret will inform more definitive efficacy trials in an individual disease. With that said, the most successful "basket trial" approach surely has been the evaluation of pembrolizumab in patients with mismatch repair deficient malignancies, which directly led to the recent FDA-approval of pembrolizumab in patients with malignancies with microsatellite instability (MSI) (42). The trial had three cohorts, including mismatch repair deficient (A) and proficient (B) colorectal cancer and then mismatch repair deficient (C) non-colorectal cancer. The findings that patients with MSI malignancies had high response rates with pembrolizumab was predicted not by a specific mutation (i.e., vemurafenb and BRAF) but rather the propensity to have a high mutational burden in the setting of MSI. The trial incorporated a two-stage statistical design aimed to limit the number of patients treated with a potentially ineffective drug but also to have sufficient statistical power to justify further study, and definitively showed significant activity in both MSI-high cohorts (A, C) and virtually no activity in the non-MSI cohort (B). The most evident limitation from the BRAF and MSI examples is the uneven accrual of patients by tumor type. With inadequate numbers of patients in some "baskets" it becomes impossible to rule in or rule out the possibility of heterogeneous treatment effects. In the case of the vemurafenib basket trial, a strong signal efficacy could only be gleaned for the Langerhans histiocytosis population (38). In the case of MSI, colorectal cancer patients constituted more than two-thirds of the total study population, with very few patients included outside of those with gastric or endometrial cancers (42). The unevenness of accrual can be addressed by allowing protocols to remain open after certain cohorts have been filled, but with basket trials being considered as an efficiency gain in drug development, this alone does not address the entire problem.

The obvious next step is the development of trials that enroll patients to one of a number of arms of a study based on molecular analysis. These types of approaches could be taken in specific diseases where a number of frontline therapies are possible based on molecular testing, or across a number of different malignancies. For example, NSCLC is a perfect example of a disease with multiple molecularly-defined categories that may benefit differently from therapy. In particular, *EGFR* mutant and *ALK* rearranged NSCLC patients tend not to benefit from anti-PD1 therapy, whereas in non-*EGFR/ALK* aberrant patients, PD-L1 staining is a powerful selection marker that predicts benefit to anti-PD1 therapy. In NSCLC, the value of molecular testing has already been established in multiple trials, including a trial that incorporated multiplex testing and then allowed investigators the discretion to utilize that testing to select therapy. Importantly, the presence of a mutation did not mandate the use of targeted therapy, however in patients who received targeted therapy, outcomes were improved (43).

The current landscape now includes a number of trials that employ broad testing with NGS platform assays such as FoundationONE to inform which cohort the patient should be enrolled in. With the development of reliable NGS assays, the challenge of identifying patients for each cohort has been addressed, but other issues remain. Perhaps the greatest challenge is developing the partnerships with industry and funding agencies to allow these studies to have the best agents get to the appropriate patients. This is not a trivial endeavor, given that each company has its own development plan for each compound/asset, and there are potential risks in offering an agent to be included on a trial in which the individual companies have very little input over subject enrollment and treatment, as well as operational control and completion of the study. Further, appropriate endpoint selection is critical as is the pre-specified identification of a level of activity that key opinion leaders and industry members would agree will justify further development. Given the remarkable amount of engineering involved in launching such a trial, it is worth taking a closer look at how the largest and most ambitious of these studies got off the ground.

Design of Multi-Arm Targeted Therapy Trials

The NCI-MATCH (Molecular Analysis for Therapy Choice; NCT02465060) launched as the largest and most ambitious multi-arm targeted therapy trial. The premise was to have an umbrella protocol, which provided a general framework that determined the molecular testing platform required (with five laboratories working in a coordinated fashion to support a high volume of sample analysis using a common DNA and RNA sequencing approach) as well as general elements used for all treatment arms (eligibility criteria, endpoints, adverse event reporting, etc.), and then each molecular subset would have its own sub-protocol, with one agent assigned per molecularly-defined subpopulation (notably, two cohorts, BRAFV600 mutations; dabrafenib and trametinib, and HER2 amplifications; pertuzumab and trastuzumab emtansine, have two agents assigned). According to clinicaltrials.gov (date accessed January 5th, 2018), 30 cohorts are open and enrolling. Importantly, the efficacy endpoints are identical for each subgroup (response rate is the primary endpoint, whereas secondary endpoints include overall survival, progression free survival, and time to progression), simplifying the statistical challenges of carrying out over two dozen cohorts. Yet, the trial also recruits multiple chairpersons for each subprotocol to run the study and guide translational endpoints. In this way, while the trial has an overall Principal Investigator, each subprotocol has a team responsible for its conduct that will steer the science and credibly claim the bulk of the academic credit.

Launched soon after NCI-MATCH, the American Society of Clinical Oncology (ASCO) opened the TAPUR (Testing the Use of Food and Drug Administration (FDA) Approved Drugs That Target a Specific Abnormality in a Tumor Gene in People with Advanced Stage Cancer; NCT02693535) study. Molecular analytics lies at the heart of this study, as it does for NCI-MATCH, and drives treatment selection for enrolled patients. Also, the statistical design is similar to the NCI-MATCH, with the primary endpoint in each cohort being response rate with overall survival the secondary endpoint. However, as opposed to NCI-MATCH, the agents to be selected from within TAPUR are all FDA-approved for an indication other than how they are to be used in TAPUR. Also, the individual agent(s) defines the cohort (e.g., multiple molecular findings may trigger eligibility to receive an agent) as opposed to the molecular abnormality defining the cohorts in NCI-MATCH. Additionally, there are other differences in the treatment selection algorithm of TAPUR. First, there is the possibility of receiving a default agent (cetuximab) in the *absence* of an *NRAS, BRAF*, or *KRAS* mutation. Second, there is the possibility of treatment selection by an investigator based on molecular abnormalities that are not defined in the protocol, but may support the use of a particular agent in the literature. This latter scenario requires the review by a study specific Molecular Tumor Board (MTB), which is a group of experts brought together by ASCO to volunteer their services to vet these situations. The TAPUR MTB is also available to investigators for consultation to discuss with the investigator their proposed treatment and/or to provide counsel on possible alternative treatment options.

Both the NCI-MATCH and TAPUR studies involve therapy selection for molecular subtypes, and are offering front line targeted therapy for a specific molecular abnormality (in this case "targeted therapy" includes immune checkpoint inhibitor therapy for selected molecular subsets in the TAPUR study). Interestingly, there are multi-arm studies investigating combination therapy for patients who have developed resistance on prior therapy. The first example was the LOGIC-2 study (NCT02159066) that enrolled patients with BRAF mutant melanoma either prior to or after failure of BRAF-targeted therapy, treated these patients with the combination of encorafenib and binimetinib (enco/bini), and at time of treatment resistance, offered therapy with enco/bini plus a third agent selected based on molecular analysis of the time of BRAF-inhibitor resistance biopsy. While this study theoretically was sound in conception, the major challenge was that none of the selected triplet therapies had been completed testing in Phase I clinical trials prior to this study, and so the recommended Phase II dose of the regimen was not known. Ultimately, this is a challenge that may not be able to be overcome. While the trial has closed to enrollment and data is not yet available, the study will have difficulty meeting its ambitious goal of defining second targeted therapy for BRAF mutant melanoma based on analysis of resistance biopsies. This is due to the fact that it likely is not feasible to give full dose triplet regimens, as was recently described in a Phase I/II study of one of the triplets (encorafenib, binimetinib, and ribociclib) (44). Still, as the knowledge of resistance mechanisms improves for targeted and immunotherapy, it is expected that many similar studies will be launched and that the next generation of trials will incorporate various molecular biomarkers of responsiveness and non-responsiveness to define treatment options in the frontline setting as well.

Conclusions

We are operating in a new era of Drug Development that emphasizes the identification of the right patient population to benefit from a drug rather than maximizing the market share by studying the effects of an agent in a more heterogeneous population. A logical extension of this Precision Medicine approach is the development of large trials that segregate patients based on molecular abnormalities, to date specific genetic (e.g., single nucleotide point mutations) or more broadly genomic (e.g., tumor mutational burden) findings, and match agent and patient. These studies provide unique challenges (statistical design, in from multiple Pharmaceutical companies, academic credit, etc.) that are clearly able to be overcome, although it remains to be seen how effective these approaches will be at bringing drugs to market or expanding the indications of an agent already approved. Whether the existing trials prove to be successful or not, the trend has been set that multi-arm trials of multiple agents that depend on molecular analysis for treatment/cohort selection are a path forward. It will be interesting to see how these trials evolve and how more innovative assays, protocol designs, and statistical approaches are applied. It seems clear that the current set of studies represents the true and very tip of the iceberg.

Disclosures

RJS serves as a volunteer for the ASCO TAPUR Molecular Tumor Board and is a translational chairperson on a proposed NCI-MATCH subprotocol. KTF is the overall Principal Investigator of the NCI-MATCH study.

References

1. Druker BJ, Sawyers CL, Kantarjian H, Resta DJ, Reese SF, Ford JM, et al. Activity of a specific inhibitor of the BCR-ABL tyrosine kinase in the blast crisis of chronic myeloid leukemia and acute lymphoblastic leukemia with the Philadelphia chromosome. *The New England Journal of Medicine*. 2001;344 (14):1038–42.
2. Flaherty KT, Puzanov I, Kim KB, Ribas A, McArthur GA, Sosman JA, et al. Inhibition of mutated, activated BRAF in metastatic melanoma. *The New England Journal of Medicine*. 2010;363(9):809–19.
3. Lynch TJ, Bell DW, Sordella R, Gurubhagavatula S, Okimoto RA, Brannigan BW, et al. Activating mutations in the epidermal growth factor receptor underlying responsiveness of non-small-cell lung cancer to gefitinib. *The New England Journal of Medicine*. 2004;350(21):2129–39.
4. Ben-Neriah Y, Daley GQ, Mes-Masson AM, Witte ON, Baltimore D. The chronic myelogenous leukemia-specific P210 protein is the product of the bcr/abl hybrid gene. *Science*. 1986;233(4760):212–14.
5. Hyman DM, Laetsch TW, Kummar S, DuBois SG, Farago AF, Pappo AS et al. (eds.). The efficacy of larotrectinib (LOXO-101), a selective tropomyosin receptor kinase (TRK) inhibitor, in adult and pediatric TRK fusion cancers. *Journal of Clinical Oncology*. 2017;35(Suppl):abstr LBA2501.
6. Garcia De Palazzo IE, Adams GP, Sundareshan P, Wong AJ, Testa JR, Bigner DD, et al. Expression of mutated epidermal growth factor receptor by non-small cell lung carcinomas. *Cancer Research*. 1993;53(14):3217–3220.
7. Shepherd FA, Rodrigues Pereira J, Ciuleanu T, Tan EH, Hirsh V, Thongprasert S, et al. Erlotinib in previously treated non-small-cell lung cancer. *The New England Journal of Medicine*. 2005;353(2):123–32.
8. Thatcher N, Chang A, Parikh P, Rodrigues Pereira J, Ciuleanu T, Von Pawel J, et al. Gefitinib plus best supportive care in previously treated patients with refractory advanced non-small-cell lung cancer: Results from a randomised,

placebo controlled, multicentre study (Iressa Survival Evaluation in Lung Cancer). *Lancet.* 2005;366(9496):1527–37.

9. Tsao MS, Sakurada A, Cutz JC, Zhu CQ, Kamel-Reid S, Squire J, et al. Erlotinib in lung cancer - molecular and clinical predictors of outcome. *The New England Journal of Medicine.* 2005;353(2):133–144.

10. Pao W, Ladanyi M, Miller VA. Erlotinib in lung cancer. *The New England Journal of Medicine.* 2005;353(16):1739–41;author reply-1741.

11. Paez JG, Janne PA, Lee JC, Tracy S, Greulich H, Gabriel S, et al. EGFR mutations in lung cancer: Correlation with clinical response to gefitinib therapy. *Science.* 2004;304(5676):1497–500.

12. Mok TS, Wu YL, Ahn MJ, Garassino MC, Kim HR, Ramalingam SS, et al. Osimertinib or platinum-pemetrexed in EGFR T790M-positive lung cancer. *The New England Journal of Medicine.* 2017;376(7):629–40.

13. Sequist LV, Yang JC, Yamamoto N, O'Byrne K, Hirsh V, Mok T, et al. Phase III study of afatinib or cisplatin plus pemetrexed in patients with metastatic lung adenocarcinoma with EGFR mutations. *Journal of Clinical Oncology: Official Journal of the American Society of Clinical Oncology.* 2013;31(27):3327–34.

14. Davies H, Bignell GR, Cox C, Stephens P, Edkins S, Clegg S, et al. Mutations of the BRAF gene in human cancer. *Nature.* 2002;417(6892):949–54.

15. Sharma A, Trivedi NR, Zimmerman MA, Tuveson DA, Smith CD, Robertson GP. Mutant V599EB-Raf regulates growth and vascular development of malignant melanoma tumors. *Cancer Research.* 2005;65(6):2412–21.

16. Wilhelm S, Carter C, Lynch M, Lowinger T, Dumas J, Smith RA, et al. Discovery and development of sorafenib: A multikinase inhibitor for treating cancer. *Nature Reviews Drug Discovery.* 2006;5(10):835–44.

17. Eisen T, Ahmad T, Flaherty KT, Gore M, Kaye S, Marais R, et al. Sorafenib in advanced melanoma: A phase II randomised discontinuation trial analysis. *British Journal of Cancer.* 2006;95(5):581–586.

18. Flaherty KT, Lee SJ, Zhao F, Schuchter LM, Flaherty L, Kefford R, et al. Phase III trial of carboplatin and paclitaxel with or without sorafenib in metastatic melanoma. *Journal of Clinical Oncology: Official Journal of the American Society of Clinical Oncology.* 2013;31(3):373–79.

19. Flaherty KT, Schiller J, Schuchter LM, Liu G, Tuveson DA, Redlinger M, et al. A phase I trial of the oral, multikinase inhibitor sorafenib in combination with carboplatin and paclitaxel. *Clinical Cancer Research: An Official Journal of the American Association for Cancer Research.* 2008;14(15):4836–42.

20. Hauschild A, Agarwala SS, Trefzer U, Hogg D, Robert C, Hersey P, et al. Results of a phase III, randomized, placebo-controlled study of sorafenib in combination with carboplatin and paclitaxel as second-line treatment in patients with unresectable stage III or stage IV melanoma. *Journal of Clinical Oncology: Official Journal of the American Society of Clinical Oncology.* 2009;27(17):2823–30.

21. Wilson MA, Zhao F, Khare S, Roszik J, Woodman SE, D'Andrea K, et al. Copy number changes are associated with response to treatment with carboplatin, paclitaxel, and sorafenib in melanoma. *Clinical Cancer Research: An Official Journal of the American Association for Cancer Research.* 2016;22(2):374–82.

22. Wilson MA, Zhao F, Letrero R, D'Andrea K, Rimm DL, Kirkwood JM, et al. Correlation of somatic mutations and clinical outcome in melanoma patients treated with carboplatin, paclitaxel, and sorafenib. *Clinical Cancer Research:*

An Official Journal of the American Association for Cancer Research. 2014;20 (12):3328–37.

23. Heidorn SJ, Milagre C, Whittaker S, Nourry A, Niculescu-Duvas I, Dhomen N, et al. Kinase-dead BRAF and oncogenic RAS cooperate to drive tumor progression through CRAF. *Cell*. 2010;140(2):209–21.

24. Poulikakos PI, Zhang C, Bollag G, Shokat KM, Rosen N. RAF inhibitors transactivate RAF dimers and ERK signalling in cells with wild-type BRAF. *Nature*. 2010;464(7287):427–30.

25. Falchook GS, Long GV, Kurzrock R, Kim KB, Arkenau TH, Brown MP, et al. Dabrafenib in patients with melanoma, untreated brain metastases, and other solid tumours: A phase 1 dose-escalation trial. *Lancet*. 2012;379 (9829):1893–901.

26. Chapman PB, Hauschild A, Robert C, Haanen JB, Ascierto P, Larkin J, et al. Improved survival with vemurafenib in melanoma with BRAF V600E mutation. *The New England Journal of Medicine*. 2011;364(26):2507–16.

27. Hauschild A, Grob JJ, Demidov LV, Jouary T, Gutzmer R, Millward M, et al. Dabrafenib in BRAF-mutated metastatic melanoma: A multicentre, open-label, phase 3 randomised controlled trial. *Lancet*. 2012;380(9839):358–65.

28. Halait H, Demartin K, Shah S, Soviero S, Langland R, Cheng S, et al. Analytical performance of a real-time PCR-based assay for V600 mutations in the BRAF gene, used as the companion diagnostic test for the novel BRAF inhibitor vemurafenib in metastatic melanoma. *Diagnostic Molecular Pathology: The American Journal of Surgical Pathology, Part B*. 2012;21(1):1–8.

29. Marchant J, Mange A, Larrieux M, Costes V, Solassol J. Comparative evaluation of the new FDA approved THxID-BRAF test with high resolution melting and sanger sequencing. *BMC Cancer*. 2014;14:519.

30. Haff LA, Smirnov IP. Single-nucleotide polymorphism identification assays using a thermostable DNA polymerase and delayed extraction MALDI-TOF mass spectrometry. *Genome Research*. 1997;7(4):378–88.

31. Su Z, Dias-Santagata D, Duke M, Hutchinson K, Lin YL, Borger DR, et al. A platform for rapid detection of multiple oncogenic mutations with relevance to targeted therapy in non-small-cell lung cancer. *The Journal of Molecular Diagnostics: JMD*. 2011;13(1):74–84.

32. Zheng Z, Liebers M, Zhelyazkova B, Cao Y, Panditi D, Lynch KD, et al. Anchored multiplex PCR for targeted next-generation sequencing. *Nature Medicine*. 2014;20(12):1479–84.

33. Johnson DB, Frampton GM, Rioth MJ, Yusko E, Xu Y, Guo X, et al. Targeted next generation sequencing identifies markers of response to PD-1 blockade. *Cancer Immunology Research*. 2016;4(11):959–67.

34. Anker P, Lefort F, Vasioukhin V, Lyautey J, Lederrey C, Chen XQ, et al. K-ras mutations are found in DNA extracted from the plasma of patients with colorectal cancer. *Gastroenterology*. 1997;112(4):1114–20.

35. Lee JH, Long GV, Boyd S, Lo S, Menzies AM, Tembe V, et al. Circulating tumour DNA predicts response to anti-PD1 antibodies in metastatic melanoma. *Annals of Oncology: Official Journal of the European Society for Medical Oncology/ ESMO*. 2017;28(5):1130–6.

36. Oxnard GR, Thress KS, Alden RS, Lawrance R, Paweletz CP, Cantarini M, et al. Association between plasma genotyping and outcomes of treatment with osimertinib (AZD9291) in advanced non-small-cell lung cancer. *Journal of*

Clinical Oncology: Official Journal of the American Society of Clinical Oncology. 2016;34(28):3375–82.

37. Adalsteinsson VA, Ha G, Freeman SS, Choudhury AD, Stover DG, Parsons HA, et al. Scalable whole-exome sequencing of cell-free DNA reveals high concordance with metastatic tumors. *Nature Communications.* 2017;8(1):1324.

38. Hyman DM, Puzanov I, Subbiah V, Faris JE, Chau I, Blay JY, et al. Vemurafenib in multiple nonmelanoma cancers with BRAF V600 mutations. *The New England Journal of Medicine.* 2015;373(8):726–36.

39. Ott PA, Bang YJ, Berton-Rigaud D, Elez E, Pishvaian MJ, Rugo HS, et al. Safety and antitumor activity of pembrolizumab in advanced programmed death ligand 1-positive endometrial cancer: Results from the KEYNOTE-028 study. *Journal of Clinical Oncology: Official Journal of the American Society of Clinical Oncology.* 2017;35(22):2535–41.

40. Ott PA, Elez E, Hiret S, Kim DW, Morosky A, Saraf S, et al. Pembrolizumab in patients with extensive-stage small-cell lung cancer: Results from the phase Ib KEYNOTE-028 study. *Journal of Clinical Oncology: Official Journal of the American Society of Clinical Oncology.* 2017;35(34):3823–9.

41. Ott PA, Piha-Paul SA, Munster P, Pishvaian MJ, van Brummelen EMJ, Cohen RB, et al. Safety and antitumor activity of the anti-PD-1 antibody pembrolizumab in patients with recurrent carcinoma of the anal canal. *Annals of Oncology: Official Journal of the European Society for Medical Oncology/ESMO.* 2017;28 (5):1036–41.

42. Le DT, Uram JN, Wang H, Bartlett BR, Kemberling H, Eyring AD, et al. PD-1 blockade in tumors with mismatch-repair deficiency. *The New England Journal of Medicine.* 2015;372(26):2509–20.

43. Kris MG, Johnson BE, Berry LD, Kwiatkowski DJ, Iafrate AJ, Wistuba, II, et al. Using multiplexed assays of oncogenic drivers in lung cancers to select targeted drugs. *JAMA.* 2014;311(19):1998–2006.

44. Ascierto PA, Bechter O, Wolter P, Lebbe C, Elez E, Miller WH, et al. (eds.). A phase Ib/II dose-escalation study evaluating triple combination therapy with a BRAF (encorafenib), MEK (binimetinib), and CDK 4/6 (ribociclib) inhibitor in patients (Pts) with BRAF V600-mutant solid tumors and melanoma. *Journal of Clinical Oncology.* 2017;25(Suppl:abstr 9518.

3

Basket Trials at the Confirmatory Stage

Robert A. Beckman and Cong Chen

Introduction

The molecular approach to disease is transforming disease biology and therapy, and a corresponding transformation is required in drug development approaches. For example, cancer drug development was originally designed with the notion that cancer was a common disease, and traditional large sample sizes for confirmatory clinical trials were feasible. But now common diseases like lung cancer are being carved up into small subsets based on their molecular characteristics, particular at the DNA level. Not only is it increasingly difficult to enroll large sample sizes from these small subsets, but the large number of subsets and large number of experimental therapies have combined to drive a combinatorial explosion of potentially worthy clinical hypotheses. The cost and patient requirements of conventional one-indication at a time development are becoming increasingly unsustainable if used exclusively.

We have alluded in the Preface to this volume to differences in preferred terminology among authors. The terminology in this chapter is as follows: a platform trial is any trial that is capable of studying either multiple drugs or multiple disease entities simultaneously (Figure 3.1). Basket trials and umbrella trials study either multiple disease entities or multiple drugs, respectively.

There are three broad approaches for developing targeted agents based on molecular predictive biomarkers.

1. Efficiency optimized single indication co-development of targeted agents and their companion or complementary diagnostics for identifying patients whose tumors are members of a molecular subset (2,3) provides a very clear hypothesis and answer, and is recommended as a foundational study in one indication when feasible. However, this will not always be feasible as discussed above.

2. "Umbrella" trials combine multiple targeted agents and molecular subgroups within a single histology (4,5) or multiple histologies, (6) providing operational efficiencies and, under some circumstances, a

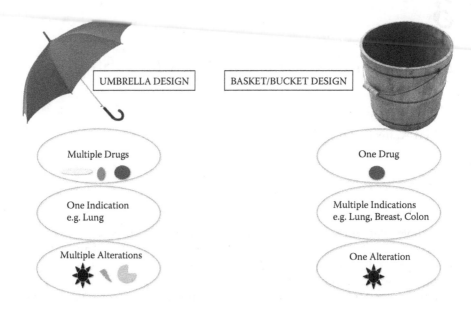

FIGURE 3.1
Schematic representation of umbrella and basket or bucket trial design. An umbrella trial allows for multiple drugs targeting multiple molecular alterations in a single indication to be tested within a single study. A basket or bucket design however, allows a single drug targeting a single molecular alteration to be tested across multiple indications. Reproduced from (1) with permission.

common control group. Umbrella trials require collaboration among multiple stakeholders, a significant challenge.

3. "Basket" or "bucket" trials feature a single targeted agent and subgroup across multiple histologic indications. The underlying assumption is that molecular classification of cancer is more fundamental than histological classification. (7) From this, it follows that similar subgroups may be studied together, and even pooled, across multiple histologies, as they may share a phenotype of potential clinical benefit from a single targeted agent. Scientific support for this assumption is a critical prerequisite for using basket trials.

While umbrella trials offer considerable operational efficiencies, basket trials offer the potential for studying multiple indications with a sample size traditionally appropriate for only one indication, a potential savings of several hundred percent in cost and patient enrollment requirements. Moreover, basket trials can easily be performed by a single sponsor. This chapter will focus on basket trials. Although this chapter focuses on oncology, basket trials may also be particularly useful in the infectious disease space, where an antimicrobial agent may be studied for infections in different areas of the body by the same organism simultaneously. Furthermore, the ability of basket trials to facilitate dramatic reductions in patient enrollment requirements can be very helpful for rare diseases when a common pathogenesis can be found across rare diseases, ie rare auto-immune diseases (8).

Basket trials have previously been used primarily in exploratory set-tings, and, if used for confirmation, in settings where there is exceptional scientific evidence, observed transformational levels of benefit from the therapy in related applications, and no or minimal other therapeutic options. Under the latter circumstances, there is justification for reducing evidentiary requirements, and indeed in the case of a pioneering basket trial of imatinib in rare tumors with the known targets of imatinib, one indication was approved based on tumor shrinkage in 1 of 4 patients in an unrandomized study (9–12). While early basket trial designs did not pool indications, but considered each indication separately, more recent designs utilize various degrees of weighted pooling based on techniques such as Bayesian hierarchical modeling (13,14) or weight hypotheses that all indi-cations are independent, or that all indications are from a common prob-ability distribution, based on the data (15). These designs generally utilize short term endpoints and are designed as Phase 2 options.

In this chapter we focus on a proposed basket trial design that may be suitable in the confirmatory setting (1,16). By far the greatest costs and patient enrollment requirements are associated with the confirmatory phase of devel-opment, and therefore the greatest impact on the problems alluded to above will come from applying the substantial savings potential of basket trials to the confirmatory phase. While application of non-rigorous designs to excep-tional situations is both valuable and justified, therapies with ordinary levels of efficacy are likely to be more common. Thus we sought to develop a confirmatory basket trial design of sufficient rigor to be generally applicable to efficacious agents without requiring exceptional circumstances.

A general approach to confirmatory basket studies would be beneficial in several regards. For patients in indications with small populations, for which development by conventional methods is not cost-effective, and thus often does not occur, access to therapies would be more likely. The featured design below also features the possibility of accelerated approval, providing even earlier access in some instances. Health authorities might have helpful datasets for evaluation of risk and benefit across molecular niche indications. For sponsors, development of niche indications would be facilitated due to lower cost and easier enrollment. A confirmatory basket trial may be a reasonable option to follow after a Phase 2 basket trial (17). Confirmatory basket trials may also be a very valuable compo-nent of an organized pipeline of linked adaptive platform trials (ie basket and umbrella trials) (18).

In this chapter we will give an overview of a general confirmatory basket trial design, (1,16) followed by a non-technical discussion of control of the false positive or type I error rate [technical details are discussed in another chapter in this volume (19)]. We then present two application examples, followed by a broad discussion of the challenges of basket trials in drug development and recommendations for managing them, including both statistical and non-statistical issues.

Overview of General Basket Design

In this design, individual histologic subtypes (indications) are grouped together for an overall randomized comparison. In order to reap the full efficiency advantage of a basket trial design, we pool indications in the final analysis so that the total sample size across multiple indications is adequate for formal confirmation by frequentist criteria. Such a design has an inherent risk, in that if indications are included for which the therapy is ineffective, they may dilute the signal from effective indications, resulting in failure of the entire basket. Accordingly, the risk of inclusion of ineffective indications is managed in multiple steps in a funnel-like design (Figure 3.2). First, the initial selection of indications must be based on significant scientific and clinical evidence, as discussed in more detail in the section on challenges of basket trials. The risk is further minimized, by *pruning*, by which we mean removal of indications determined to be high risk based on external data, or that do not show significant evidence of efficacy at an interim analysis, prior to the final pooled analysis. Pruning using data internal to the study creates complications with regard to controlling the type I error rate, and an overview of this is given in the next section. Furthermore, pruning based on internal study data may contribute to a small estimation bias, i.e., a slight tendency to overestimate the benefits associated with approved indications (20).

The recommended study design is randomized, each indication with its own control group, unless there is a common standard of care, in which case a shared control group may be used for the relevant indications. The strong preference for a randomized controlled design follows from the desire that the design be generally applicable in the confirmatory setting. Single arm designs using a concurrent registry control may be considered, preferably only in instances involving ultra-rare tumors with no standard of care, or in which a transformational effect featuring durable responses and a large survival benefit are expected (12). Concurrent registries control for several factors that affect the validity of historical controls, related to improvements over time in diagnostic sensitivity (resulting in patients being diagnosed and classified with less actual disease over time, also known as stage migration) and supportive care (resulting in less favorable outcomes in historical datasets). However, it is a far greater challenge to overcome selection bias, the tendency of clinical research physicians to

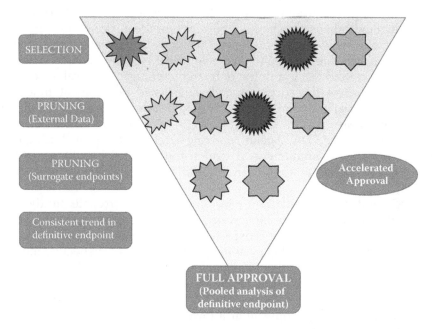

FIGURE 3.2

Flow chart of design concept for basket studies. Indications are selected, and may be pruned based on external data from the class, from off-label use of the therapy, or from a maturing exploratory study. Within the study, an accepted surrogate endpoint is used to either prune indications or qualify them for accelerated approval. Remaining indications are then pooled for evaluation of a final approval endpoint. If this pooled analysis is negative, the study fails. If the pooled analysis is positive, remaining indications are evaluated for a consistent trend in the definitive endpoint consistent with a positive benefit-risk balance. Indications displaying these characteristics are qualified for full approval. In the example in the figure, five indications are selected initially, one is pruned based on external data, two are pruned based on internal surrogate marker data, and the rest proceed to full approval. Pre-specified adaptations are applied to control the false positive rate under the global null hypothesis (i.e., all indications ineffective) and to maintain study power (not shown). Reproduced from (1) with permission.

select patients who will do well, resulting in an overestimate of benefit in single arm trials. This issue can be partially mitigated by matching algorithms, but physicians have a considerable ability to assess patients in an intuitive manner that is difficult to quantify and thus challenging to adjust for. The use of registry data should be pre-agreed with health authorities.

Each indication cohort would be sized for individual accelerated approval based on a predetermined surrogate endpoint (i.e., response rate, RR, or progression free survival, PFS) reasonably likely to predict clinical benefit (i.e., overall survival, OS). It is critical that the surrogate endpoint be more sensitive than the final clinical benefit endpoint, i.e., the expected effect size for an effective therapy should be greater for the interim surrogate endpoint than for the final clinical endpoint. Thus, the individual indications may be fully powered for the more sensitive interim endpoint, and when pooled at the end will have adequate sample size for the less sensitive final endpoint. We note that the endpoints named above should be viewed as examples only, representing a typical case. For example, either of the surrogate endpoints listed here can at times be primary approval endpoints (21,22). This approach is an accepted route to accelerated approval in the United States (23), requiring pre-discussion and agreement with the FDA. Agents receiving accelerated approval using this approach have a commitment to demonstrate clinical benefit using the final clinical benefit endpoint, and would receive full approval at that point.

Tumor indications failing to meet the interim surrogate hurdle for accelerated approval would be "pruned" (removed from the basket). In so far as the surrogate endpoint is expected to correlate to some degree (albeit imperfectly) with the final clinical endpoint, the risk of ineffective indications being included in the final pool is mitigated. For the remaining indications, the patients who contributed data at the interim analysis will be included in the final analysis, which may affect the false positive rate, resulting in the need to operate at a lower nominal false positive rate to control the resulting false positive rate of the pooled study, amounting to a statistical penalty for the re-use of internal study information.

Additional indications may be pruned based on external data such as maturing early stage data involving the definitive clinical benefit endpoint (2), real world data from off-label use of the therapy (discretionary use by physicians for non-approved indications, permitted in the United States) (8), or data from other agents in the class. Pruning based on external data may be done before or concurrently with pruning based on internal data, does not affect false positive rate, and does not incur a statistical penalty. Moreover, use of maturing data from previous early stage studies allows the definitive endpoint to govern adaptation, removing uncertainties due to imperfect correlation between interim and definitive endpoints.

After pruning, sample size readjustment is required to maintain the power of the final pooled analysis. The sample size adjustment strategy must be pre-specified, pre-agreed with health authorities, and ideally should be managed by an independent data monitoring committee. Chen, et al. (16) compared several sample size adjustment strategies and noted that the most aggressive strategy provided the best maintenance of reasonable power with increasing ineffective indications in the study prior to pruning. This strategy consisted of increasing the numbers of patients in the remaining indications to keep the size of the final pooled analysis as originally planned, which corresponds to a larger total study sample size than would have occurred without pruning. With this option the power is clearly superior (i.e., false negative rate lower) with pruning than without (16). For pruning to be effective in mitigating the risk of pooling, the bar for being included in the final pooled analysis is set relatively high. As such, pruning does not show that the indication is not worthy of further investigation, only that the indication is too high risk to be included in the basket.

The remaining indications would be eligible for full approval if the pooled analysis for the definitive clinical benefit endpoint reached statistical significance at the reduced nominal type I error level required by the design. Individual indications would not be required to show statistical significance but rather to demonstrate a sufficient trend for the definitive clinical benefit endpoint to be judged as having a positive benefit risk balance (pre-agreed with health authorities for each indication). Those indications not showing a sufficient consistent trend would not be approved, a final "pruning" step. Other data sources could potentially be used to make this judgement in borderline cases.

The above design concept can also be varied to use the definitive clinical endpoint to govern pruning at the interim analysis. In this case, typically the bar for passing the pruning step at interim must be set lower because only a small amount of data concerning the final endpoint will have accumulated. The bar for passing pruning and the fraction of available definitive endpoint information available at interim are important design parameters in this instance. We will consider an application example of this type later in this chapter.

Finally, in situations where single arm studies and response rate pivotal endpoints are appropriate, the design may be applied using an adaptation of the Simon 2-stage design paradigm (24). An application example is given in Beckman et al. (1).

Pruning, Random High Bias, and False Positive Rate Control

In order for a confirmatory basket trial to meet acceptance from health authorities, it will be necessary for the false positive rate of the pooled analysis to be rigorously controlled. Thus the false positive rate (type I error) is of particular interest in the context of a confirmatory basket trial.

Pruning of indications using data from within the study may inflate the false positive rate of the pooled analysis. In the setting where all indications are ineffective (termed the global null hypothesis), there will, due to the play of chance, still be random variation of the observed interim therapeutic effect around the expected average of zero. If, in the global null case we "prune" those indications randomly showing a negative or no therapeutic effect, and retain those randomly showing a positive therapeutic effect, we are in effect "cherry picking" those indications that got off to a good start. As this preliminary data is included in and thus will partly correlate with the final result, there is a greater chance that the remaining indications will randomly generate positive final data, resulting in a false positive result. This effect is termed "random high bias."

A counterbalancing effect is due to the fact that ineffective indications are more likely than effective indications to be screened out at the pruning step. These indications then must be removed according to the study design, termed "binding futility." Binding futility will tend to lower the false positive rate. The overall effect on the false positive rate depends on the exact study design and depends in a complex way on the interplay of random high bias and binding futility.

Fortunately, it is possible to calculate exactly how much the false positive rate of the pooled analysis is increased by random high bias, or decreased by binding futility, and to adjust the nominal false positive rate of the study such that the actual false positive rate of the final study pooled analysis remains in control after adjustment for these effects (16). In order to do this, we need to know the rules for pruning, the number of indications pruned, and which indications they were, given that the sample sizes may vary from indication to indication, as well as the percent of the events collected at interim if the interim analysis is based on the same endpoint as the final. We calculate the chance, if all indications truly have no therapeutic effect, of pruning the indications suggested for pruning by random chance and then of observing an apparently positive effect in the pooled analysis of the remainder by random chance. We then sum over the possible pruning scenarios. Usually the resulting false positive rate will be greater than the desired false positive rate due to inflation by random high bias, and we must pay a penalty by lowering the nominal false positive rate of the study until the actual false positive rate of the pooled analysis adjusted for random high bias is as desired. The false positive rate control assumes that the interim stopping rules and other adaptation rules are strictly followed. The rules for these adaptations can be prospectively pre-specified and administered by an independent data monitoring committee. Although a statistical penalty must be paid for pruning based on internal data, the benefit of being able to investigate multiple indications in one study far outweighs the penalty. If indications are pruned due to data external to the study, there is no concern about random high bias affecting the pooled analysis, and no need for a statistical penalty. Hence, it may be possible to improve the performance of this design using external data sources such as real world data (8).

It should be noted that the false positive rate control in (16,19) applies only to the case in which all indications are ineffective and not to the « family wise error rate », including cases where the basket contains a heterogeneous mixture of ineffective and effective indications. In this case, if an ineffective indication or indications escapes pruning, a heterogeneous mixture of effective and ineffective indications may proceed to the second step in which indications are evaluated based on a pooled result. As we have previously noted in this chapter, the ineffective indications may dilute the overall pooled result, resulting in a false negative with respect to the effective indications. Conversely, if the effective indications dominate the average result, the pool of indications may be approved, resulting in a false positive result with respect to the ineffective indications (25).

Thus heterogeneity is a risk in basket trials. We note however that this risk is not unique to basket trials, since every pivotal clinical trial population is heterogeneous based both on characteristics suspected to be important, and characteristics whose importance was unfortunately never suspected. Typically, subgroup analysis for known predictive and prognostic factors is performed, and since these subgroup analyses are underpowered, they provide qualitative information only. If the health authority believes heterogeneity with respect to a given characteristic may affect the result based on subgroup analysis of a conventional study, it might result in a narrowing of the approved label, or in severe cases denial of approval.

Several authors have proposed methods for detecting heterogeneity based on interim data (14,15). Simon discusses the application of his method for detecting heterogeneity at the interim stage and its application to this design in this volume (17). Detection of statistically significant heterogeneity at interim, while underpowered, could provide some degree of risk mitigation, particularly if it resulted in additional pruning until the heterogeneity fell below a pre-agreed threshold.

Cunanan and colleagues have demonstrated that the *family wise* false positive rate of some basket trial designs may be higher than expected, and have advocated that these family wise false positive rates be characterized by simulation and disclosed to the community. (26) We agree, but point out that basket trials may require their own definitions of and/or thresholds for the false positive rate. For example, if a basket trial contains six indications, it is replacing six individual trials that would have been performed if they were feasible. These six individual trials collectively would have approximately a six-fold higher chance of at least a single false positive result than a single trial would. Therefore, we believe basket trials with N indications should be allowed family wise false positive rates of approximately N times 2.5% (the threshold for approval for individual trials), i.e., approximately 15% if there are six indications. In ongoing research, we are studying the family wise false positive rate of our design under various conditions and the effect of various simple risk mitigation strategies.

Application Examples

Below we give two application examples of the generalized confirmatory basket trial. The first uses PFS as the interim and OS as the final endpoints, respectively. A second example involves OS as interim and final endpoints.

A single arm design involving tumor response rate (RR) as interim and final endpoints is discussed in (1).

In the first example, we assume median PFS on the control therapy is 3 months, median OS is 7 months. We further assume a moderate but imperfect correlation between PFS and OS (0.5).

We study six indications, powering each on an improvement in PFS from 3 to 6 months at interim. We enroll 110 patients in each indication, collecting 88 PFS events shortly after all patients are enrolled. Each indication has 90% power for PFS and a one-sided type I error of 2.5%, standard for confirmatory studies. Indications meeting the PFS endpoint will be included in the final pooled analysis, and may be eligible for accelerated approval.

After pruning, the sample size of the remaining indications is adaptively increased to maintain a sample size of 660 in the final pooled analysis and an OS endpoint is evaluated in the pooled remaining indications. For example, if half the indications are pruned, an additional 330 patients are added. The false positive rate (prior to adjustment for pruning) is set at 0.8%, which is 2.5% after adjustment for pruning. The power is approximately 90% for detecting an increase in OS from 7 to 10 months (the exact power depends on the number of positive indications in the basket).

> In summary, in this randomized example, a 660–990 patient randomized confirmatory study has the potential to lead to accelerated and full approval of up to six indications. This is about 1–1.5 times the number of patients in a standard confirmatory oncology trial of a single indication.

In a second example, we employ an interim analysis of OS for pruning rather than utilizing a surrogate endpoint, and OS is also the final endpoint. This paradigm is equally applicable if another endpoint such as PFS or RR is a suitable final endpoint. The characteristics of this design can be more easily calculated in that there is no need to assume a particular level of correlation between an interim endpoint and a definitive endpoint. Instead the two endpoints are identical and the level of correlation depends in a simple way on the fraction of the total data available at interim, and the sample size readjustment strategy. (16) Depending on the rates of enrollment and the survival time, adequate OS information to support an interim analysis may not occur in some instances until after all indications are fully enrolled.

We plan the study for six indications, enrolling 375 patients to observe 300 OS events. We assume a very significant benefit of experimental therapy, improving median survival from 6 to 10 months. We will perform an interim analysis after 150 deaths have occurred. An indication is permitted to continue if a 10% apparent advantage in OS is seen in the experimental arm relative to control. This low threshold for continuing is required due to the small amount of available OS data at interim. Other-wise, too many effective indications would be rejected. As a consequence of the low pruning bar, 40% of ineffective indications will be permitted to continue. The sample size is increased such that the indications which continue have a total of 300 OS events in the pool. For example, if half of the indications are terminated, it will be necessary to enroll another 188 patients to replace their events and maintain study power. Thus, the study may contain 375 + 188 = 563 patients if the interim analysis occurred after enrollment was complete.

The nominal false positive rate before pruning must be set at 0.5% to control the actual false positive rate at 2.5%. The study power ranges from 84% (if three of the six indications were really inactive) to 99% (if all 6 indications were active) for confirming the relatively large assumed benefit.

> In summary, in this example, a randomized confirmatory study con-taining 375–563 patients has 84–99% power to confirm efficacy (and potentially lead to full approval) for 3–6 indications assuming a rela-tively large OS benefit.

Other Challenges of Basket Trials and Recommendations for Overcoming Them

In this section, we discuss other challenges of basket trials, particularly in the confirmatory setting, and recommendations for overcoming the chal-lenges and/or mitigating the risks. The emphasis in this section is on issues or problems with additional dimensions beyond statistics.

Risks of Pooling

Pooling entails risks of both false positives and false negatives if the set of indications pooled contains both effective and ineffective indications. If the ineffective indications dilute a signal from the effective indications, the pool is rejected, and there are false negatives concerning all the effective indications. Conversely, if the effective indications are sufficient to lead to approval of the pool even in the presence of ineffective indications, a false positive will occur with respect to the ineffective indications. To some extent, these risks are generic to clinical research, as any population is an amalgam of subpopulations. We are just more used to tolerating the sub-populations within populations defined by histol-ogy than within populations defined by a biomarker. In populations defined by a biomarker, histology, traditionally the defining character-istic, is only a covariate.

Heterogeneity is the fundamental cause of this risk, and can be evaluated at the pruning step, and even at the end of the study, by statistical methods referenced above. (14,17) However, the fundamental basis for pooling indications must be scientific, not statistical. If pooling is based on a biomarker hypothesis, i.e., that a given therapy will be beneficial to patients who share a common biomarker across traditional histologically defined indications, there should be extensive laboratory and clinical evidence supporting this biomarker hypothesis. This should include a well-understood biochemical mechanism, appropriate mechanistic studies, genetic confirmation of mechanism by gene knock-in or knock-out if applicable, and confirmed biomarker-dependent efficacy *in vitro* and *in vivo* across several histologies. At a minimum, there should short term evidence from non-randomized clinical studies linking short-term outcomes to pharmacodynamic effects on the biomarker defined target in several indications, as well as clinical confirmation that pharmacodynamically significant exposure to the therapy is achievable in all proposed populations. An efficient way to obtain this kind of data might be within a Phase II non-randomized basket trial (17). If there is real-world data from use of other agents in the class, or off-label for the proposed experimental agent, this data should be consistent with the biomarker hypothesis (8). In the ideal case, there would be randomized Phase 2 clinical data supporting the inclusion of all proposed indications, and one lead indication that actually achieved approval in the biomarker defined subset, supporting the biomarker hypothesis and providing an approved companion diagnostic (1). This lead indication can be achieved by optimized conventional methods (2), and then the basket trial becomes an efficient way to broaden the approval across many other disease states. In the case of vemurafenib in *b-RAF* mutated solid tumors, approval in melanoma was the lead indication, and this was used to justify a much more aggressive basket design than the rigorous one proposed herein (12).

Even with all the evidence listed above, there may still be surprises. Vemurafenib, a b-RAF inhibitor, whose efficacy in *b-RAF* mutated tumors was supported by considerable preclinical evidence and an approval in melanoma, is ineffective in *b-RAF* mutated colorectal cancer (27). This was not anticipated; rather the colorectal cancer feedback loops leading to this effect were discovered in an effort to explain the negative clinical data (28,29). There is still a degree to which histology influences sensitivity to therapy. Some authors believe that considering combinations of mutations will enable better prediction of tissue specific effects (30).

Given the above, careful selection of indications based on scientific and clinical evidence can mitigate, but not eliminate, the risks of pooling. Pruning, based on data either external or internal to the study, further minimizes the risks. Use of external data does not incur a statistical penalty. Two sources of external data are real-world data (8), which may be updated prior to the pruning step, and maturing Phase 2 randomized studies of the same agent. In particular, a development program may be designed to make the randomized Phase 2 studies as similar to the randomized Phase 3 basket study as possible, for example using the same inclusion criteria and at least some of the same investigative sites. At the time of the pruning step, randomized data on the final clinical endpoint may be available from the external Phase 2 studies to supplement the data on the interim endpoint from the Phase 3 basket trial itself. (2) Statistical evaluation for heterogeneity may be conducted at the pruning step (17), or even after study completion, and outlier indications removed. Qualitative or semi-quantitative risk benefit analysis may be performed on each remaining indication after study completion (1).

Companion Diagnostic Assay

In order to identify patients in the biomarker-defined subset, there must be a clinical laboratory test that has been validated both for its analytical properties in laboratory studies as well as for its actual predictive value in clinical studies. This test is called the "companion diagnostic." If a lead indication has previously been approved for the biomarker-defined subset in another histologic type, the companion diagnostic would generally have been simultaneously approved for that purpose.

However, even if there is a previously approved companion diagnostic in one histologic sub-type, one cannot assume that its analytical properties against laboratory standards will be independent of tissue type. Rather, for each histology, these analytic properties must be validated in the laboratory, and if sensitivity, specificity, and (where applicable) linearity are not validated, a customized variant of the original companion diagnostic may need to be created.

While some companion diagnostics, such as those that look for mutations, may give a binary result, others, such as those that quantify expression of a gene, give continuous results. For those companion diagnostics with a continuous readout, a cutoff must be established between "biomarker positive" and "biomarker negative" patients, another important goal that should be accomplished based on Phase 2 studies before the confirmatory Phase 3 basket trial is initiated (31). Further, gene expression levels are frequently normalized to the expression levels of "housekeeping genes," i.e., genes whose expression level is believed to be relatively constant. However, these "housekeeping genes" may vary from tissue to tissue, and should be optimized in the laboratory as part of customizing the companion diagnostic assay for each tissue.

Tissue Acquisition and Processing

Uniform and rapid tissue acquisition and processing is essential to obtain consistent results from a companion diagnostic assay. Consistent results are essential to enroll comparable populations with respect to biomarker status across histological subtypes and even across investigative sites within a single histologic subtype. If these goals are not met, additional variability will be introduced.

Academic medical centers are currently organized by histology, not by biomarker subsets. To achieve uniformity in this area, cooperation may have to occur between divisions, such as the lung and breast cancer divisions, which may not have extensive experience working together.

Based on the above considerations, we recommend that a full time pathologist be engaged for a confirmatory basket study to establish and maintain standards for optimal tissue acquisition and processing, to educate investigative sites, and to facilitate strict adherence to these practices.

Clinical Validity of the Biomarker Hypothesis

In order to validate the companion diagnostic for new indications as a test that can distinguish between patients who will and will not benefit from the therapy, biomarker-negative patients must also be enrolled. It is desirable to keep the number of biomarker-negative patients as small as possible, and in some indications it may not be ethically feasible to enroll them. If the lead indication supports the biomarker hypothesis and companion diagnostic assay, we propose that a single biomarker negative cohort be made with small contributions of biomarker-negative patients from those indications for which this is ethically feasible, normally those for which the randomized design is an add-on of the experimental therapy to a base of standard of care. We propose this biomarker negative randomized sub-study be powered on the more sensitive interim endpoint.

High Screen Failure Rate

If the biomarker-defined subset of interest for the study is uncommon, most of the screened patients will be rejected by the screen. These patients will have invested precious time and energy in the screening process without a chance to benefit from the study directly. Given this circumstance, we recommend that patients be offered broad-based screening for other biomarkers, for example, next generation sequencing, as part of the screening process. This will expedite their identification of another suitable study.

Imperfect Correlation between Interim and Final Endpoints

This risk is unavoidable. We propose two mitigations. The first recommendation, already alluded to, is to utilize maturing data on the primary endpoint from earlier Phase 2 studies for pruning (1,2). The second recommendation is to set thresholds for the data on the final endpoint in each individual indication that will be required to constitute a "consistent trend" towards a positive risk-benefit analysis in that indication in the final analysis. Any indication not meeting its threshold for a "consistent trend" in the final endpoint will be removed from the approved dataset. These thresholds should be pre-agreed with health authorities, taking into account regional variations (32).

Conclusions

We have outlined a general histology agnostic "basket study" that can enable grouping and simultaneous development of a therapy in multiple indications with a common predictive biomarker hypothesis. Such a design entails screening and removal of indications of lower likelihood to succeed based on maturing external data and on internal surrogate data or interim definitive endpoint data, the possibility of individual accelerated approval of indications based on an approved surrogate endpoint or on interim definitive endpoint data, pooling of the definitive endpoint across indications for approval, and the demand for a favorable numerical trend in the definitive endpoint in each approved indication. In contrast to previous designs, this design incorporates the rigor of concurrent control groups and control of the false positive rate under the assumption of all indications being ineffective. Thus this design may be suitable for confirmatory studies of effective therapies without requiring that they be transformational. Attention must be paid to the selection of indications and to the risk of diluting positive indications with negative ones in the pooled analysis, to protect the validity of the conclusions. Generalized control of the false positive rate is an area of ongoing research.

The proposed confirmatory basket trial design has the potential to lead to considerable resource savings, either utilized alone or as part of an overall PIPELINE of platform trials (18). It can facilitate development in molecular niche indications where accrual for a standalone confirmatory trial is challenging, resulting in earlier and enhanced patient access to effective therapy in these settings.

Acknowledgments

This work originated from the Drug Information Association (DIA) workstream on small populations and rare diseases, pathway design subgroup. The small populations/rare diseases workstream is in turn a subgroup of the DIA Adaptive Design Scientific Working Group. We are indebted to the following members of the pathway design subgroup and small populations/rare diseases workstream: Ohad Amit, Zoran Antonijevic, Christine Gause, Sebastian Jobjornsson, Rasika Kalamegham, Lingyun Liu, Robert T O'Neill, Sue Jane Wang, Samuel Yuan, and Yi Zhou.

Conflict of Interest Disclosure

RAB is a stockholder in Johnson & Johnson, Inc., and consults for Astra-Zeneca and EMD Serono. He is the founder and Chief Scientific Officer of Onco-Mind, LLC, founded to foster study of the effect of intratumoral heterogeneity and evolutionary dynamics on optimal personalized treatment strategies for cancer.

CC is a full time employee of Merck & Co., Inc., and may benefit from expedited drug approvals based on the proposed basket design of clinical trials.

References

1. Beckman RA, Antonijevic Z, Kalamegham R, Chen C Adaptive design for a confirmatory basket trial in multiple tumor types based on a putative predictive biomarker. *Clin. Pharmacol. Ther.* 2016; 100:617–625.
2. Beckman RA, Clark J, Chen C Integrating predictive biomarkers and classifiers into oncology clinical development programmes. *Nat. Rev. Drug Disc.* 2011; 10:735–749.
3. Ondra T, Jobjörnsson S, Beckman RA, Burman CF, König F, Stallard N, Posch M Optimized adaptive enrichment designs. *Stat. Meth. Med. Res.* 2017. doi:10.1177/0962280217747312.
4. Barker AD, Sigman CC, Kelloff GJ, Hylton NM, Berry DA, Esserman LJ I-SPY2: An adaptive breast cancer trial design in the setting of neoadjuvant chemotherapy. *Clin. Pharmacol. Ther.* 2009; 86:97–100.
5. Kim ES et al. The BATTLE trial: Personalizing therapy for lung cancer. *Cancer Disc.* 2011; 1:44–53.
6. Kaiser J Biomedicine. Rare cancer successes spawn 'exceptional' research efforts. *Science.* 2013; 340:263.
7. Ciriello G, Miller ML, Aksoy BA, Senbabaoglu Y, Schultz N, Sander C Emerging landscapes of oncogenic signatures across human cancers. *Nat. Genet.* 2013; 45:1127–1133.
8. Guinn DA, Madhavan S, Beckman RA Harnessing real world data to inform platform trial design. In *Platform Trials: Umbrella Trials and Basket Trials*, Antonijevic Z, Beckman RA, editors, CRC Press; Boca Raton, FL, 2018.
9. Meador CB, Micheel CM, Levy MA et al. Beyond histology: Translating tumor genotypes into clinically effective targeted therapies. *Clin. Cancer Res.* 2014; 20:2264–2275.
10. Lacombe D, Burocka S, Bogaerts J, Schoeffskib P, Golfinopoulosa V, Stuppa R The dream and reality of histology agnostic cancer clinical trials. *Mol. Onc.* 2014; 8:1057–1063.
11. Sleijfer S, Bogaerts J, Siu LL Designing transformative clinical trials in the cancer genome era. *J. Clin. Oncol.* 2013; 31:1834–1841.
12. Demetri G, Becker R, Woodcock J, Doroshow J, Nisen P, Sommer J Alternative trial designs based on tumor genetics/pathway characteristics instead of histology. *Issue Brief: Conference on Clinical Cancer Research* 2011; http://www.focr.org/conference-clinical-cancer-research-2011.

13. Berry SM, Broglio KR, Groshen S et al. Bayesian hierarchical modeling of patient subpopulations: Efficient designs of phase II oncology clinical trials. *Clin Trials*. 2013; 10:720–734.
14. Cunanan KM, Iasonos A, Shen R et al. An efficient basket trial design. *Stat. Med.* 2017; 36:1568–1579.
15. Simon RM, Geyer S, Subramanian J, Roychowdhury S The Bayesian basket design for genomic variant-driven phase II trials. *Seminars Onc.* 2016; 43:13–18.
16. Chen C, Li N, Yuan S, Antonijevic Z, Kalamegham R, Beckman RA Statistical design and considerations of a phase 3 basket trial for simultaneous investigation of multiple tumor types in one study. *Stat. Biopharm. Res.* 2016; 8:248–257.
17. Simon RM Primary site-independent clinical trials in oncology. In *Platform Trials: Umbrella Trials and Basket Trials*, Antonijevic Z, Beckman RA, editors, CRC Press; Boca Raton, FL, 2018.
18. Trusheim M, Shrier AA, Antonijevic Z et al. PIPELINEs: Creating comparable clinical knowledge efficiently by linking trial platforms. *Clin. Pharmacol. Ther.* 2016; 100:713–729.
19. Chen C, Beckman RA Control of type I error for confirmatory basket trials. In *Platform Trials: Umbrella Trials and Basket Trials*, Antonijevic Z, Beckman RA, editors, CRC Press; Boca Raton, FL, 2018.
20. Li W, Chen C, Li X, Beckman RA. Estimation of treatment effect in two-stage confirmatory oncology trials of personalized medicines. *Stat. Med.* 2017; 36:1843–1861.
21. United States Food and Drug Administration Guidance for Industry: Clinical trial endpoints for the approval of cancer drugs and biologics, 2007; www.fda. gov/downloads/drugs/guidancecomplianceregulatoryinformation/gui dances/ucm071590.pdf
22. European Medicines Agency. Guideline on the evaluation of anticancer medicinal products in man, 2013; www.ema.europa.eu/docs/en_GB/document_li brary/Scientific_guideline/2013/01/WC500137128.pdf
23. United States Food and Drug Administration. Guidance for Industry Expedited Programs for Serious Conditions – Drugs and Biologics, 2014; www.fda.gov/ downloads/drugs/guidancecomplianceregulatoryinformation/guidances/ ucm358301.pdf
24. Simon RM Optimal two-stage designs for Phase II clinical trials. *Control. Clin. Trials*. 1989; 10:1–10.
25. Yuan SS, Chen A, He L, Chen C, Gause CK, Beckman RA On group sequential enrichment design for basket trial. *Stat. Biopharm. Res.* 2016; 8:293–306.
26. Cunanan KM, Iasonos A, Shen R, Hyman DM, Riely GJ, Gönen M, Begg CB Specifying the true- and false-positive rates in basket trials. *JCO Precision Oncol.* 2017; 1:1–5.
27. Prahallad A et al. Unresponsiveness of colon cancer to BRAF(V600E) inhibition through feedback activation of EGFR. *Nature*. 2012; 483:100–103.
28. Solit DB, Jänne PA Translational medicine: Primed for resistance. *Nature*. 2012; 483:44–45.
29. Chandarlapaty S et al. AKT inhibition relieves feedback suppression of receptor tyrosine kinase expression and activity. *Cancer Cell*. 2011; 19:58–71.
30. Tabchy A, Eltonsy N, Housman DE, Mills GB Systematic identification of combinatorial drivers and targets in cancer cell lines. *PLoS One*. 2013; 8:e60339.

31. Jiang W, Freidlin B, Simon R Biomarker-adaptive threshold design: A procedure for evaluating treatment with possible biomarker-defined subset effect. *J. Natl. Cancer Inst.* 2007; 99:1036–1043.

32. Marschner IC Regional differences in multinational clinical trials: Anticipating chance variation. *Clin. Trials.* 2010; 7:147–156.

4

Harnessing Real-World Data to Inform Platform Trial Design

Daphne Guinn, Subha Madhavan, and Robert A. Beckman

Introduction

Current drug development is dependent on traditional clinical trials for data generation. Clinical trials are experiments designed to ask specific questions with defined endpoints. The evaluated patient population is often narrow and excludes patients with common comorbidities that will be given the drug in the clinical setting.[1] While clinical trial data provides standard evidence for regulatory decision-making, these data represent only a subset of the population and therefore are insufficient to inform everyday clinical decision-making. Traditional clinical trials also require large sample sizes for sufficient power, which may not be feasible when studying rare diseases or small biomarker defined subsets of a disease. These deficiencies in the current development paradigm highlight a need for exploring alternative data sources that can provide evidence that cannot be collected in a traditional clinical trial setting.

Data collected outside of traditional clinical trial sources have been defined as real-world data (RWD), which can be obtained from a variety of sources that relate to patients' healthcare experiences.[2] Thus, RWD sources are diverse and can be stratified based on the source and each source's level of pragmatism.[1] These data may be collected from observational studies, registries, case reports, electronic health records (EHR), and administrative claims data[2] (Figure 4.1). RWD can provide important information about factors associated with the clinical care setting that may affect treatment effect and outcomes.[3] To provide meaningful information, RWD sources must be carefully evaluated for data quality, including any biases associated with data collection. Many of the sources that are associated with patient clinical care, such as the EHR, may be plagued with missing or incomplete data because of the lack of standardization in the type and method of data collected during a patient's visit with a healthcare provider. In addition, the most relevant information may be in free text fields such as provider notes that are difficult to mine in a high throughput

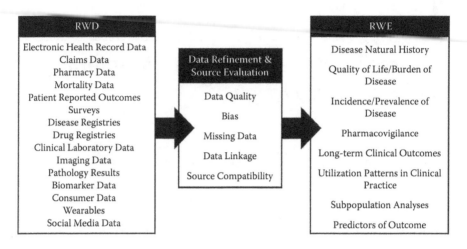

FIGURE 4.1
RWD Sources to Produce RWE.

automated fashion. Understanding the strengths and weakness of the RWD source allows for evaluating its ability to produce meaningful evidence.

Real-world evidence (RWE) can be defined as the clinical evidence that is derived from an analysis of the RWD.[2] For example, RWE can be generated by collecting and analyzing clinical data from EHR and claims databases to inform long-term clinical outcomes associated with an approved therapy. There are many advantages to using RWD sources for evidence generation. RWD is considered to be more generalizable, as it is often collected without specific research questions in mind. It could represent a broad intersection of patients, which would allow researchers to address questions about the impact a therapy has had on both modifying the disease trajectory or affecting patient quality of life.

Often, drug development in rare diseases or biomarker defined subsets of a disease, where recruiting sufficient patients can be a costly challenge.[4] Identifying eligible patients through EHRs or registries could streamline patient recruitment. Moreover, while the randomized controlled trial is the standard for clinical trial evidence, a control arm may not be ethical for severe diseases if there is no current standard of care. In such a case, RWD may be used to construct a historical control arm in selected instances, and with attention to additional confounding factors, which affect the use of historical controls. It is clear that diverse sources of RWD could be used to answer questions that cannot be addressed through traditional methods.

Real-World Data for Evidence Generation

Many stakeholders recognize how RWD could transform medical product development and are discussing how RWD can be best applied.[5,6] This modernization of considered data sources was highlighted in the 21st Century Cures Act,[7] which requires regulators to review drug development tools that will provide novel methods and pathways to facilitate drug approval.[7,8] It also specifically supports the submission of information related to the patient experience and real-world evidence.[7,8] The use of RWD sources was also supported in the most recent FDA Prescription Drug User Fee Act (PDUFA) VI,[9] which prompted the FDA to identify goals and timelines for producing guidance to industry on how best to integrate RWD into research for regulatory decision making.[5,10] RWD sources could be informative in both the pre- and post-market phases of development (Figure 4.2). While some of these applications are already being used in novel programs, others are still theoretical.

In the pre-market stage of development, RWD can be used to explore the natural history of disease. Epidemiological methods are used to determine disease incidence and prevalence, which can assist medical product developers in defining the disease population of interest, information critical for defining unmet need.[11,12] It provides the basis for narrowing the indication that will be sought in the label. Furthermore, patient recruitment is a well-known challenge, and unsuccessful recruitment can lead to trial failure.[13] RWD sources could provide estimates for the number of patients with a particular disease at certain clinical sites, allowing sponsors to determine how many sites are needed for the study and which sites have a sufficient patient volume. For example, sales figures for a standard of care drug were more accurate than investigator estimates in predicting actual enrollment rates in a study of metastatic ovarian cancer patients (Beckman, RA,

Pre-Market		Post-Market	
Disease Natural History	Historical Control	Pharmacovigilance	Label Expansion or Modification
Disease Incidence or Prevalence	Trial Site Selection	Subgroup Analysis	Prescribing and Usage Patterns
Indication Selection	Estimating Effect Sizes	Long Term Risk/ Benefit Analysis	Impact on Disease

FIGURE 4.2
Uses for RWD for Evidence Generation in Medical Product Development.

unpublished) RWD associated with therapy in the clinical setting could be used to estimate the degree of clinical benefit associated with a therapy and hence the sample size needed to appropriately power the clinical trial.

Another consideration when designing the clinical study is the type of control that will be utilized. Many trials testing targeted therapies or assessing an experimental therapy in a rare disease are single-armed, perhaps because recruitment in a rare patient population is difficult or the disease does not have an adequate standard of care. In order to produce adequate evidence, developers may employ a matched historical control of patients receiving standard of care or palliative therapy to compare their intervention.[5,14] When using a historical control, there are three major sources of bias which one must attempt to minimize. First, the progressive improvement of standard of care as well as supportive measures means that a historical control from the past may underperform relative to a control from the present. Second, the historical control from the past may underperform because of "stage migration," i.e., over time, patients with lesser disease may be diagnosed with having a particular stage due to improvements in diagnostic sensitivity compared to the past. Third, "selection bias" could mean that healthier patients are enrolled in an active clinical trial rather than as a historical control; selection bias may occur both due to visible sources (trial inclusion criteria) and invisible sources (investigator bias). The historical control could be composed of individual patient data taken from RWD sources, rather than only relying on previously published clinical trial data.[15] If the control is recent, it may minimize the first two sources of bias. However, selection bias is harder to minimize, especially in that RWD by its nature is in a realistic clinical setting and the patients may have more comorbidities and increased risk factors for poor outcomes compared to patients selected for a clinical trial. Awareness of these risks is helpful when comparing RWD to clinical trial data.

In some cases, evidence derived from RWD sources may be used for regulatory decision-making. This could be considered for rare diseases that are difficult to study through traditional clinical development methods. When considering approval of a new drug, regulators may take data derived from non-traditional sources if they can be legitimized and provide enough information to prove a positive benefit-risk relationship. It more likely that this information would be considered alongside information collected from traditional clinical trials.

In the post-market setting, RWD has been widely used for post-market safety surveillance and pharmacovigilance. The collection of information from claims and EHR databases has allowed for the identification of safety signals. In the FDA Amendments Act of 2007, it was mandated that an active surveillance system for safety evaluation be created, and in May 2008, the FDA launched the Sentinel Initiative.[16] Sentinel uses retrospectively collected private healthcare information from EHRs, administrative claims, and registries in a distributed data network to study potential safety signals that may arise associated with regulated medical products.[6,16]

RWD sources, such as claims or EHR databases, could be systematically explored to identify indications that could be effectively treated with a previously approved drug. They may also be useful in discovering how drugs are prescribed in clinical practice, providing information about drug utilization, commonly used drug combinations, and dosing regimens. All this information could inform a clinical program aimed at label expansion or modification.[5,6]

Currently, many groups are interested in creating new sources of RWD to inform clinical practice and drug development. This may be through creation of registries, such as the RISE (Rheumatology Informatics System for Effectiveness) registry created by the American College of Rheumatology and Amgen, to facilitate research through the collection of health information captured from the EHR to support clinical care and payment.[17,18] The American Society of Clinical Oncology also has developed an innovative approach to promote the use of big data to improve health care through the creation of ASCO CancerLinQ.[19] CancerLinQ collects information from participating physicians' EHR systems to support clinical decision-making and answer research questions.[19,20] Another method for RWD collection is to perform a prospective trial using existing infrastructure associated with routine clinical care or a registry system. These pragmatic trials can be an administrative and cost efficient way to perform clinical research and produce RWD.[21] The Thrombus Aspiration in ST-Elevation Myocardial Infarction in Scandinavia (TASTE) trial is an example of a trial that used a registry platform to efficiently randomize patients and collect data for a large multicenter, prospective, open-label trial.[22] The trial was able to collect information about thrombus aspiration, where previous underpowered traditional trials had failed.[23] Another example is the PCORNET ADAPTABLE (Aspirin Dosing: A Patient-centric Trial Assessing Benefits and Long-term Effectiveness) trial, which is assessing two different daily doses of aspirin for prevention of heart attack or stroke.[24] This trial is patient-focused and has used patient feedback to develop all aspects of the design and implementation. Pragmatic clinical trial designs could be useful in generating data for label expansion or modification, when traditional trials cannot be efficiently executed.[5]

Novel methods for RWD generation are being explored through the creation of registries and developing methods for extracting and analyzing EHR and claims data. Technological advancements in sensors and wearables will also aid in modernizing clinical drug development by enhancing the ability to monitor disease and patient experience.[25] The data that is and will be collected from existing and novel sources will allow researchers to better understand disease and improve how medical products are developed. RWD can be utilized in all stages of drug development, from hypothesis generation to post-market surveillance. It has the potential to be transformative in addressing the deficiencies and improving efficiency of clinical trial design and development.

Utilizing Real-World Data to Inform Innovative Platform Trial Designs

RWD can be used to inform innovative trial designs. Pre-trial planning aimed at increasing trial efficiency and probability of success can optimize innovative trial designs. These designs can incorporate one more indication, therapeutics, or molecular markers.[26] In particular, basket trial designs explore the use of one targeted therapeutic in many indications that share a common molecular marker,[26] and by pooling several indications together, considerable increases in development efficiency can be achieved. With basket trials, there are many complex statistical considerations that must be investigated, such as type I error, study power, and estimation bias.[27–29] These considerations are particularly critical when using basket designs in the confirmatory phases of clinical development.[27] At present, basket designs have been primarily used in the exploratory phase and have not been utilized to produce confirmatory evidence, except in cases where agents have shown extraordinary efficacy in diseases with a high unmet need. For example, in the B2225 study, a basket trial design, imatinib, a kinase inhibitor, was simultaneously tested in rare solid tumor and hematological malignancies with KIT, PDGFRA, or PDGFRB mutations.[30] Based on the results, along with other published studies, imatinib was approved for use in four novel indications.[31] Another example is the Phase II VE-BASKET trial where vemurafenib, previously approved by the FDA for *BRAF* V600 melanoma, was evaluated in non-melanoma cancers that contain the *BRAF* V600 mutation.[32] The trial comprised rare cancers or small biomarker defined subsets of more common cancers. The results led the FDA to approve vemurafenib for the treatment of Erdheim-Chester disease, a rare blood disorder, with the *BRAF* V600 mutation.[33] In both of these examples, the drug was previously approved, safety and efficacy was well-established, and the studied indications were rare diseases with few or no approved therapeutic options. The basket trial designs in both examples did not employ randomization or a matched control group. The resulting label expansions were obtained using non-traditional data under extraordinary circumstances. The previous designs do not provide the statistical rigor or study power to produce evidence for drugs that may be effective, but not transformative in studied indications. Since the confirmatory phase of development requires far more patient and financial resources than exploratory phases, the ability to routinely utilize basket trials in the confirmatory phase would have a transformational effect on drug development.

The Confirmatory Basket Trial

Beckman, et al. proposed a basket trial design that could be used in the confirmatory setting for any effective agent.[27] This general confirmatory basket trial (CBT) design was intended to have the statistical rigor needed to be used for producing evidence for regulatory submission. The design can used to test a single targeted agent in diseases that share a common molecular marker with either a matched control group for each indication or a common control group, if all the diseases had a common standard of care. This type of design is considered in four stages: targeted therapy selection, indication selection, individual analysis of an interim clinical endpoint in each indication, and a pooled analysis of a final clinical endpoint across indications (Figure 4.3).[27]

The experiment planning begins when a therapeutically targetable genetic abnormality or disease pathogenesis is identified in multiple indications. Since the design is aimed to produce confirmatory evidence, the selected drug or drug class should be well studied to present sufficient understanding of the drug-target interaction. Following therapeutic selection, indications with the shared abnormality or disease pathogenesis are chosen. Indications are required to be at a similar stage of clinical development, so there is sufficient evidence to support a confirmatory trial and

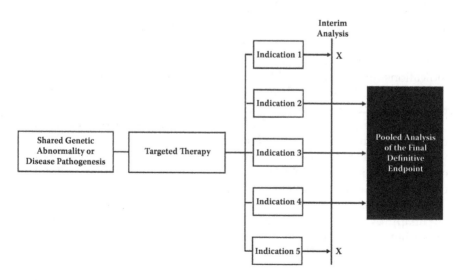

FIGURE 4.3
General Confirmatory Basket Trial Design. Adapted from[27]

potential regulatory submission. After initial indications are selected, the clinical endpoints must be determined. In this particular design, there is an interim endpoint and final definitive endpoint. The interim endpoint must be highly selective and predictive of therapeutic benefit. The interim endpoint may be different between the selected indications. It will likely be a disease-defined response variable or progression-free survival. Only the indications that show statistical superiority to control at interim will be included in the final analysis. Those that do not meet the pre-specified interim threshold will be selectively removed or "pruned" from the trial.[27] The remaining indications will complete the trial and a final pooled analysis of all the remaining indications using a final clinical benefit endpoint will assess trial success.

The selection of an interim endpoint that is predictive of the final endpoint is critical for the success of the trial, otherwise a positive interim result could lead to inclusion of an ineffective indication in the final pooled analysis. Such an indication could dilute signals from effective indications in a pooled analysis, resulting in a false negative trial. The final pooled endpoint must be a clinical benefit endpoint suitable for regulatory approval. It may be a time to worsening endpoint, such as time to relapse or time to next therapy. In oncology trials, it likely would be overall survival. Even if the pooled result is positive, each indication will require a positive trend and benefit-risk ratio to be approvable.[27] This design could provide an innovative and cost effective solution for producing confirmatory evidence for rare or biomarker defined indications.

RWD Sources to Inform CBT Design

This CBT design could be utilized for novel drug development and could be ideal for label expansion for a previously approved drug. In fact, it is preferable for label expansion in that the risk is reduced if one or more indications already have validated the drug and companion diagnostic in other settings. Rather than only utilizing data from traditional clinical trials to inform the confirmatory trial design, RWD sources could be used for decision-making. EHRs, claims databases, and disease or patient registries could be the most informative sources about drug utilization in the real world. Each of these data sources present challenges and opportunities for exploring information on populations and drug utilization that is not captured through traditional clinical research methods.

Following an initial drug approval, clinicians may prescribe a drug for an unapproved indication, dose, or schedule, which is called off-label prescribing. Typically, sponsors cannot market off-label use, but off-label use data are often reported in the literature. Off-label prescribing makes up approximately 20% of all prescribing and is most prevalent in indications that may not have an approved standard of care or options after treatment failure.[34] It is particularly common in pediatrics, oncology, and rare diseases.[34–36] Some clinical guidelines or drug compendia may support the use of an off-label drug based on the published literature, which could lead to coverage by payers.[37] Clinical information associated with off-label prescribing collected from RWD sources could be utilized for hypothesis generation and planning label expansion clinical programs.

The EHR can be a rich source of information, providing the clinical experience and outcomes associated everyday patient care.[38] It contains information about a patient's medical history, therapeutics prescribed, procedures performed, and associated procedural results.[38,39] One of the unique resources within the EHR are healthcare provider notes. These notes contain the provider's assessment and comments about the patient's condition, environment, and lifestyle. To date, provider notes are recorded in an unstructured format and thus are not easily searchable.[40] Many researchers and data vendors use natural language processing to distill information contained in the notes, but this processing is costly and some-times the provider's intent is lost in the analysis.[40–42] Currently manual chart review is the best way to discover clinical outcomes, but it is burdensome and time-consuming. Often electronic records do not give a comprehensive picture of a patient's medical history, given that many U.S. healthcare systems are open, meaning patients see clinicians in different systems, and records are not easily shared across systems.[39] Even if patients forward their EHRs to new providers, the EHR systems may not be compatible; therefore, the data is not electronically accessible. If the EHR is not linked to claims or pharmacy database, then it may not have complete information about prescribed medications from all providers.[38] The EHR alone does not contain information about when a patient fills a prescription, therefore tracking drugs taken outside of the clinical setting is difficult and information about therapeutic compliance is lacking. The most complete information will be found for drugs that are given in the hospital or infusion center, such as those administered intravenously. While the EHR serves as a clinical snapshot, it can be greatly improved by addressing the identified inadequacies. Although there are many obsta-cles concerning EHR data completeness, it can be an invaluable source when assessing clinical outcomes associated with off-label drug therapy in a broad patient population receiving medical care.

Given the inadequacies of EHRs for capturing complete patient informa-tion, administrative claims data may provide a more complete, longitudi-nal view of patient care, while insured.[43] While covered by a particular payer, all medical claims for a patient would be captured from all health-care providers in a structured format.[43] Claims databases contain dates of service, diagnosis and procedure codes, and details about the medication prescribed and when those prescriptions were filled.[44] This information could be used to understand what dose, schedule, and combination of prescribed drugs are commonly prescribed off-label in clinical practice. It can also provide some information on adverse events through evaluating patterns in diagnosis codes, procedural codes, and prescribing.[45] The disadvantage of using claims data is that without linkage to an EHR, there is no clinical information associated with the services. It cannot provide information on disease severity, patient lifestyle, environmental factors, or over-the-counter medication use.[44] Therefore, the researcher cannot utilize this source to predict therapeutic response or determine potential cofounding variables. It is best used for informing trial designers about disease incidence and prevalence and off-label use rates in particular disease populations. It could be potentially used to estimate time to worsening or time to next therapy clinical endpoints based on an algorithm using diagnostic codes and medications prescribed.

Finally, registries are a potential source of RWD. Registries can be created for a variety of reasons by professional associations, pharmaceutical companies, or patient advocacy groups and can be diverse sources of data.[46] Some registries are intended not only to collect clinical information, but also to promote the collection of patient reported information.[46–48] This information may be gathered through direct patient reporting or it may be captured through questionnaires associated with a clinical visit.[48,49] Currently, there is little standardization for how patient reported outcomes are captured.[46] When utilizing registry data, analyzing the data capture methods and source is critical for assessing completeness and usability. Registries that contain patient reported and clinical information related to off-label use could inform indication and endpoint selection for label expansion. It would allow drug developers to design studies with endpoints that are clinically relevant and important to patients.

Each of these sources provides another dimension to the patient experience. The ideal RWD source would contain structured and unstructured clinical care information from the EHR, structured longitudinal diagnosis, procedural, and medication information from administrative claims databases, and patient reported information associated with therapy use often found in disease or patient driven registries.

Integrating RWD into CBT Design for Label Expansion

The RWD associated with off-label use is a promising source for informing a basket trial that aims to provide evidence for a label expansion. Off-label use data collected from these sources could be incorporated into CBT planning and decision-making at all stages (Figure 4.4). Building upon the original general CBT design,[27] researchers could integrate RWD along with published literature into the CBT decision making process. Each step is focused on ensuring that trial has the highest likelihood of success by careful selection of the drug, indications, and clinical endpoints. The CBT planning begins by selecting a targeted therapy that has been previously FDA approved for at least one indication. The drug must have sufficient evidence indicating efficacy as well as an approvable benefit-risk profile. It

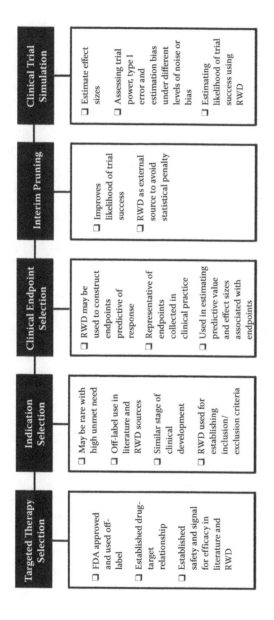

FIGURE 4.4
RWD Integration to Inform CBT Design Elements for Label Expansion.

should also have been used off-label in a variety of diseases. This information may be found in the published literature, but RWD sources may be more informative for rare populations. Following drug selection, indications that share a common, targetable molecular marker, and which have been widely treated off-label will be evaluated. Indication selection is critical and only those with the highest likelihood of success are included to reduce the chance of a false negative trial due to dilution of positive signals in the final pooled analysis. The indications may be rare, or they may be small biomarker defined subsets of a disease; typically there will be a practical difficulty with enrolling them for a confirmatory trial individually. The selected indications must be at a similar stage of confirmatory development, so there is sufficient information about safety and a signal for efficacy. The prevalence of off-label use in the indications of interest would be explored in the literature and in RWD sources. This information would be useful in narrowing down the patient populations of interest, by determining the type of patients that generally respond based on provider assessment, laboratory values, pathology, and imaging and those comorbidities or common variables that should be exclusionary. The final requirement for indication selection would be that the indications would need to share a poolable final endpoint to be included in the basket trial.

Following initial indication selection, possible interim and final endpoints are chosen. Some trial endpoints are not representative of what is generally collected and monitored during clinical care. Consulting RWD sources when selecting endpoints may allow for the development of alternative clinical endpoints that may complement or even replace traditional clinical endpoints. In the CBT design, interim and final endpoints are chosen. The interim endpoint is collected at an early time-point and should be predictive of the final endpoint. It may be a response composite endpoint collected from several clinical measures. Many trials use quantitative scoring scales or laboratory measures to determine the interim response. RWD sources could inform what clinical measures are most important for determining a patient response. The success of the CBT is determined by a final pooled analysis of the remaining indications. Therefore, all the selected indications must share the same final definitive endpoints. The endpoint could be response measurement at a longer time point or it could be a measure of time to worsening. This endpoint may be defined differently for each disease, but must be similar enough to be pooled. In many diseases, sensitive and specific clinical endpoints have yet to be discovered. To improve clinical trial efficiency, easily collected and valid endpoints are needed in many diseases. Reviewing RWD sources for how providers and patients define and track the disease of interest could improve clinical endpoint selection.

The CBT design has an interim pruning step, to ensure that only indications that are likely to succeed are included. Pruning implies selective removal of indications that do not meet the pre-specified threshold for the interim endpoint. Typically, pruning would be done by looking at the ongoing internal trial data at an interim time point to determine if indications should be pruned. A statistical penalty to control the false positive rate must be incurred when internal trial data is analyzed for interim pruning.[27,28] As a novel use, RWD information updated since the study design stage could be collected and used to inform interim pruning, and by using an external data source, no statistical penalty would be incurred. For RWD to be successfully used, the selected interim endpoint would need to be easily extracted from the RWD source. Methods for extracting the structured and unstructured data related to the endpoint would need to be developed prior to the interim time point.

All design components can be assessed using clinical trial simulation. Clinical trial simulation utilizes mathematical modeling to test trial scenarios to inform which elements will be most likely to lead to a successful trial.[50] The data related to safety and efficacy is collected from RWD sources and is used to estimate the drug effect size and hazard ratio in each indication. The trial metrics, such as power, false positive rate, benefit-cost ratio, and estimation bias,[27–29] would be assessed in simulations using trial data generated from RWD sources versus data taken from traditional literature sources, which serves as the control. The objective is to use RWD to improve design consideration by aiding in the selection of indications most likely to succeed, the selection of sensitive and specific interim and final clinical endpoints, and by diminishing statistical penalties for use of internal data for removing indications at interim. Utilizing diverse data sources and simulation will assist researchers in planning complex CBT designs that aim to produce confirmatory evidence for regulatory submission.

Considerations for the Future

The current focus on using RWD to generate evidence for decision-making is highlighting the advantages associated with utilizing alternative data sources, but has also emphasized the pitfalls associated with current data collection and analysis methods. Many of these RWD data sources were designed to facilitate a business interaction and not to serve as a research resource.[39] To produce fit-for-purpose RWD sources that can produce RWE, we need to consider each stakeholder; including patients, healthcare providers, researchers, sponsors, payers, and regulators; as well as the protections and incentives that will be necessary to move the field forward. Each stakeholder has separate concerns about patient privacy, data quality, and logistics related to capture and entry. Each of these can only be addressed by experimentation and finding

Innovative ways to improve our electronic data capture and sharing. There must also be standardization, so that once disparate sources can be accessed through a common data model. Simplifying the capture, collection, and analysis of RWD will improve all phases of medical product development and promote innovation. When considering the complexity and infrastructure necessary for planning and executing innovative clinical trials, such as platform and basket trials, it is clear that utilizing pre-existing data and systems could improve the likelihood of success. One method for increasing efficiency could be creating a trial ecosystem that allows for combining the best innovative designs, while integrating RWE for decision making into a streamlined development process.[51] Both RWD and innovative trial designs have the ability to reduce cost and time associated with gaining FDA approval for multiple indications, especially in diseases with a clear unmet need. Improving the efficacy of clinical trials and of evidence generation will lead to be more cost- and patient-efficient systems for modern drug development.

References

1. Jarow JP, LaVange L, Woodcock J. Multidimensional evidence generation and FDA regulatory decision making: Defining and using "real-world" data. *JAMA.* 2017; 318(8): 703–704.
2. U.S. Food and Drug Administration. *Use of real-world evidence to support regulatory decision-making for medical devices: Guidance for industry and food and drug administration staff.* Silver Spring, MD: FDA; 2017.
3. Sherman RE, Anderson SA, Dal Pan GJ, et al. Real-world evidence – What is it and what can it tell us? *N Engl J Med.* 2016; 375(23): 2293–2297.
4. Rimel BJ. Clinical trial accrual: Obstacles and opportunities. *Frontiers in Oncology.* 2016; 6: 103.
5. Berger M, Daniel G, Frank K, et al. *A framework for regulatory use of real-world evidence.* Washington, DC: Duke Margolis Center for Health Policy; 2017.
6. Downey A, Gee AW, Claiborne AB. *Real-world evidence generation and evaluation of therapeutics: Proceedings of a workshop.* Washington, DC: National Academy of Sciences; 2017.
7. United State Congress. 21st Century Cures Act. 2016; www.congress.gov/bill/114th-congress/house-bill/34/text#tocHBC0DF02539024F65AEF0DD6A88063188.
8. Kesselheim AS, Avorn J. New "21st century cures" legislation: Speed and ease vs science. *JAMA.* 2017; 317(6): 581–582.
9. U.S. Food and Drug Administration. Center for drug evaluation and research. Prescription Drug User Fee Act (PDUFA) – PDUFA VI: Fiscal years 2018–2022. www.fda.gov/ForIndustry/UserFees/PrescriptionDrugUserFee/ucm446608.htm.
10. U.S. Food and Drug Administration. PDUFA reauthorization performance goals and procedures fiscal years 2018 through 2022. www.fda.gov/downloads/ForIndustry/UserFees/PrescriptionDrugUserFee/UCM511438.pdf.

11. Manack A, Turkel C, Kaplowitz H. Role of epidemiological data within the drug development lifecycle: A chronic migraine case study. In: N Lunet ed *Epidemiology – Current Perspectives on Research and Practice*; 2012. www.intecho pen.com/books/epidemiology-current-perspectives-on-research-and-prac tice/role-of-epidemiological-data-within-the-drug-development-lifecycle-a-chronic-migraine-case-study

12. Williams RJ, Tse T, DiPiazza K, Zarin DA. Terminated trials in the clinicalTrials. gov results database: Evaluation of availability of primary outcome data and reasons for termination. *PLoS One*. 2015; 10(5): e0127242.

13. Baldi I, Lanera C, Berchialla P, Gregori D. Early termination of cardiovascular trials as a consequence of poor accrual: Analysis of clinicalTrials.gov 2006–2015. *BMJ Open*. 2017; 7(6).

14. Viele K, Berry S, Neuenschwander B, et al. Use of historical control data for assessing treatment effects in clinical trials. *Pharmaceut Stat*. 2014; 13(1): 41–54.

15. Desai JR, Bowen EA, Danielson MM, Allam RR, Cantor MN. Creation and implementation of a historical controls database from randomized clinical trials. *JAMIA*. 2013; 20(e1): e162–e168.

16. The Sentinel Initiative: A National Strategy for Monitoring Medical Product Safety. www.fda.gov/Safety/FDAsSentinelInitiativeucm2007250.htm, 2017.

17. Lakhanpal S. RISE registry data now available for research purposes. *Rheumatologist*. 2017. www.the-rheumatologist.org/article/rise-registry-data-now-available-research-purposes/

18. American College of Rheumatology. RISE (qualified clinical data registry). 2017; www.rheumatology.org/I-Am-A/Rheumatologist/Registries/RISE.

19. Sledge GW, Miller RS, Hauser R. CancerLinQ and the future of cancer care. *ASCO Educational Book*: 430–434; 2013. doi:10.1200/EdBook_AM.2013.33.430

20. American Society of Clinical Oncology. ASCO CancerLinQ. cancerlinq.org/research-database, 2017.

21. Sugarman J, Califf RM. Ethics and regulatory complexities for pragmatic clinical trials. *JAMA*. 2014; 311(23): 2381–2382.

22. Fröbert O, Lagerqvist B, Gudnason T, et al. Thrombus aspiration in ST-elevation myocardial infarction in Scandinavia (TASTE trial). A multicenter, prospective, randomized, controlled clinical registry trial based on the Swedish angiography and angioplasty registry (SCAAR) platform. Study design and rationale. *Am Heart J*. 2010; 160(6): 1042–1048.

23. Fröbert O, Lagerqvist B, Olivecrona GK, et al. Thrombus aspiration during ST-segment elevation myocardial infarction. *N Engl J Med*. 2013; 369(17): 1587–1597.

24. ADAPTABLE, the Aspirin Study – A patient-centered trial. http://theaspirin study.org/. Accessed December 19, 2017.

25. Pantelopoulos A, Bourbakis NG. A survey on wearable sensor-based systems for health monitoring and prognosis. *IEEE Transactions on Systems, Man, and Cybernetics, Part C (Applications and Reviews)*. 2010; 40(1): 1–12.

26. Woodcock J, LaVange LM. Master protocols to study multiple therapies, multiple diseases, or both. *N Engl J Med*. 2017; 377(1): 62–70.

27. Beckman RA, Antonijevic Z, Kalamegham R, Chen C. Adaptive design for a confirmatory basket trial in multiple tumor types based on a putative predictive biomarker. *Clin Pharmacol Therapeut*. 2016; 100(6): 617–625.

28. Chen C, Li X, Yuan S, Antonijevic Z, Kalamegham R, Beckman RA. Statistical design and considerations of a phase 3 basket trial for simultaneous investigation of multiple tumor types in one study. *Stat Biopharm Res.* 2016; 8(3): 248–257.

29. Yuan SS, Chen A, He L, Chen C, Gause CK, Beckman RA. On group sequential enrichment design for basket trial. *Stat Biopharm Res.* 2016; 8(3): 293–306.

30. Heinrich MC, Joensuu H, Demetri GD, et al. Phase II, open-label study evaluating the activity of imatinib in treating life-threatening malignancies known to be associated with imatinib-sensitive tyrosine kinases. *Clin Canc Res.* 2008; 14 (9): 2717.

31. Blumenthal. FDA perspective on innovative trial designs toaccelerate availability of highly effective anti-cancer therapies. Presentation at *AACR* annual meeting, San Diego 2014.

32. Hyman DM, Puzanov I, Subbiah V, et al. Vemurafenib in multiple nonmelanoma cancers with BRAF V600 mutations. *N Engl J Med.* 2015; 373(8): 726–736.

33. *FDA approves zelboraf (vemurafenib) for Erdheim-Chester disease with BRAF V600 mutation press release*; 2017. www.roche.com/media/releases/med-cor-2017-11-07b.htm

34. Radley DC, Finkelstein SN, Stafford RS. Off-label prescribing among office-based physicians. *Arch Intern Med.* 2006; 166(9): 1021–1026.

35. Levêque D. Off-label use of targeted therapies in oncology. *World J Clin Oncol.* 2016; 7(2): 253–257.

36. Bazzano ATF, Mangione-Smith R, Schonlau M, Suttorp MJ, Brook RH. Off-label prescribing to children in the United States outpatient setting. *Acad Pediatr.* 2009; 9(2): 81–88.

37. Green AK, Wood WA, Basch EM. Time to reassess the cancer compendia for off-label drug coverage in oncology. *JAMA.* 2016; 316(15): 1541–1542.

38. Weiskopf NG, Weng C. Methods and dimensions of electronic health record data quality assessment: Enabling reuse for clinical research. *JAMIA.* 2013; 20 (1): 144–151.

39. Cowie MR, Blomster JI, Curtis LH, et al. Electronic health records to facilitate clinical research. *Clin Res Cardiol.* 2017; 106(1): 1–9.

40. Liu F, Weng C, Yu H. Natural language processing, electronic health records, and clinical research. In: RL Richesson, JE Andrews eds. *Clinical Research Informatics.* London: Springer London; 2012:293–310.

41. Chapman WW, Nadkarni PM, Hirschman L, D'Avolio LW, Savova GK, Uzuner O. Overcoming barriers to NLP for clinical text: The role of shared tasks and the need for additional creative solutions. *JAMIA.* 2011; 18(5): 540–543.

42. Townsend H. Natural language processing and clinical outcomes: The promise and progress of NLP for improved care. *J AHIMA.* 2013; 84(2): 44–45.

43. Weber GM, Mandl KD, Kohane IS. Finding the missing link for big biomedical data. *JAMA.* 2014; 311(24): 2479–2480.

44. Chan EW, Liu KQ, Chui CS, Sing C–W, Wong LY, Wong ICK. Adverse drug reactions – examples of detection of rare events using databases. *Br J Clin Pharmacol.* 2015; 80(4): 855–861.

45. Wahl PM, Rodgers K, Schneeweiss S, et al. Validation of claims-based diagnostic and procedure codes for cardiovascular and gastrointestinal serious adverse events in a commercially-insured population. *Pharmacoepidemiol Drug Saf.* 2010; 19(6): 596–603.

46. Gliklich R, Dreyer N, Leavy M. *Registries for Evaluating Patient Outcomes: A User's Guide*. 3rd ed. Rockville, MD. Agency for Healthcare Research and Quality; 2014.
47. Basch E. New frontiers in patient-reported outcomes: Adverse event reporting, comparative effectiveness, and quality assessment. *Annu Rev Med*. 2014; 65(1): 307–317.
48. Van De Poll-Franse LV, Horevoorts N, Eenbergen MV, et al. The patient reported outcomes following initial treatment and long term evaluation of survivorship registry: Scope, rationale and design of an infrastructure for the study of physical and psychosocial outcomes in cancer survivorship cohorts. *Eur J Cancer*. 2011; 47(14): 2188–2194.
49. Okun S, Goodwin K. Building a learning health community: By the people, for the people. *Learn Health Syst*. 2017; 1(3): e10028-n/a.
50. Hummel J, Wang S, Kirkpatrick J. Using simulation to optimize adaptive trial designs: Applications in learning and confirmatory phase trials. *Clin Investig*. 2015; 5(4): 401–413.
51. Trusheim MR, Shrier AA, Antonijevic Z, et al. PIPELINEs: Creating comparable clinical knowledge efficiently by linking trial platforms. *Clin Pharmacol Therapeut*. 2016; 100(6): 713–729.

5

Impact of Platform Trials on Pharmaceutical Frameworks

Zoran Antonijevic, Ed Mills, Jonas Häggström, and Kristian Thorlund

Introduction

The pharmaceutical industry is experiencing great challenges in trying to maintain their profitability. Most governments and private payers are increasingly challenging pricing of approved products. As a result of this trend we are seeing that sponsors are trying to maximize efficiency of product development. There is an increased focus on quantitative methodologies and optimization, as well as an increased interest in the utilization of platform trials as a replacement to series of independent trials, where applicable. While relevant methods have been developed, more work on proper implementation of these methods and concepts is needed. This chapter will define Pharmaceutical Frameworks (PF) and specify how Platform Trials fit there. First, the concept of PF and its elements will be described in a format of a glossary where related concepts are prospectively defined. At the high level, the role of PFs is to provide elements and procedures that enable optimization at the Pharmaceutical program and portfolio levels. Most concepts mentioned in this chapter are not necessarily new, the greater focus is on describing procedures necessary for implementation of these concepts. Finally, for the purpose of this book the chapter explains how to set-up PFs that involve Platform Trials.

Perceived Risk vs. Objective Risk

The pharmaceutical industry has often been labeled as "risk averse." The pharmaceutical industry's aversion to risk has also been identified as one of the key reasons for being slow at embracing new, yet very intuitive development approaches; such as adaptive designs, and more recently, platform clinical trials. As with most risk assessments, "risk" in this context is referring to a perceived risk, and not necessarily some true and objective risk. Sticking with the example of adaptive trials, it is clear that the perceived risks of such designs say 10 or 20 years ago (versus present year 2018) was far exaggerated. In fact, adopting certain innovative adaptive designs in the past would have mitigated several risks that one is exposed to with the more familiar and conventional two-arm parallel RCT.

Development Options and Operating Characteristics

At the beginning of any project or program, one has to define the vision, frame the problem, and develop and evaluate new or alternative options to achieve the vision and solve the problem. When deciding upon the optimal option, a key objective is typically to avoid high perceived risk. One therefore has to assess operating characteristics of candidate development options over the range of possible scenarios. Operating characteristics provide more objective measurements to compare development options based on risk, or inversely on Probability of Success (PoS). The most relevant aspect of overall PoS to this chapter is Probability of Technical and Regulatory Success (PTRS). In addition to providing assessments of PTRS, summary of operating characteristics can also include cost, development time, and financial measurements; such as expected Net Present Value (eNPV) or Return on Investment (RoI). Derivation of Operating Characteristics has become a common practice in the Pharmaceutical Industry recently, and it is an essential component of Pharmaceutical Frameworks.

Bayesian Updating

To assess any parameter over the course of development one needs relevant data and applicable methodology. The most intuitive and probably best suited methodology is *Bayesian updating*. Bayesian updating starts with an initial belief or some preliminary information from which a Bayesian *prior distribution* is generated. For example, at early stages this distribution can be derived from historic success rates or from subject matter expert opinion. Naturally, more data becomes available later in the development stage. These data can be from clinical trials or from the real world. They can be internal to the program, or relevant external data. As new information is generated, Bayesian methods are used to calculate a *posterior distribution*, as a combination of prior belief and newly accumulated information. Bayesian updating is primarily focused on the PTRS, as this parameter is the key driver of the development and can be impacted by both internal and external information.

Objective Decision Criteria

Pharmaceutical Framework decisions should follow two key principles: (1) be evidence-driven, and (2) use prospectively defined decision criteria. This is not to say that some level of subjectivity should not be applied in decision-making, but only after available information is assessed in an objective way.

Optimality

One of the most important characteristics of decision criteria is optimality. Optimal criteria assure maximum output under a set of constraints. Optimality at program vs portfolio level involves different concepts.

At the program level optimization is directly related to *value of information*. Gathering more information (larger sample size) can improve PTRS, but requires a larger budget and more development time. Since PTRS naturally has a ceiling, at some point new information will be contributing to limited improvements in PTRS and one will be experiencing diminishing returns. Therefore, the question if/when additional information is worth the investment has to be asked. From the optimization standpoint we need to re-frame the question to: *what is the optimal level of information?* At the program level eNPV is generally considered the most suitable parameter for optimization as it incorporates all three factors mentioned above: cost, duration of development, and PTRS. A number of papers have been published that describe trade-offs between collecting more information vs. saving in cost and time.[1,2,3,4]

At the portfolio level, we have a more complex question. The dilemma is not only how much to invest but also where to invest. Here one has to assess the *opportunity cost* which entails selection of the "best" choice for where (and how much) to invest among a number of alternatives. The "best" is referring to the alternative that results in the maximum output per unit invested. Given that we now have a different type of problem, the eNPV is no longer an appropriate outcome for optimization. At the portfolio level, one should use the Productivity Index, which is essentially (financial) benefit of investment divided by the cost of investment, or as some call it, "Bang for Buck."

Pharmaceutical Frameworks

Program Level Framework

Program-Level Framework (PLF) is illustrated in Figure 5.1. PLF accompanies Evidence Generation that involves collection and qualitative assessment of information related to product development. It serves as a quantitative tool to help develop the optimal strategy. Two key parameters that affect optimality at the program level are statistical design and decision criteria. Note that the term "program," rather than "product" level optimization is used. A product can be considered for multiple

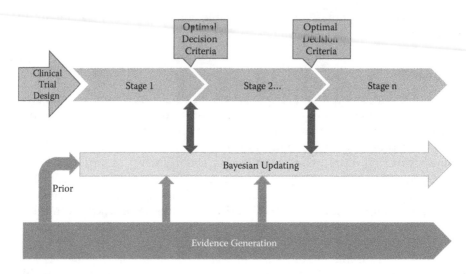

FIGURE 5.1
Program Level Framework

indications, which itself creates a small portfolio of indications, or can create a basket type of platform. This will be discussed later in the chapter.

Evidence generation begins with defining the value and objectives of the program. This is followed by gathering relevant, mostly qualitative, evidence. Several differentiated development options are then specified. Evidence generation may initially be conducted at the product level, but once indications of interest are selected the optimization that is described in this section is done at a program level. PLF is first applied to assess key quantitative parameters for each option: PTRS, cost, duration of development, and eNPV. When options are drafted and compared, selected parameters (e.g., sample size) can be refined such that the eNPV for the program is maximized. This could be the last step in defining the baseline quantitative strategy. PLF then needs to be set-up to allow for a swift assessment when strategy needs to be adjusted as result of any significant new information.

The first Bayesian prior is derived from information gathered during the initial Evidence Generation. For example, the subject matter experts can develop their opinion on how the industry PTRS average needs to be adjusted, given the evidence gathered. The adjusted industry average then serves as the initial Bayesian prior.

Bayesian updating begins with the arrival of any new information. This new information can be (1) internal, i.e, the data gathered from within the development program itself, or (2) external, such as the competitor information or changes in market trends. After each information readout Bayesian information can be updated, and at each stage the posterior distribution becomes the prior distribution for the next stage. Please note that stages in Figure 5.1 do not need to be Phases 1, 2, 3, as there will be data readouts at interim analyses. Even if an interim analysis is blinded, the action after analysis reveals information, and can be used for Bayesian updating. Clinical trials data are not the only source of information that can be used for Bayesian updating as other, usually external events, have impact on development strategy.

The newly derived PTRS and corresponding eNPV can then trigger re-evaluation of development strategy depending where exactly the program is. For example, if Phase 2 results importantly affect PTRS and eNPV, adjustments to Phase 3 strategy and design can be made. If, on the other hand, significant new information is obtained during Phase 3, major strategy or design adjustments may not be possible.

Portfolio Level Framework

Expanding a PF to the portfolio level elevates the complexity and requires understanding of additional concepts. Since a pharmaceutical portfolio includes multiple programs contributing to the value of a portfolio, it incorporates consideration beyond parameters discussed above.

First, budget limits are not set at the program, but at the portfolio level. This makes decisions interrelated and increases the complexity of decision making. Further, given budget constraints, not all planned programs and clinical trials can be executed. One needs to focus on the programs expected to bring the greatest revenues per unit invested, that is addressed by "product prioritization." Product prioritization is done by ranking products by eNPV, and selecting as many top products as it can fit under the portfolio-level budget constraints. Clearly, this approach does not maximize the portfolio-level Productivity Index. In order to do that, one also has to determine the optimal level of investment into each program. As such, the optimal solution requires that optimal design elements and optimal decision criteria are specified at the portfolio level as illustrated in Figure 5.2. Portfolio optimization can bring substantial productivity improvements over product prioritization.

Another challenge is how to establish the communication between program and portfolio optimization since program and portfolio level decisions involve different decision makers. Program-level decision makers have a vested interest in their program, while portfolio-level decision makers have a broader vision of the company's portfolio. What is the best strategy for any individual program may not be the best strategy for the portfolio as a whole. Persinger describes this problem and proposes strategies how to address it.[5] In general, portfolio level reviews have to be conducted on a regular basis to assess if portfolio-level decisions need to be revisited.

Every program within the portfolio will have its own PLF. A need for major adjustment in program level strategy is communicated to portfolio level decision makers, particularly if desired adjustments require additional

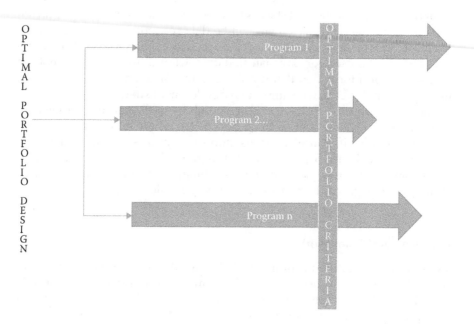

FIGURE 5.2
Portfolio Level Framework

resources. Inversely, portfolio level reviews may identify needs for changes in overall portfolio strategy that can impact individual projects.

Pharmaceutical Frameworks that Include Platform Trials

The emergence of platform trials brings another dimension to both program and portfolio level planning. Let's first clarify platform trials nomenclature that will be used in this chapter:

- Basket trial involves one product with multiple indications
- Umbrella trial involves multiple products targeting one indication.

Both basket and umbrella trials create mini-portfolios within the larger company's portfolio, with a different effect. The premise is that platform trials can improve the efficiency over one-at-a-time trials by (1) having correlated outcomes, and/or (2) sharing concurrent controls. Platform trials can improve various other administrative efficiencies that are discussed in other chapters of this book.

Basket

Since basket trials involve only one product, it is possible that basket-level decisions are the responsibility of people in charge of that product, and not the responsibility of portfolio-level decisions makers. This model is illustrated in Figure 5.3. Let us assume that in this model there is a defined product level budget. The first objective is then to provide optimal solution that will maximize the output over the range of indications. This model clearly does not provide the optimal solution for the company portfolio as a whole, since it is hierarchical. The first level is the product-level decision of what indication(s) will be developed, and the level of investment for each indication is specified. This product then goes to portfolio level decision making with other products that are under consideration.

An alternative is that each indication within the basket is treated as a separate program for the purpose of optimization. The basket design is still there to improve the overall efficiency of development, but previously described portfolio-level optimization is implemented. This process is identical to that illustrated in Figure 5.2, and provides the optimal solution.

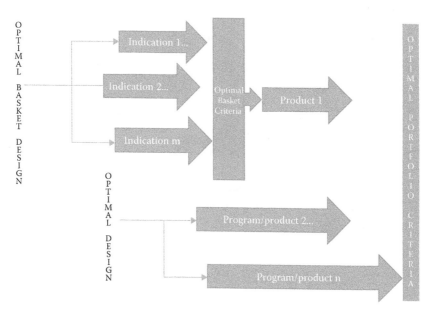

FIGURE 5.3
Framework that Includes Basket Trial

Umbrella

Since umbrella design involves multiple products within the portfolio, the default would be that each one is treated as the independent product, and previously described portfolio optimization process that is illustrated in Figure 5.2 is implemented.

An alternative is to form a sub-portfolio of products within the umbrella, and optimize at this level first. In this model the first step is product selection from within the umbrella. Selected products then proceed into portfolio level optimization with other products in the portfolio. This process is described in Figure 5.4. This optimization is hierarchical and does not lead to the optimal solution for a company's portfolio as a whole.

Perpetual Clinical Trial

A new concept of direct relevance to PF is aimed at reducing the time and costs associated with conducting multi-arm trials, called Perpetual Clinical Trials, which also discussed in Chapter 10.[6] Perpetual clinical trials aim to support the investment in basket and platform designs by ensuring that infrastructure built can be carried over into future clinical questions. This mandates that investigators conducting these large-scale studies can plan

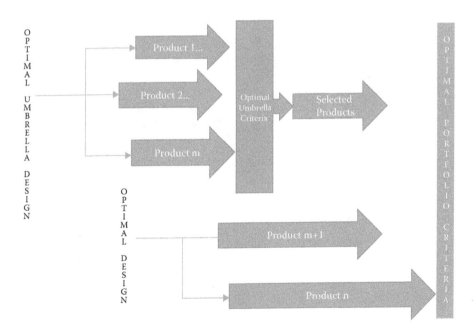

FIGURE 5.4
Freamework that Includes Umbrella Trial

for alternative populations and clinical questions such that when the basket or platform trial has sufficiently answered the initial questions of interest, follow-up questions and refinement of clinical indications can be further studied. This approach requires planning for the future and should assume that multiple trials will need to be conducted on either a population or a drug. It also requires a perpetual optimization of clinical trials, programs, and portfolios, which should be the ultimate objective of PF. This is not just a statistical or methodological issue, but improves patient and staff retention in clinical trials such that the expertise developed over the course of a trial can be maintained for future clinical trials.

Summary and Conclusions

This chapter describes program and portfolio level Pharmaceutical Frameworks and how formation of these frameworks is necessary for delivering optimal solutions. The chapter then describes how to set-up frameworks when company's portfolios include platform trials. In general, the process illustrated in Figure 5.2 provides the optimal solution at the company level portfolio, regardless if the portfolio includes platform trials or not.

References

1. Antonijevic Z, Pinheiro J, Fardipour P Lewis R. 2010. Impact of dose selection strategies used in phase II on the probability of success in phase III. *Statistics in Biopharmaceutical Research* 2, 469–486.
2. Patel N, Bolognese J, Chuang–Stein C, Hewitt D, Gammaitoni A Pinheiro J 2012. Designing phase 2 trials based on program-level considerations: A case study for neuropathic pain. *Drug Information Journal* 46 (4), 439–454.
3. Antonijevic Z, Kimber M, Manner D, Burman C–F, Pinheiro J Bergenheim K 2013. Optimizing drug development programs: Type 2 diabetes case study. *Therapeutic Innovation and Regulatory Science* 47 (3), 363–374.
4. Marchenko O, Miller J, Parke T, Perevozskaya I, Qian J Wang Y 2013. Improving oncology clinical program by use of innovative designs and comparing them via simulations. *Therapeutic Innovation & Regulatory Science* 47 (5), 602–612.
5. Persinger C 2015. Challenges of portfolio management in pharmaceutical development. In *Optimization of Pharmaceutical R&D Programs and Portfolios; Design and Investment Strategy*. Springer International PublishingCham, Switzerland, 71–83.
6. Mills E, Häggström J Thorlund K 2018. Highly efficient clinical trials: A resource-saving solution for global health. In *Platform Trials Designs in Drug Development; Umbrella Trials and Basket Trials*. CRC Press, Boca Raton, FL, USA.

Part II
Stakeholders

6

Friends of Cancer Research Perspective on Platform Trials

Jeffrey D. Allen, Madison Wempe, Ryan Hohman, and Ellen V. Sigal

Introduction

In 2012, an Institute of Medicine Report titled "A National Cancer Clinical Trials System for the 21st Century: Reinvigorating the NCI Cooperative Group Program" emphasized the critical need for a public clinical trials system. This report stated four goals for the modernization of the traditional clinical trial system: 1) to improve the speed and efficiency of the design, launch, and conduct of clinical trials; 2) to incorporate innovative science and trial design into cancer clinical trials; 3) to improve prioritization, selection, support, and completion of cancer clinical trials; and 4) to incentivize participation of patients and physicians in clinical trials.[1] This report, and others, inspired collaborative efforts by Friends of Cancer Research (*Friends*), the National Cancer Institute (NCI), the Food and Drug Administration (FDA), the Foundation for the National Institutes of Health (FNIH), leaders in biotechnology, patient advocates, and the Southwest Oncology Group (SWOG) to develop a "master protocol" clinical trial called Lung-MAP for the study of squamous cell lung cancer treatments.

Upon creation, the goal of the Lung Master Protocol (Lung-MAP) was to quickly identify and test new targeted treatments and immunotherapies for squamous cell lung cancer, and, if effective, move those drugs to FDA approval. This goal was especially critical in the squamous cell cancer (SCCA) disease setting, a disease setting that had previously seen minimal developments in targeted, effective therapies. Although limited progress had been achieved in the treatment of SCCA prior to Lung-MAP, screening for potential therapeutic targets in the disease was rapidly gaining interest, with as much as 63% of SCCA having an identifiable therapeutic target. Moreover, a number of molecular subtypes of the disease had been identified, enabling researchers to treat specific groups of patients with different targeted agents. The Lung-MAP trial sought to capitalize on this knowledge, simultaneously evaluating several targeted therapies in patients who had been previously screened for a series of related molecular abnormalities. The increase in

modern medical technology utilization, coupled with perennial inefficiencies of the traditional clinical trial system, mandated this innovative
response by stakeholders such as *Friends* in the squamous cell cancer
disease setting and continues to drive innovative trial designs by clinical
trial sponsors across a host of other disease settings.

The clinical trial system from which the Lung-MAP trial emerged has
evolved as technological and scientific advancements, providing researchers with opportunities to better understand the biological underpinnings of
disease. Furthermore, a series of legal and policy decisions made over
many decades have laid the foundation for the modern biomedical
research enterprise. In 1935, for example, the Supreme Court of Michigan
first authorized controlled clinical investigations on the condition of
informed consent, a concept that has become central to the ethical conduct
of all subsequent clinical research.[2] Another advancement took place in
1962 with the passage of the Kefauver-Harris Drug Amendments to the
Food, Drug, and Cosmetic Act, which ushered in the modern era of clinical
trials. The Kefauver-Harris Amendments mandated that drug approval be
based on evidence from "adequate" and "well-controlled" studies, and in
doing so established parameters around the type of research that could be
used to support claims of safety and effectiveness of new treatments.[3,4]
Similar to the changes in the medical field, this evolution was a response to
emerging science and was intended to maintain patient safety and the
integrity of the clinical trial system.

Despite the many advancements in clinical research that have been
made to date, progress has been slow in the critical area of multi-
stakeholder collaboration. Many entities, both public and private,
remain hesitant to participate in the promising solution of collaborative,
multi-party, large scale research endeavors. Collaborative clinical trial
design and master protocols, however, are a critical solution to the
current problems faced by the traditional clinical trial system. The
remainder of this chapter will focus on defining the shortcomings of
the existing clinical trial system and highlighting the improvements that
collaborative clinical trial design could bring to the efficiency and
expense of clinical research.

Shortcomings of the Traditional Clinical Trial System

As diagnostic medicine and the demands on the clinical trial system have
evolved, pharmaceutical companies and other organizations have had to
adapt to different technologies and increased regulatory requirements.
Challenges brought on by these changes include increased costs, difficulties in accruing patients, and impediments in the translatability of research
to clinical practice.

Costs

First, the cost of conducting a clinical trial in the traditional clinical trial system has become highly burdensome for many clinical trial sponsors. The total costs associated with the implementation of a clinical trial can reach anywhere between $300 and $600 million.[5] Yet despite the extensive financial investment in clinical trials, many drugs never even make it to market. In fact, it is estimated that only 8% of all drugs complete clinical trials and receive FDA approval.[6] Resources invested in the other 92% of drugs that do not complete trials or do not receive approval, therefore, may never see any financial returns.

The costs of bringing a new drug to market are dependent upon many factors, such as the number of patients being accrued, the number and location of research sites, and the complexity of the trial protocol.[5] These costs are especially burdensome for clinical trial sponsors wishing to investigate treatments for rare diseases or for biomarker-positive subgroups. The latter trials often include advanced screening techniques aimed at identifying a particular subset of patients for enrollment in their trial, which both increases the number of patients needed to be screened and adds cost through the use of sophisticated diagnostic testing platforms. There are additional explanations for increasing clinical trial costs, such as the shift in management strategies for several conditions from acute strategies to chronic strategies. In light of the increasing expense of conducting clinical research, it is evident that the current clinical trial system needs to adapt to manage these financial burdens.

Problems with Patient Accrual

The traditional clinical trial system also faces significant problems with patient accrual. In fact, it is estimated that less than 2% of adult cancer patients participate in United States clinical trials.[7] As the science and technology behind molecular diagnosis has evolved and the definitions of diseases, particularly within the field of oncology, have narrowed, it has become increasingly more difficult for clinical trial sponsors to accrue patients for trials of increasingly rare biomarker targeted treatments. In fact, studies have emphasized that, under the traditional clinical trial structure, trials randomize the 1%–5% of consenting, eligible patients and spend anywhere from 5 to 10 years struggling to increase "lagging accrual."[8] Those clinical trials unable to sustain this long, drawn-out process due to a lack of resources, are forced to close early, wasting already invested resources and leaving research questions unanswered.

Other trials able to run until completion are often faced with another problem: the time lapse between the proposal of the trial and its completion may render the results no longer scientifically relevant. Because many trials are being conducted simultaneously, it is likely that trial results from other clinical trials may alter the standard of care or produce other results necessitating a change in the protocol being used in an individual trial. In the case of an already enrolled trial, patients may be permitted to cross over to the experimental arm of the study, but the results of the study may no longer be relevant.

Translatability to Clinical Practice

Translating clinical trial results into clinical practice is another difficulty of the traditional clinical trial system. This difficulty results in part from the lack of community physician involvement in clinical research. While an estimated 80% of cancer patients are treated in non-academic practices, the comparatively low community physician involvement in the conduct of clinical research decreases incentives for physicians to refer patients to clinical trials. In addition, a lack of participation may reduce the likelihood of physicians to adopt the findings of clinical research in their daily practice.[5] By some estimates, it may take over a decade to incorporate new research results into clinical practice.[9] Additionally, it is estimated that on average, American adults receive only 54.9% of recommended care.[10]

Collaborative Clinical Trial Design: The Master Protocol

The aforementioned challenges of the traditional clinical trial system have instigated an innovative response by stakeholders in the research, regulatory, and drug development community. These stakeholders have developed a new framework for conducting clinical research, one that improves the trial efficiency, speeds up recruitment, and avoids unnecessary duplication in the development of study protocols. Trials such as the Lung-MAP clinical trial embody this new approach, solving many of the problems presented by the traditional clinical trial system and benefitting a diversity of stakeholders.

Before detailing the efficiencies of master protocol clinical trials, however, it is imperative to first understand what is meant by the term "master protocol" clinical trial design. By definition, a master protocol involves a coordination of efforts by numerous drug development stakeholders to evaluate multiple treatments, in multiple patient groups or disease settings, within the same overall trial structure.[11] This singular trial structure is designed to answer multiple research questions and may involve comparisons of competing therapies or the parallel analysis of different therapies.

The benefits of master protocol trials are derived primarily from their unique design: an overarching, consistent framework that can be implemented, or amended, as needed to answer a multitude of research questions. Use of a common protocol allows sponsors to more efficiently initiate clinical trials, accrue patients, and translate their findings into clinical practice. Additionally, this infrastructure offers a significant opportunity for the immediate matching of patients to clinical trials and the receipt of otherwise unavailable genomic screening technologies and experimental therapies. These benefits will be further explored for the duration of this section.

Efficient Initiation of Clinical Trials

The use of a common, baseline study protocol and consistent infrastructure in master protocol clinical trials allows pharmaceutical companies or other clinical trial sponsors to more efficiently initiate investigations of their experimental therapies. Within a master protocol, the development, regulatory review, and approval of sub-study designs typically occurs when the master protocol trial is first initiated. This process involves a number of time-consuming and labor-intensive steps such as protocol review, trial site activation processes, and administrative processes that, on average, take over a year to complete.[12] For the sub studies in a master protocol clinical trial, however, these steps have often already been completed. This allows new sub-study concepts to be developed using the base master protocol and to be activated and enrolling patients on an accelerated timeline compared to if the sub-study had been set up as an independent clinical trial.

Patient Accrual

Master protocols typically activate multiple sub-studies governed by a common protocol. This can provide more options for patients that begin the screening process for participation as compared to a traditional clinical study. In the case of Lung-MAP, initial screening is performed using a next generation sequencing test to sequence a patient's tumor. Based on those results it is determined whether the patient matches to an enrolling biomarker-defined sub-study to which they would be assigned. If a potential participant isn't matched to an existing biomarker sub-study, they are assigned to the "non-match" sub-study. The non-match sub-study in Lung-MAP tests immunotherapy regimens in a non-biomarker defined population. This approach ensures that there is a treatment sub-study available for all patients that are enrolled in the Lung-MAP study. In addition, it allows for a patient to receive a biopsy just once to determine their course of treatment, as opposed to pursuing studies on a trial by trial basis until they match specific biomarker criteria, in the case of trials testing a targeted therapy.

Broad-based screening of large numbers of patients for multiple targets, as is done in the Lung-MAP study, has the added benefit of lowering the screen failure rate for the trial (compared to independently conducted targeted therapy trials) and provides a sufficient "hit rate" to engage patients and physicians. For example, if a clinical trial is being conducted to test a drug directed toward a specific alteration that occurs in only 5% of the population, only one out of every 20 patients screened would result in a patient being matched to a study. High levels of screen failures such as these may deter patients and physicians to participate in a research study, as well as increase the costs and time of the study itself. Other opportunities for patient accrual available to master protocols include the pre-screening of patients in a community center for assignment to the master protocol clinical trial upon further progression of their disease using other treatment options. This pre-screening front loads the necessary screening process, thereby eliminating the usual time lag between screening and treatment arm assignment after disease progression.

Community Sites

The involvement of community sites in master protocol clinical trial designs is also advantageous to clinical research. Because many clinical trials are operated in academic research centers and not in the community centers, there is less competition for patient accrual among clinical trials at these community sites.[13] Additionally, the infrastructure established by a master protocol clinical trial creates a standing research network in the community, allowing sub-studies to consistently enter and accrue patients efficiently for their trials. Having a master protocol in place, therefore, could reduce the burden on community sites that can come with regularly implementing new trials from the start each time. Interested practices could align their processes with the master protocol and be an activated site for their patients as needed.

The involvement of community sites in master protocol trials also represents a positive step towards increasing the translatability of clinical research findings to clinical practice. In contrast to the traditional clinical trial system, where community-practicing physicians must typically refer patients away from their care to participate in clinical trials, master protocols can more easily involve community practitioners in the process of referring patients to trials and monitoring their care. Results from the clinical trial, therefore, are more likely to influence their treatment decisions in the future, bringing about greater translatability of research. As Dr. Janet Woodcock, the Director of the FDA Center for Drug Evaluation and Research (CDER), has emphasized, the generation of relevant research based in clinical practice must actively involve community practitioners in the clinical trial process.[5] Under the current clinical trial system, the divergence between community practitioners and academic researchers serves as a major barrier to the successful translation of study results into clinical practice.[5] Master protocols, however, help bridge this gap through their direct engagement with community medical centers. These trials also provide physicians in a community setting with access to promising experimental agents that would most often only be available through trials at larger medical centers, which allows them to offer more comprehensive care to their patients. By extending access to these trials to community settings, master protocols can expand the trial population's cultural, racial, socioeconomic, and geographic diversity, resulting in a trial that more accurately represents the population that may ultimately be treated with a subsequently approved agent. The Lung-MAP study, for example, has almost 750 sites open for the conduct of its master protocol clinical trial (http://lung-map.org/locations). The patients accrued to the trial have been from over 200 different sites, and the majority of patients have been treated at sites outside of lead academic participating sites.

Patient Access

Perhaps one of the greatest efficiencies of the collaborative clinical trial system is its increased benefit to patients seeking access to genomic screening technologies and experimental therapies. Rather than being forced to undergo multiple screening attempts and to move from trial to trial before ever being matched with a trial and treatment arm, patients who are screened for inclusion in a master protocol study need only be tested once to have a high likelihood of eventually participating in the study. The variety of patient subgroups that are evaluated over the course of a master protocol, as well as the use of non-match sub studies greatly increases patients' chances of receiving a study treatment. Moreover, patients who participate in master protocols are given access to a broad-based screening technology such as Next Generation Sequencing (NGS), which efficiently screens patients for a multitude of genomic markers and matches them to treatment arms based upon this information. For many patients, particularly patients at community sites, broad-based screening technologies would not be accessible in the absence of a clinical trial. Additionally, the treatments being studied at these community sites would most likely not all be accessible to these patients in the absence of the master protocol clinical trial if each one required the separate set up and conduct of individual clinical trials.

Challenges for Master Protocols

Although collaborative clinical trials solve many of the problems of the traditional clinical trial system, they also are accompanied by a number of new, different challenges. These challenges include the management of extensive patient information, complicated logistical planning across multiple sites and sub studies, and the need to adapt to the changes in medical science that require investigators to keep pace with new standard of care treatments. Each of these challenges was faced during the course of implementing the Lung-MAP study. As additional master protocols are explored in the future, it will be important to address these unique challenges upfront to avoid unnecessary delays and to capitalize on the benefits that the master protocol model has to offer both to patients and the broader researcher enterprise.

Management of Patient Information

Screening technologies such as NGS used in clinical trials have dramatically increased the efficiency of the molecular diagnosis of disease. Many of these technologies are capable of sequencing the entire human genome within a single day, profiling molecular alterations that could increase a person's risk for disease or predict the likelihood of response to treatment. This increased volume of information, although beneficial, also poses various challenges to laboratories and clinical trial sponsors responsible for its storage and distribution.

Lung-MAP relies on NGS to screen patients towards the different biomarker-defined sub studies. Without capitalizing on the ability of NGS platforms to assess numerous molecular alterations simultaneously, Lung-MAP and other biomarker directed master protocols would not be possible. However, questions can arise with the use of NGS testing in clinical trials, particularly regarding how patients access the results of tumor sequencing. In most cases, patients want access to their genomic data to the fullest extent possible.[14] In fact, previous legal complaints have been filed by patients in instances when their genomic data was withheld from them.[15] Most would agree that patients have ownership of their data and test results should be made available to them, but the data generated by NGS testing requires meaningful interpretation by highly specialized experts. In order to make this information understandable for the vast majority of patients, genetic counselors and other trained individuals may be needed to interpret the data or to put the information into a comprehensive report. As the use of NGS becomes more widespread, access to genetically trained experts may be limited in some of the practices that are seeking to utilize this technology. While this may not be a reason to withhold patient data, it may be a complicating factor for master protocols that are intended to expand into community based sites that may not have genetic counselors or other staff onsite to help facilitate access to and interpretation of these data sets.

An additional consideration for study sponsors is the timing of the release of test results to patients. As previously described, NGS testing can identify many alterations that may be beyond the scope of the intended trial. With the rapid expansion of trials exploring the use of

targeted therapy, NGS testing performed for one trial may uncover alterations that may be under study in a separate research initiative. The
question of when test results should be provided to participants was one
that Lung-MAP leadership had to consider. In the case of Lung-MAP, the
centralized institutional review board (IRB) that was reviewing the protocol as the baseline review for most participating sites ultimately determined that full test results should be provided as part of the determination
of which study arm the patient was qualified for and not delayed until
after they had had started or even completed the study. The IRB determined that it would be coercive to require patients to complete a trial in
order to have access to the data provided by the sequencing of the tumor.

Another example of a collaborative trial that utilizes NGS screening at
the outset, the NCI Molecular Analysis for Therapy Choice trial (NCI-
MATCH) has a pre-determined process for providing the results of genetic
screening. In NCI-MATCH, genetic results are communicated to the doctor
and patient, and are included in the patient's medical record at the site as
soon as they are available. The information is reported in a clinical report
that, similar to Lung-MAP, is provided at the time the trial arm that the
patient qualifies for is presented. This report includes information on the
molecular alterations of interest as well as the non-actionable alterations
that were identified with the assay. For the overall study population, no
genetic counseling services are provided. However, since the launch of the
trial a sub-study has been embedded that invites patients to provide
feedback on any anxiety or questions that they had prior to testing and
upon receipt of the results, and remote genetic counseling by a team of
credentialed counselors is provided.[16] Both Lung-MAP and NCI-MATCH
have implemented processes without any notable problems, but as more
master protocols are developed and rely on larger volumes of related and
unrelated genomic data prior to the start of the trial, communication of this
data with trial participants is something that should be planned for.

Responding to Emerging Data

Clinical trials often represent the cutting edge of biomedical research. This
is particularly true for master protocols that are designed to accelerate the
development of new products and make those successful new drugs
available to patients sooner. With thousands of clinical trials being conducted concurrently, the results of one can have significant impacts on
other trials in similar settings. For example, if a clinical trial yields results
that alter the standard of care for a particular disease, on-going trials for
that population may have trouble completing accrual, or may even become
unethical if they are using a randomized design with a control that has
been deemed outdated. In cases such as this, the trial would either need to
be modified in design or discontinued. A change in treatment landscape
has been shown to account for 8% of discontinued clinical trials.[17]

However, this may be a challenge that is more frequently encountered for master protocols that function as a standing clinical research network over a longer period of time than the average clinical study.

Lung-MAP encountered a significant shift in the treatment landscape early on, which required a significant modification of the overall master protocol. In 2015, the checkpoint inhibitor nivolumab was approved for the treatment of patients with advanced squamous NSCLC who had progressed on or after platinum-based chemotherapy.[18] This was the patient population that the initial version of Lung-MAP was enrolling. In that original design, for each of the biomarker-defined sub-studies, patients were to be randomized to the experimental targeted therapy or docetaxel, which was the standard of care at the time the trial launched. When nivolumab was approved for these patients, it essentially replaced docetaxel as the recommended standard treatment for these patients, thereby making docetaxel an outdated treatment option. Lung-MAP has since modified the study design to recognize this, and has undergone other modifications to the design in order to keep pace with the current evidence in treating NSCLC.

Responding to the current medical landscape is not a challenge unique to master protocols, but it is one that those developing master protocols should pay particular attention to and take measures to recognize how new research in the field may affect the master protocol and plan processes for modifications as needed. Because master protocols are the foundation for numerous different sub-studies that may all be affected by emerging data, both internal and external to the trial, changing aspects of a master protocol is likely to be more complicated than in a traditional clinical trial.

Conclusion

The traditional clinical trial system is beset by a number of inefficiencies, which, if not addressed, will hamper biomedical research and stifle innovations that could lead to transformative new treatments. Costs of doing research are exorbitant, patient accrual is often inadequate to meet the needs of research objectives, and results of clinical trials often fail to be adopted into widespread practice in a timely manner. These challenges necessitate an innovative response from a range of stakeholders, including government, private industry, academia, and patient groups. These groups have begun to provide answers in the form of large-scale, collaborative master protocol clinical trials. These trials aim to improve the efficiency of trial development and activation, incorporate innovative science and trial design, improve the completion of trials, and incentivize the participation of patients and physicians. Although these trials are accompanied by their own new challenges, as seen in the case of Lung-MAP, they are an innovative and effective alternative to the current slow, costly, and burdensome clinical trial system that exists today.

References

1. Overview of Conclusions and Recommendations. Institute of Medicine. 2010. *A National Cancer Clinical Trials System for the 21st Century: Reinvigorating the NCI Cooperative Group Program*. Washington, DC: The National Academies Press. doi: 10.17226/12879.
2. "Fortner v. Koch, 261 N.W. 762, 272 Mich. 273 – CourtListener.com." *CourtListener*. www.courtlistener.com/opinion/3523231/fortner-v-koch/.
3. Office of the Commissioner. "Consumer Updates – Kefauver-Harris Amendments Revolutionized Drug Development." *U.S. Food and Drug Administration Home Page*. Office of the Commissioner. www.fda.gov/ForConsumers/ConsumerUpdates/ucm322856.htm.
4. *[USC10] 21 USC 355: New Drugs*, uscode.house.gov/view.xhtml?req=%28adequate%2BAND%2Bwell-controlled%29%2BAND%2B%28%28title%3A%2821%29%29%29&f=treesort&fq=true&num=0&hl=true&edition=prelim&granuleId=USC-prelim-title21-section355.
5. Institute of Medicine (US) Forum on Drug Discovery, et al. "Challenges in Clinical Research." *Transforming Clinical Research in the United States: Challenges and Opportunities: Workshop Summary*. U.S. National Library of Medicine. 1 Jan. 1970. www.ncbi.nlm.nih.gov/books/NBK50888/.
6. The Drug Development and Approval Process. *The Drug Development and Approval Process: FDAReview.org*, www.fdareview.org/03_drug_development.php.
7. Mannel RS, Moore K. "Research: An Event or an Environment?" *Gynecologic Oncology*, 134(3). 2014: 441–442.
8. Lai TL, LavoriPW. "Innovative Clinical Trial Designs: Toward a 21st-Century Health Care System." *Statistics in Biosciences*, 3(2). 2011: 145–168.
9. Dilling JA, et al. "Accelerating the Use of Best Practices: The Mayo Clinic Model of Diffusion." *Joint Commission Journal on Quality and Patient Safety*. U.S. National Library of Medicine, Apr. 2013. www.ncbi.nlm.nih.gov/pubmed/23641536.
10. Mcglynn EA, et al. "The Quality of Health Care Delivered to Adults in the United States." *New England Journal of Medicine*. 2003. www.nejm.org/doi/full/10.1056/NEJMsa022615#t=article.
11. Woodcock J, LaVange L. "Master Protocols to Study Multiple Therapies, Multiple Diseases, or Both." *New England Journal of Medicine*, 377. 2017: 62–70. doi: 10.1056/NEJMra1510062
12. Lamberti MJ, Chakravarthy R, Getz KA. Assessing Practices & Inefficiencies with Site Selection, Study Start-Up, and Site Activation. *Applied Clinical Trials Home*, 5(Nov). 2017, www.appliedclinicaltrialsonline.com/assessing-practices-inefficiencies-site-selection-study-start-and-site-activation?pageID=1.
13. Baquet CR, et al. "Clinical Trials: The Art of Enrollment." *Seminars in Oncology Nursing*, U.S. National Library of Medicine, Nov. 2008, www.ncbi.nlm.nih.gov/pubmed/19000600.

14. "Should Patients Have Full Access to Their Genomic Data?" *Front Line Geno-mics.* www.frontlinegenomics.com/opinion/3385/should-patients-have-full-access-to-their-genomic-data/.
15. Zeughauser B, et al. *U.S. Department of health and human services office for civil rights health information privacy complaint.* 19 May 2016. www.aclu.org/sites/default/files/field_document/2016.5.19_hipaa_complaint.pdf+.
16. "NCI-MATCH Trial (Molecular Analysis for Therapy Choice)." *National Cancer Institute.* www.cancer.gov/about-cancer/treatment/clinical-trials/nci-supported/nci-match.
17. Williams RJ, et al. "Terminated Trials in the ClinicalTrials.gov Results Data-base: Evaluation of Availability of Primary Outcome Data and Reasons for Termination." *PLoS One.* Public Library of Science, 2015. www.ncbi.nlm.nih.gov/pmc/articles/PMC4444136/.
18. "Press Announcements – FDA Expands Approved Use of Opdivo to Treat Lung Cancer." *U.S. Food and Drug Administration Home Page.* www.fda.gov/NewsEvents/Newsroom/PressAnnouncements/ucm436534.htm.

7

Regulatory and Policy Aspects of Platform Trials

Rasika Kalamegham, Ramzi Dagher, and Peter Honig

I. Introduction

Platform trials, including umbrella trials, basket trials, and some hybrid models that integrate elements of both, are increasingly being used in drug development. Multiple factors are contributing to this phenomenon including the explosion in our knowledge of molecular targets, a better understanding of the biological underpinnings and natural history of diseases, the desire on the part of multiple stakeholders to conduct development more rapidly and more efficiently, and the relatively limited pool of patients available for enrollment in clinical trials (1).

Regulators are also taking an increasing interest in these trials as they seek to play a more active role in guiding drug development as partners and collaborators, not just as reviewers of data. The availability of regulatory tools to allow acceleration of development and drug review, including the possibility of registration directed filings based on phase 1/2 data in the U.S., Europe, and elsewhere have also contributed to an increased interest in these trials (2,3).

In this chapter we will review the framework for demonstration of efficacy and safety, and the role of clinical trials generally in this process, as well as the potential role of platform trials in accelerating and optimizing drug development, registration, and post-marketing assessment. We will also review special considerations related to platform trials and drug diagnostic co-development, combination therapies, and pediatrics. Where appropriate, special considerations related to the regulatory framework in the U.S., EU, and Japan will be highlighted. Finally, we will comment on regulatory and policy initiatives which portend future considerations in the use of platform trials for regulatory purposes.

II. Historical Development of the Randomized Controlled Trial

a. General Considerations

The ascendency and acceptance of the randomized controlled trial (RCT) as a 'gold standard' that can inform regulatory decision making regarding the efficacy and safety of a medical product or intervention dates back to the 1962 amendments to the U.S. Food Drug & Cosmetic Act (FD&CA) (4). Prior to that time, many medicinal products were cleared for marketing by the FDA with little to no evidence to support their clinical utility beyond uncontrolled and poorly conducted clinical observations. For drugs with very large and immediate treatment effects where the natural history of untreated disease was well appreciated (e.g., antibiotics for streptococcal infections), this posed less of a problem, but there were still unanswered questions about the durability of efficacy and long term safety. However, for many other drugs, the effectiveness was often in question. This led congress, in the aftermath of the thalidomide tragedy, to amend the FD&C Act to require 'substantial evidence' to support the claims of effectiveness for new drugs. The Act further went on to require 'adequate and well controlled studies' to support such claims. At the time of enactment, the precise operating definition and characteristics of an adequate and well-controlled study were not universally understood or accepted as they are today.

b. DESI and the Origins of the Modern Clinical Trial

A key provision of the 1962 Amendments required the FDA to conduct a review of the medical effectiveness of 3,000–4,000 drugs introduced to the U.S. market between 1938 and 1962. The effort began in earnest in 1966 and was conducted in several stages. The FDA enlisted the assistance of the National Academy of Sciences and many outside experts in a series of public evaluations. This was the Drug Efficacy Study Implementation (DESI) and it evaluated over 3,000 separate products and over 16,000 therapeutic claims. By 1984, final action had been completed on 3,443 products; of these, 2,225 were found to be effective, 1,051 were found not effective and eventually removed from the market (5).

The impact of DESI effort cannot be underestimated in helping FDA and the clinical research community to understand and define the characteristics of the 'adequate and well-controlled' clinical experiment and ultimately led to current FDA regulations that define the hallmarks of an adequate and well controlled study (6). The regulations and accompanying guidance are clearly derivative from the DESI experience in that they state that the purpose of conducting clinical investigations of a drug is to distinguish the effect of the drug from other influences such as spontaneous change in the course of the disease, a placebo effect, or bias, and go on to explicitly define the design features which include, amongst others, a clear statement of the objectives and prospectively articulated description of the planned data analysis methods, use of a concurrent control or justification for use of non-concurrent historical controls, expected use of well-accepted bias control methods such as randomization and blinding, and that the clinical investigation be conducted under generally accepted international Good Clinical Practice Guidelines (GCP) (7). GCP is now an internationally harmonized standard that is intended to ensure strict guidelines on the ethical aspects of a clinical study by requiring appropriate documentation of informed consent and institutional and regulatory oversight of clinical investigations. It also imposes high regulatory expectations and comprehensive documentation of protocol development and amendments, record keeping, training, and facilities by defining the roles and responsibilities of the clinical trial sponsors, clinical investigators, and clinical study monitors. Sponsor quality assurance and regulatory inspections ensure these standards are achieved and that the data submitted in support of regulatory decision making have the expected data quality standards and that human subject protections have been provided.

c. Continued Evolution of Evidentiary Requirements

Although the 1962 FD&C amendments did not explicitly require that the effectiveness of a drug be replicated, the FDA has traditionally required more than one adequate and well-controlled study to approve a new molecular entity. The scientific basis for this legal standard is derivative of the need to have independent substantiation of clinical results to protect against false positive findings that may potentially arise from unidentified, undetected systemic or conscious biases that may lead an incorrect conclusion. The requirement for replication may also protect against flawed findings that may result from the clinical trial design's features (e.g., disease definitions, inclusion/exclusion criteria, concomitant treatments) as well as investigator-specific issues (e.g., large single center driving the results of the trial) and, to a lesser extent, outright fraudulent data. In 1997, the FD&C was amended as the FDA Modernization Act (FDAMA) to revised Section 505 to make it clear that substantial evidence of effectiveness could be derived from one adequate and well controlled trial when accompanied by confirmatory evidence. The FDA issued guidance that articulated the situations in which this paradigm may be applicable and the more precise expectations of 'confirmatory evidence' (8). The guidance identified and defined potential sources of confirmatory evident as including, but not necessarily limited to:

- Phase 2 clinical trials in the same disease state
- Results from trials in other phases of the same disease
- Results from other investigations in the same disease using different clinical endpoints

- Results from other populations or from studies in closely related diseases
- Results from trials in less closely related disease, but where the general purpose of the therapy is similar
- Results from studies using different formulations, doses, regimens, or routes of administration
- Results from investigations using pharmacologic and/or pathophysiologic endpoints.

Many considered this to be a conservative interpretation of the intention of the amendments that, in practice, was largely applied to supplemental indications or extrapolation of clinical results to formulation changes through pharmacokinetic/pharmacodynamic (PK/PD) modelling. However, the FDA did acknowledge at the time that the adequacy, quantity, and quality of the data, including on whether to rely on a single pivotal adequate and well controlled trial, was inevitably a matter of scientific judgement and implicitly in the context of unmet medical need by articulating the following criteria for reliance on a single trial:

- A single, multi-center study of excellent design that provides highly reliable and statistically strong evidence of an important clinical benefit on survival or irreversible morbidity and . . ..
- A situation in which confirmation of the result in a second pivotal trial would be practically or ethically impossible.

Further characteristics of a persuasive clinical trial include: relatively broad patient inclusion criteria; diverse study populations with regards concomitant or prior treatment, disease stage, age, gender, race and other baseline demographics; multiple endpoints that measure different aspects of disease or disease burden each showing relevant and statistically significant benefits. Finally, it should be noted that the FDA guidance calls for a single pivotal trial to have a statistically very persuasive finding (i.e., very low p-value) to protect against Type I (False Positive) inferential error. In addition to the substantial experience in oncology, several non-oncology drugs have received initial full approval based on a single pivotal trial including ticagralor and prasugrel for cardiac event risk reduction following acute coronary syndrome (ACS) and both are excellent examples of a single pivotal trial that have the desired clinical and statistical features described above (9,10).

d. Emergence of Adaptive Designs

The cost of developing a new medicine continues to increase and much of this overall cost is attributable to the daunting cost of late stage failures and the rising costs of Phase 2 and 3 registration trials. There are many strategies and tactics being employed to reduce attrition rates and to increase the predictability of the clinical safety and efficacy of new mole-cules that are beyond the scope of this chapter. However, there are also numerous efforts to increase the efficiency and decrease the overall unit costs of clinical trials that are intended to inform regulatory approval decisions. The most commonly discussed and currently employed technique falls under the general term of adaptive clinical trials.

Adaptive trial design is employed both in exploratory and confirmatory clinical trials and both employ the fundamental concept of using accumulating data to inform modification of the ongoing trial without undermining the validity or integrity of the results. Possible adaptation tactics include, but are not limited to:

- Sample size adjustments
- Patient allocation to treatment arms
- Addition or deletion of treatment arms and/or doses
- Addition or deletion of study visits/procedures
- Modification of inclusion/exclusion criteria
- Modification of statistical analysis plan including selection of primary and ordering of secondary endpoints
- Combining phases (e.g., seamless phase 2/3 transitions)

The benefits of such approaches are obvious, including more efficient and cost-effective drug development, decreased burden to patients who may be receiving ineffective or suboptimal drugs or doses, enhanced patient acceptance and increased participation in clinical trials, and rapid access to patients of new approved therapeutics. There are, of course, challenges to preserving study integrity while adapting a trial based on accumulating clinical evidence from the same. The FDA issued draft guidance on the subject and clearly articulated the critical distinction between adaptations based on un-blinded results versus adaptations based on blinded assessment of non-comparative data. In the latter cases, clinical trialists are generally on firm ground when using adaptation strategies such as a sample size re-estimation based on blinded analysis of data variance, discontinuation rates, outcome event rates, time course of outcomes, etc. The use of un-blinded interim analyses to support adaptations requires special care to preserve bias control including thoughtful limitation of the knowledge of the interim results. The technique most frequently employed to preserve trial integrity is the use of an external Data Monitoring Committee that can guide adaptation decisions based on pre-specified and clinical and statistically robust criteria (e.g., early stopping for futility or overwhelming efficacy, dropping of ineffective doses, etc.). The disadvantage of this approach is that the sponsor is not aware of the data details that are the basis of the DMC recommendation. An alternative approach would be to use an internal DMC (iDMC) that is privy to un-blinded data and inform clinical trial adaptations. The advantage of this approach is that experienced internal personnel have insight into the totality of the data which can instill increased internal confidence in the decision. This approach is potentially more acceptable for exploratory or non-pivotal clinical trials but may be problematic for trials intended to support regulatory decision making and licensure. The use of interim data from an ongoing clinical trial while preserving and continuing to conduct the clinical trial has been successfully used to support regulatory decisions in the field of hypoglycemic agents. Current FDA guidance requires new diabetes drugs to demonstrate no adverse effect on cardiovascular outcomes in order to be licensed. Ongoing cardiovascular outcome trials (CVOTs) have had planned interim analyses that have been analyzed by a small firewalled internal DMC and submitted to the FDA. Extreme care must be taken to ensure the integrity of the firewall between the internal un-blinded individuals and the blinded clinical trial team and it should be recognized that this approach has not been universally successful (11,12).

e. Future of Innovation in Clinical Trials, Evidence Generation, and Statistical Methods

Clinical trial modernization attempts continue to be a priority for industry, academia, and regulatory agencies. On the heels of the passage of the 21st Century Cures Act by the U.S. Congress in 2016 and the Food and Drug Administration Reauthorization Act (FDARA) in 2017, there is impetus for determining an appropriate path forward for the use of totality of evidence including real world evidence (RWE) to support regulatory decision making on the effectiveness of new therapies. The FDA is charged with developing guidances on the subject which will likely reinforce the limitations of the use of existing data particularly with regard to the impact of residual bias due to lack of traditional mechanisms such as randomization and blinding on the outcome of retrospective analyses. Regulators and industry are, however, enthusiastic about the potential use of more pragmatic clinical trials that use data obtained in the normal course of clinical practice under the rubric of a clinical trial protocol that employs conventional bias control techniques. The more widespread use and acceptability of electronic medical records as a source of patient level data add to the potential near term value and viability of such RWE approaches (13).

As previously stated, randomization is a key feature of RCTs and is done to create balanced groups with regard to known and unknown background characteristics to ensure that any observed clinical and statistical inferences are likely to be due to the assigned interventions. Analyses of interventions therefore have traditionally analyzed the groups as initially assigned in an Intention to Treat (ITT) manner which preserves the assumption of equal distribution of potential influencing and confounding variables across treat-ment groups and that all patients take the drug as expected throughout the course of the trial. This, of course, is not always possible as patients drop out of trials due to adverse events, lack of expected treatment response, cross-over to or added use of rescue therapy, lack of continued interest in participation, and a host of other reasons. These are commonly grouped under the term 'post-randomization intercurrent events' and pose a chal-lenge to clinical and statistical interpretation of the treatment effects. Clin-icians, statisticians, and regulators have debated the appropriate methods to handle missing data with no ideal solution being adopted. The International Conference on Harmonization (ICH) is attempting to resolve and harmonize regulatory approaches by revising the ICH E9 document on Statistical Principles for Clinical Trials to include adoption of a common definition and characteristics of clinical trial estimand which would include a precise articulation of the study objective (i.e., what is to be estimated) taking into account intercurrent events which also inform the net benefits of the inves-tigational treatment (14). In short, the estimand approach requires careful definition of the population to be studied, the variable to be measured and when, the intervention effect (including intercurrent events) to be measured, and the summary measure for the variable on which the treatment effect will be based. Choices on the above four attributes should inform trial design and conduct, but also interpretation of the clinical and statistical relevance of the findings. When this approach is adopted by international regulators, it will require sponsors and trialists to more carefully and prospectively consider how to handle intercurrent events in both oncology and non-oncology trials.

Novel trial designs such as platform, basket, and tools such as Bayesian approaches to adaptation are gaining acceptability from trialists and regula-tors as a way to increase the efficiency and effectiveness of drug development. These will be discussed in the following sections. However, it should be remembered that the fundamental features of 'adequate and well-controlled' clinical trials intended for regulatory purposes such as provision for bias control, the use of concurrent or well-characterized historical controls, the prospective definition of objectives, independent adjudication of endpoints, statistical handling, as well as Good Clinical Practice (GCP) will apply.

III. Role of Platform Trials in Accelerating and Optimizing Drug Development, Registration, and Post-Marketing

a. Current Regulatory Pathways and Mechanisms Available to Leverage

Classically, clinical development had been characterized as a linear process beginning with phase 1 trials designed for dose finding and early assess-ment of safety, phase 2 trials designed to assess safety and activity, and phase 3 trials designed to provide more definitive evidence of safety and effectiveness. In this paradigm, submission of applications for marketing authorization of new agents to health authorities had to await accumulation of data across these stages of development, often iteratively and including the need for definitive outcome results from multiple phase 3 trials providing evidence of safety and effectiveness before filing. Even after submission, filings were often at substantial risk of prolonged review timelines and the need for multiple cycles of review.

Recognizing the need to improve trial and development efficiencies, especially for patients with serious and unmet medical needs, efforts led by multiple stakeholders including patient advocates, academia, industry, and government over the last 2 decades have resulted in several programs being incorporated into the regulatory framework through legislative statute and regulation to accelerate development, review, and approval of new medicines. The public health impact of cancer, HIV/AIDS, and other areas of substantial unmet need have served as catalysts for these efforts, along with the explosion in our understanding of the underlying biology and drivers of pathogenesis in these areas. Key programs are summarized here, with focus on the U.S,. EU, and Japan. It should be noted that these programs have been put in place as a complement and response to the emerging trends summarized above and should be viewed as tools within a broader development strategy, not as individual ends in and of themselves. In some ways, the use of these tools is blurring the lines between the three traditional phases of clinical development, and at some point one may view clinical development as a continuum leading to a threshold of evidence justifying initial approval and further life cycle management of individual agents and combinations, all with the goal of improving health on an individual and collective basis.

Orphan drug programs have been in place for several decades in the U. S., EU, and Japan . These programs are designed to encourage innovative medicines development in disease areas with small populations and areas where research is considered very challenging so that the costs of development and access would not justify investment without incentives offered within orphan programs. The requirements and general incentives in each market are summarized in Table 7.1. The incentives and requirements vary by region depending on the regulatory framework. For example in Europe and Japan, orphan designation relies not only on prevalence considerations, but also the potential for a new agent to impact medical practice within the field of available existing therapies (15,16). In addition, orphan designation in Europe can affect drug pricing considerations and not just serve as an incentive for research and development . In Japan, drugs with orphan designation are often reviewed within a shorter review timeline once a marketing application (JNDA) is submitted. More recently, orphan designation has been successfully applied to subsets of disease areas, especially sub-sets of non-small cell lung cancer defined by molecular

TABLE 7.1

Orphan Designation Criteria and Implications

Region	Orphan Criteria	Implications of Orphan Designation
U.S.	Disease or condition affects less than 200,000 persons in the U.S. or Affects more than 200,000 persons in the U.S. but there is no reasonable expectation that cost of development and availability will be recovered from U.S. sales	Tax credits for clinical testing Waiver of user fees when filing a new drug or biologic application 7 years marketing exclusivity
EU	Intended for treatment, prevention, or diagnosis of a life-threatening or chronically debilitating disease Prevalence must not be more than 5 in 10,000 or unlikely that marketing in the EU would generate sufficient returns to justify the needed investment No approved satisfactory method of diagnosis, prevention or treatment or of significant benefit	Reduction of fees 10 years marketing exclusivity Micro, small or medium sized enterprises (SME) eligible for further incentives
Japan	Prevalence less than 50,000 within Japanese territory For rare and serious incurable diseases No other treatment available or clinically superior to other available treatments	Tax credits Research grants for clinical and non-clinical studies Post-approval reassessment period 10 years instead of 4

pathways such as ALK and ROS. Given these considerations, it can be deduced that depending on the design and results, platform trials can have a role in generating data supportive of orphan designation, either through generation of data supporting a subset approach to defining the population within a broader disease type (such as in defining lung cancer populations based on molecular criteria that extend beyond clinical and histologic considerations as has been done in the U.S. and Japan), or at least in generating early evidence of activity through assessment of surrogate endpoints to justify the potential role of a new agent within the existing field of available treatments (this is especially important when seeking orphan designation in Europe and Japan).

In the following section we will review programs that have been put in place to more directly expedite the development and review process. Table 7.2 summarizes key USFDA program requirements and their implications including Fast Track Designation, Accelerated Approval, Breakthrough Therapy Designation, the Regenerative Medicine Advanced Therapy Designation, and Priority Review Designation. Analogous programs relevant in the EU and Japan will be discussed in text. Subsequently

TABLE 7.2

U.S. Regulatory Tools for Acceleration of Development, Review, and Approval

Tool/Program	Criteria/Requirements	Implications
Fast Track Designation	Potential to address an unmet need; level of evidence for FTD depends on stage of development Development plan that has a likelihood of demonstrating the agent's potential	Potential for rolling submission Potential for priority review
Accelerated Approval	For serious or life-threatening diseases Meaningful advantage over available therapies Effect on a surrogate endpoint reasonably likely to predict clinical benefit	Often allows for initial approval based on phase 2 data or an interim endpoint assessed in phase 3 Subject to post-approval confirmation
Breakthrough Therapy Designation	Preliminary clinical data demonstrates potential for significant improvement	Fast Track features plus focus from senior FDA staff and with multi-center collaboration within FDA Potential for priority review
Regenerative Medicine Advanced Therapy Designation	Cell therapy, tissue engineering, human cell and tissue products Intended to treat, modify, reverse, or cure a serious or life-threatening condition Preliminary clinical data demonstrates potential	Similar to fast track and breakthrough therapy designations
Priority Review	Significant improvement in safety or effectiveness	Shorter review timeline (approximately 4 month advantage over standard review timeline)

we will review how platform trials, when conducted as part of a comprehensive development program, can be used to leverage on or more of these tools and we will discuss some examples.

Fast track designation (FTD) was included as a provision of the FDA Modernization Act of 1997 (17). It is intended to facilitate development and review of drugs and biologics for serious or life threatening diseases. The drug or biologic of interest must have the potential to address unmet medical needs in such serious conditions. A notable feature of FTD is that the criteria may be met with data generated depending on the stage of development at the time of Fast Track application. For example, an application for FTD can be made as early as the time of the initial investigational drug application (IND) to initiate human testing, and in that case preclinical laboratory and animal data alone may be used to justify FTD (18). When FTD is requested at later stages of development, some clinical data would be expected as part of the justification, such as phase 1/2 data. If FTD is granted, sponsors would be allowed the opportunity to submit a New Drug Application in portions over time, a process referred to as a 'rolling submission,' as opposed to the typical situation where FDA requires all key components of of a NDA application to be filed at the same time.

In 1992, the Accelerated Approval (AA) (subpart H/E) provisions were promulgated, largely in response to the public health crisis of cancer and HIV/AIDS. Under these provisions, the FDA has the authority to approve drugs or biologics for serious life threatening diseases based on surrogate endpoints reasonably likely to predict clinical benefit (19). Also under these provisions, confirmation of benefit is expected based on conduct of confirmatory trials, which ideally would be ongoing at the time of initial AA. In oncology, the most common approach in leveraging these regulations has been to obtain initial AA based on non-randomized phase 2 trials evaluating objective response rate (ORR) as a primary endpoint in advanced cancer populations, and confirmation of benefit in randomized phase 3 trials evaluating time to event endpoints in less refractory patient groups (20). In some cases in oncology, and in many cases of HIV drug development, the a phase 3 trial would provide evidence to support AA, and subsequently the same trial would provide more conclusive outcomes to confirm clinical benefit in the same population. More recently and when evaluating new agents in combination with standard of care, randomized phase 2 trials in oncology have also been used to obtain AA (21). This regulatory tool and these precedents over the last 2 decades provide a supportive environment for possible use of platform phase 2 trials (either randomized or non-randomized multi-cohort trials) not only for signal detection but also for marketing authorization in some cases. Even if many platform trials may not, in and of themselves, provide adequate evidence of efficacy and safety to support registration under the AA regulations, they can play an important enabling role such as in further validation of potential surrogate endpoints. In Europe, similar provisions were promulgated under Conditional Marketing Authorization provisions (CMA). These are similar to the U.S. AA provisions, but differ in that they only apply to new drug applications and not supplemental applications in follow on indications. In addition, the EU regulations do not refer to surrogate endpoints reasonably likely to predict clinical benefit but more generally to approval based on preliminary evidence (22). In Japan, regulations supporting early conditional approval were also introduced in 2017, although the Japan Health Authorities have accepted marketing applications based on phase 2 data in some circumstances previously.

Building on these tools, breakthrough therapy designation (BTD) provisions were put in place in 2012 in the U.S. via the Food and Drug Administration Safety and Innovation Act (FDASIA) Section 902 (23). This designation is granted based on preliminary *clinical* evidence that the agent in question can represent a substantial leap in a particular population compared to available standard treatments. If granted, BTD allows a sponsor to apply for rolling submission, places the agent in the list of high priority assets not only for sponsors but also for FDA leadership, allows for frequent interactions between the sponsor and FDA intended to facilitate and speed the time from BTD to filing and approval, and triggers close collaboration within and across relevant centers within FDA as needed, such as between the Center for Drug Evaluation and Research (CDER), the Center for Biologics (CBER) and the Center for Devices and Radiologic Health (CDRH), which has the authority to regulate diagnostics. Given that clinical evidence of substantial activity is needed to justify BTD, it is conceivable that results from ongoing or completed platform trials could support requests for BTD, regardless of whether the results themselves reach a threshold supporting filing a marketing application. Similar programs to BTD have been introduced recently outside the U.S., namely the PRIME designation program in the EU and Sagikake in Japan (24,25). As part of the 21st Century Cures Act, a regenerative medicine advanced therapy (RMAT) designation is also now available for promising cellular and tissue engineering products (26). Finally, priority review is a designation which determines the length of the review process from NDA or supplemental NDA filing to FDA action. Whether a submission receives a priority or standard review timeline is determined at the time of filing and is based on whether a significant improvement in safety or efficacy over standard treatment is demonstrated.

b. Health Authority Views on Platform Trials and Their Potential Use

In general, health authorities have been supportive of the use of platform trials in medicines development (3). Their guidance and expectations for the design, execution, and analysis depend on multiple factors including the role intended for the platform trial within the overall development program in terms of stage of development, and whether the results are intended to be exploratory or whether they will be a component of a set of data and study results supporting a marketing application. For example, when using molecular markers to identify patients for inclusion in these trials, the expectations and requirements from health authorities depend on whether trial results are going to be used in an exploratory fashion only to help inform additional investigation, or whether trial results are planned to be used for registration purposes. Similarly in measuring outcomes, the intended use will guide health authority expectations. For exploratory studies health authorities can exhibit substantial flexibility in how response outcomes are measured captured and interpreted. In contrast, if results of response or progression endpoints in these trials are to be used for regulatory purposes, mechanisms to ensure additional consistency and rigor in data capture, adjudication, and interpretation are to be expected.

In oncology, reliance on imaging usually necessitates a charter for imaging review and adjudication as well as a clear and a priori defined analysis plan.

c. Case Studies

Some examples of platform trials that are being used in ways that have potential regulatory implications are summarized in Table 7.3. The investigation of serial studies to predict your therapeutic response with imaging and molecular analysis-2 (I-SPY 2) trial is an example of an adaptive platform trial to identify treatments for breast cancer in the setting of neoadjuvant treatment. Women with early high risk breast cancer defined by three biomarkers have been enrolled (hormone receptor status, HER2 status, and MammaPrint risk score). As of March 2017, 12 therapies from nine sponsors had been evaluated. Some assets have advanced for further study, including some that are investigational and others that are already marketed for other indications (27). Given that the agents being assessed include approved and investigational agents, this is an example of a mixed premarket/post-market use of such a trial. The potential relevance of the pathologic Complete Response (pCR) endpoint relates to the ability to evaluate pCR at the time of surgical resection, after a course of neoadjuvant treatment has been given. Ultimately, it is important to evaluate

TABLE 7.3

Examples of Platform Trials with Regulatory Implications

Platform Trial	Key Features	Regulatory Implications
I-SPY2	Several interventions evaluated in a platform for one disease (high risk early breast cancer)	Validation of pathologic CR rate in the neoadjuvant setting using both approved and investigational agents
Pembrolizumab approval in MSI-H and dMMR solid tumors	Tumor agnostic indication based on efficacy in 5 non-randomized trial including one basket trial and overall safety profile of an approved agent	Part of a submission package to justify a tumor agnostic indication under Accelerated Approval provisions Lack of a companion diagnostic
TAPUR	Evaluation of several approved agents based on patient profiling	Post-market use of a platform

I-SPY 2 = investigation of serial studies to predict your therapeutic response with imaging and molecular analysis – 2
MSI-H = microsatellite-instability high
dMMR = mis-match-repair-deficient
TAPUR = the targeted agent and profiling utilization registry study

across multiple experiences whether a difference in pCR rate will translate into longer term tangible benefits. Therefore the relevance of ISPY relates not only to the ability to evaluate multiple agents, but also to the ongoing assessment of pCR, an endpoint previously considered exploratory in nature in populations of breast cancer patients receiving neoadjuvant treatment. The FDA initially expressed public interest in the pCR endpoint as a possible surrogate reasonably likely to predict benefit in 2010. Prior to that, the endpoints used as the basis of approvals in early breast cancer had been disease free survival or overall survival. However, relying exclusively on these outcomes creates an estimated gap of 5–10 years between approvals for metastatic breast cancer and subsequent approval for use in earlier stages of disease. Over the next few years, as interest grew, FDA led an international effort to pool data from more than 12,000 women enrolled in neoadjuvant trials, and the first approval of a neoadjuvant drug for high risk early breast cancer occurred in 2013 with the accelerated approval of pertuzumab (which was also a test treatment in I-SPY2) on the basis of pCR rates and safety data from two neoadjuvant trials with a commitment to conduct a large randomized trial to confirm that pertuzumab reduces the risk of recurrence or death (28). In I-SPY2, the approval of pertuzumab necessitated a substitution for trastuzumab in the HER-2 positive setting, and the master protocol for the trial allowed for this change in practice to be addressed with a design modification as the trial was ongoing. Thus, this is an example of a platform trial design that has helped validate a novel surrogate endpoint.

Platform trials are increasingly being used in the immuno-oncology space given the multiple questions being addressed around the role of biomarker status in patient selection, dose and schedule, and role of combinations in optimal modulation of the immune response. The potential to demonstrate early signs of efficacy across multiple tumor types was a key driver as well. Although platform trials may not often serve as standalone trials to support an assessment of positive risk-benefit supporting a marketing application, they are already demonstrating the role they can play in marketing applications. A recent example is FDA's approval of pembrolizumab for patients with unresectable or metastatic, microsatellite-instability high (MSI-H) or mis-match-repair-deficient (dMMR) solid tumors, regardless of tumor site or histology (29). This approval is considered a first for a tumor agnostic indication and represents a situation where a threshold of evidence was reached to justify that the molecular features are at least equally important if not more important than clinical/histologic considerations in determining natural history, treatment, and outcome. Although the filing included data from five individual studies, it should be noted that one of those studies, referred to as KEYNOTE-158, is a basket trial investigating a number of rare tumor types and including a cohort that enrolled any colorectal solid tumor characterized by high microsatellite instability. Of note, an independent central radiologic review has been a component of the design and data capture approach to assessment of the primary endpoint of objective response rate in KEY-NOTE 158. This approval was also notable for lack of a simultaneous approval of a companion diagnostic test for MSI-H or dMMR, although the Agency did require a post-marketing commitment for the sponsor to develop an In Vitro Diagnostic (IVD) test to determine biomarker status and eligibility for treatment. In this supplemental application, the identification of biomarker eligibility was prospectively determined in most patients using local laboratory-developed tests. In this case, FDA has acknowledged the limitations of this approach and rationalized the decision making based on the very high unmet need in a set of tumors including a group of rare malignancies, the known safety profile, the substantial effect on response and durability of response, and the substantial experience over decades in the prior use of MSI-H or dMMR testing as a prognostic determinant for colorectal cancer recurrence. It should be recognized that this approach relied on a unique set of circumstances and cannot be assumed to apply in most cases.

Although much of the attention around platform trials involves their role in pre-market assessment, these trials can play an important role in the post-marketing setting. We have already discussed I-SPY2 as a platform trial evaluating a mix of premarket and approved agents. In addition, the targeted agent and profiling utilization registry study (TAPUR) sponsored by the American Society of Clinical Oncology (ASCO) is specifically evaluating a number of approved agents in populations that were not part of the approved indications (30). The goal of TAPUR is to systematically capture outcomes data such that the benefit-risk profile can be further elucidated.

Platform trials have the potential to play a more direct and important role in the post-market setting. Confirmatory basket trials could be considered where individual histologic subtypes are grouped together each with its own control group or with a common control arm. This will be discussed further in Section V below on future considerations.

Although FDA has been historically more proactive in supporting and promoting the use of platform trials in the development setting, EMA is also evolving its approach to leverage these trials. Some of the reluctance in Europe was not related to any specific concern around platform trials in general, but rather concerns about the potential use of phase 2 trials (especially non-randomized trials) to support marketing authorization, as well as the need to clarify the approach to randomization in the platform setting where applicable. Given the considerations discussed above including the conditional marketing authorization mechanism that has now been available in Europe for over a decade with several precedents for approvals of new agents under this mechanism (22), the EMA environment is expected to continue to progress, and this is manifested by recent workshops co-sponsored by EMA and updates to its guidances (31,32).

IV. Special Considerations

a. Drug-Diagnostic Development

Most platform trials to date in oncology have focused on populations with molecular markers for which one or more diagnostic tests have already been validated and marketed. In addition, many of the populations being included in oncology platform trials are enrolled after receiving initial diagnosis and marker assessment and multiple treatments. In these cases drug-diagnostic codevelopment may not be particularly challenging as in the first case, there may not be a need for a novel diagnostic kit but rather validation of an existing kit in the new clinical setting. In the second case, if the treatment being assessed is targeting the same molecular marker that was identified at baseline, then a similar clinical validation approach may be satisfactory or verification of a biomarker using an FDA approved diagnostic test at enrollment may suffice. However, if a biomarker or panel of markers for which there is not a precedent pre-market approved test (PMA) or FDA approved diagnostic test is being evaluated, then one is faced with a situation where there needs to be parallel attention to the clinical assessment as well as the full development of diagnostic kit information to justify a full/new PMA, including consistency of screening performance, predictability of outcome, manufacturing, and other considerations. Therefore in such cases the new diagnostic test will have to be analytically and clinically validated in order to submit a PMA. These issues need to be considered when designing platform trials that involve patient selection based on molecular markers, especially if the ultimate intent is to use results from such trials as part of a registration package. Moving beyond the use of a single biomarker, assay, or test is the use of next-generation sequencing (NGS) based tests that can detect multiple biomarkers of clinical significance. NGS technologies are moving from being employed primarily in clinical research settings to settings where they are used to determine the course of treatment for patients, thus paving the way for their incorporation into standard of care (33). An advantage of NGS-based tests is the potential for a single test to deliver information on multiple tumor variants, saving time and tissue samples, and creating greater efficiencies. One of the greatest advantages of employing these tests in platform trial designs is the potential to rapidly discover and clinically validate biomarkers of significance and to allow sponsors to further refine target patient populations. The recent FDA approvals of two NGS-based tests that can be used as companion diagnostics paves the way for more such approvals (34,35).

b. Combination Therapies

As we gain a better understanding of the pathogenesis and molecular drivers of serious and life-threatening diseases, it has become evident that using an add-on approach where one new single agent is evaluated as an addition to existing therapy or as a single replacement for existing therapy is not likely to result in breakthrough therapies in most cases. Many circumstances will likely require assessment of novel-novel combinations of agents with complementary mechanisms of action either given simultaneously or in a rational sequence. For new interventions with novel combinations, health authorities expect a demonstration of the role of individual agents in the overall risk-benefit profile of the combination. In the classic development paradigm described at the beginning of this chapter, this would have required very large phase 3 trials with upwards of 4 or more arms (placebo or standard control, agent A, agent B, and combo) after an exhaustive set of phase 1 and 2 studies. Multiple stakeholders including regulators around the globe have recognized that such an approach is not usually feasible. Instead, demonstration of the individual clinical effects in well-designed phase 1 and 2 trials can translate into more practical phase 3 trials (A plus B versus standard as an example). Here, platform trials could play an important role in streamlining development and approval. In the immune-oncology space, several sponsors are now conducting phase 3 trials with such designs in the advanced/metastatic renal carcinoma setting and this is likely to expand to other tumor areas.

c. Pediatrics

Patients under 18 years of age have been traditionally excluded from adult trials. However pediatric development could be expedited by inclusion of some pediatric patients in trials with adults, as opposed to relying entirely on separate pediatric trials that can be difficult to initiate, complete, and interpret. At least in oncology and where appropriate, there is support from the FDA for including patients 12 years and older in adult trials if certain criteria are met. This can be followed with clinical evaluation in younger children. Here, adaptive trial designs may have a role. For example, basket trials could include pediatric expansion cohorts (36). This could be especially feasible where evidence to support extrapolation including PK/PD assessments may be more readily available. A recent example is a planned extension to the NCI-MATCH trial (Molecular Analysis for Therapy Choice) to include a pediatric component with multiple arms designed to assess targeted therapies in pediatric and adolescent patients with solid tumors that have progressed on initial therapy and with mutations of interest in over 160 genes. Patients can stay on treatment and can also move to another arm of the trial if the treatment targets another genetic abnormality identified in the tumor. At this point the study is intended as a screening tool to evaluate early signals of activity. As of July 2017, the MATCH trial had 19 treatment arms evaluating 14 different agents (37)

V. Conclusions and Future Trends

It is evident that to date, regulatory and development interest in the design, execution, and interpretation of platform trials has largely been focused on oncology. Reasons for this include the substantial unmet need, the precedence and familiarity with use of surrogate endpoints not only for exploratory purposes but also for regulatory purposes, and the substantial knowledge available in selecting patients based on molecular criteria that transcend clinical-histologic considerations. However, there are still ways in which platform trials can be more fully leveraged both in oncology and beyond. Some of the possibilities include the following;

a. Allowing pooling of samples if the variant signature is shared across various histologies: This would address practical challenges such as the limited patient population that can be enrolled into clinical studies. This issue is likely to be further amplified as we discover rare variants of clinical significance in specific disease settings.

b. Allowing novel statistical approaches that enable transitioning from exploratory to confirmatory/registrational studies: Basket trials have largely been used for exploratory biomarker discovery and early detection of activity. Qualitative alternative designs and novel designs that allow for confirmation of benefit should be embraced. These studies may incorporate use of common control arms, or use of information on natural history of disease as controls for non-randomized trials, especially in the case of rare populations. Ultimately, the goal of performing these studies is to provide patients in niche indications with enhanced access to novel therapies, facilitate full development and approval, and enhance the ability of regulatory authorities to fully evaluate risk and benefit in these settings (38).

c. Data management and prioritization: Leveraging new information about disease biology and utilizing new techniques such as NGS-based testing in the design and conduct of platform trials is an attractive option to allow development of therapies for molecularly-defined sub-populations. However, employing these techniques, especially in the context of seamless studies that attempt to discover and validate biomarkers and to employ biomarker based stratification can result in generation of vast amounts of data. Health authorities should work with other stakeholders to help define minimal and essential data standards to avoid collection of extraneous data that can drive up costs and lead to other inefficiencies.

d. Gaining experience in additional disease areas: In addition to enhancing the use of platform trials in oncology especially for marketing and in the post-market setting, steps should be taken to more proactively plan for the use of platform trials in other disease areas. Areas being considered include infectious diseases, neuro-degenerative diseases, orphan metabolic conditions, and inflammation/immunology. The ability to leverage platform trials in these settings will depend on the successful construction of the necessary networks to support startup and completion. There are already signs of progress on this issue. One example is an emerging network for assessment in pediatric and neonatal populations. The FDA is also contributing to this effort; in a draft guidance to industry on Gaucher Disease as a model issued in December 2017, the FDA has proposed a multi-trial multi-company superiority/non-inferiority platform trial design as a possible solution to the many challenges facing drug development in this rare disease (39).

e. Small molecule and biologic combinations: To optimize the emerging knowledge of biology, it will be necessary not only to combine or sequence multiple small molecules as part of a treatment approach, but also to develop combinations of small molecules and biologics. Combining small molecules with strict dosing regimens with biologics that may have a broader range of doses and schedules will pose challenges especially if the combination will have to be sequenced and scheduled differently within different baskets in a study. However, this challenge must be addressed in order to leverage the efficiencies that these trial designs offer to explore better treatment options.

f. From platform trials to platform development: The design, analysis, and interpretation of platform trials should evolve to recognize the broader trends in drug discovery and development, where data generation must meet the expectations of multiple stakeholders including patients and payers (40). This will likely include further reliance on novel and composite endpoints, prospective planning for data pooling in order to interpret study results in the broader context of public health and not just with respect to populations studied in individual trials, and assessment of different interventions such as surgery, radiation, vaccines, drugs, and antibodies in a matrixed way to provide rigorous evidence to allow a clearer picture for proper care across a patient's journey from diagnosis forward.

Disclaimer

Dr. Kalamegham is an employee of Genetech, Inc, Dr Dagher and Dr Honig are employees of Pfizer, Inc. The views expressed here are those of the authors and do not necessarily represent those of Genentech or Pfizer.

References

1. Prowell TN, Theoret MR, Pazdur R. Seamless Oncology – Drug Development. *NEJM* 2016; 374 (21): 2001–2003.
2. Elsaber A, Regenstrom J, Vetter T, et al. Adaptive Clinical Trial Designs for European Marketing Authorization: A Survey of Scientific Advice Letters from the European Medicines Agency. *Trials* 2014; 15: 383.
3. Woodcock J, LaVange LM. Master Protocols to Study Multiple Therapies, Multiple Diseases, or Both. *NEJM.* 2017; 377 (1): 62–70.
4. Kefauver-Harris Amendments Revolutionized Drug Development. www.fda.gov/ForConsumers/ConsumerUpdates/ucm322856.htm
5. DESI. www.nasonline.org/about-nas/history/archives/collections/des-1966-1969-1.html
6. 21 Code of Federal Regulations Subpart D Section 314.126. Adequate and Well Controlled Trials. www.accessdata.fda.gov/scripts/cdrh/cfdocs/cfcfr/cfrsearch.cfm?fr=314.126
7. International Conference on Harmonisation Guideline on Good Clinical Practice (ICH E6). www.ich.org/products/guidelines/efficacy/article/efficacy-guidelines.html
8. Providing Clinical Evidence of Effectiveness for Human Drug and Biological Products. www.fda.gov/downloads/Drugs/GuidanceComplianceRegulatoryInformation/Guidances/UCM072008.pdf
9. Wiviott SD, Braunwald E, McCabe CH, et al. Prasugrel versus Clopidogrel in Patients with Acute Coronary Syndromes. *NEJM* 2007; 357: 2001–2015.
10. Wallentin L, Becker RC, Budaj A, et al. Ticagrelor versus Clopidogrel in Patients with Acute Coronary Syndromes. *NEJM* 2009; 361: 1045–1057.
11. Diabetes Mellitus – Evaluating Cardiovascular Risk in New Antidiabetic Therapies to Treat Type 2 Diabetes. www.fda.gov/downloads/Drugs/GuidanceComplianceRegulatoryInformation/Guidances/UCM071627.pdf
12. U.S. FDA Advisory Committee Meeting: Canagliflozin. www.accessdata.fda.gov/drugsatfda_docs/nda/2013/204042orig1s000riskr.pdf
13. Sherman RE, Anderson SA, Dal Pan GJ, et al. Real-World Evidence – What Is It and What Can It Tell Us? *NEJM* 2016; 375: 2293–2297.
14. International Conference on Harmonisation. Guideline on Statistical Principles for Clinical Trials (E9R1). www.ich.org/products/guidelines/efficacy/article/efficacy-guidelines.html
15. Institute of Medicine (U.S.) Forum on Drug Discovery, Development, and Translation. Breakthrough Business Models: Drug Development for Rare and Neglected Diseases and Individualized Therapies: Workshop Summary. Washington, DC, National Academies Press, (US), 2009. https://www.ncbi.nlm.nih.gov/books/NBK50977/, 10.17226/12219.

16. The Committee for Orphan Medicinal Products and the European Medicines Agency Scientific Secretariat. European Regulation on Orphan Medicinal Products: 10 Years of Experience and Future Perspectives. *Nature Reviews Drug Discovery* 2011; 10: 341–349.

17. Food and Drug Modernization Act of 1997, Public Law 105–115, 111 STAT.2296 (1997), 21 U.S.C.301

18. Guidance for Industry: Fast Track Drug Development Program-Designation, Development, and Application Review. www.fda.gov/cder/guidance/2112fnl.pdf, posted November, 17, 1998

19. 21 Code of Federal Regulations 312.80.

20. Johnson JR, Ning YM, Farrell A, et al. Accelerated Approval of Oncology Products. The Food and Drug Administration Experience. *JNCI* 2011; 103 (8): 636–644.

21. Beaver JA, Amiri-Kordestani I, Charlab R, et al. FDA Approval: Palbociclib for the Treatment of Postmenopausal Patients with Estrogen Receptor Positive HER-2 Negative Metastatic Breast Cancer. *Clinical Cancer Research* 2015; 21: 4760–4766.

22. Martinalbo J, Bowen D, Camarero J, et al. Early Market Access of Cancer Drugs in the EU. *Annals of Oncology* 2016; 27 (11): 96–105.

23. Horning SJ, Haber DA, Selig WKD, et al. Developing Standards for Breakthrough Therapy Designation in Oncology. *Clinical Cancer Research* 2013; 19 (16): 4297–4303.

24. Enhanced Early Dialogue to Facilitate Accelerated Assessment of PRIority MEdicines (PRIME). EMA/CHMP/57760/2015.

25. Kondo H, Hata T, Ito K, et al. The Current Status of Sakigake Designation in Japan, PRIME in the European Union, and Breakthrough Therapy Designation in the United States. *Therapeutic Innovation and Regulatory Science* 2017; 51 (1): 51–54.

26. FDA. Regenerative Medicine Advanced Therapy Designation (RMAT). www.fda.gov/BiologicsBloodVaccines/CellularGeneTherapyProducts/ucm537670.htm

27. Park JW, Liu MC, Yee D, et al. For the I-SPY Investigators. Adaptive Randomization of Neratinib in Early Breast Cancer. *NEJM* 2016; 375 (1): 11–22.

28. Amiri-Kordestani L, Wedam S, Zhang L. First FDA Approval of Neoadjuvant Therapy for Breast Cancer: Pertuzumab for the Treatment of Patients with HER2-Positive Breast Cancer. *Clinical Cancer Research* 2014; 20 (21): 5359–5364.

29. Lemery S, Keegan P, Pazdur R. First FDA Approval Agnostic of Cancer Site – When a Biomarker Defines the Indication. *NEJM* 2017; 377 (15): 1409–1412.

30. TAPUR: Testing the Use of Food and Drug Administration (FDA) Approved Drugs that Target a Specific Abnormality in a Tumor Gene in People With Advanced Stage Cancer (TAPUR). clinicaltrials.gov/ct2/show/NCT02693535

31. EMA-ESMO Workshop on Single-Arm Trials in Oncology. *ESMO*. www.esmo.org/.../Workshops.../EMA-ESMO-Workshop-on-Single-Arm-Trials-in-Oncology

32. Guideline on Strategies to Identify and Mitigate Risks for First-in-Human and Early Clinical Trials with Investigational Medicinal Products. EMEA/CHMP/SWP/28367/Rev.1. July, 20, 2017.

33. IOM (Institute of Medicine). *Evolution of Translational Omics: Lessons Learned and the Path Forward*. Washington, DC, The National Academies Press, 2012.

34. FDA Approves Test to Detect Mutations in 324 Genes, Two Genomic Signatures. Second to be Approved with Proposed Coverage under FDA/CMS Parallel Review Program. www.fda.gov/NewsEvents/Newsroom/PressAnnouncements/ucm587273.htm

35. Premarket (PMA) Approval for Oncomine Dx Target Test. www.accessdata.fda.gov/scripts/cdrh/cfdocs/cfpma/pma.cfm?id=P160045

36. Beaver JA, Ison G, Pazdur R. Reevaluating Eligibility Criteria-Balancing Patient Protection and Participation in Oncology Trials. *NEJM* 2017; 376 (16): 1504–1505.

37. NCI-MATCH Trial (Molecular Analysis for Therapy Choice). www.cancer.gov/about-cancer/treatment/clinical-trials/nci-supported/nci-match

38. Beckman RA, Antonijevic Z, Kalamegham R, et al. Adaptive Design for a Confirmatory Basket Trial in Multiple Tumor Types Based on a Putative Predictive Biomarker. *Clinical Pharmacology and Therapeutics* 2016; 100 (6): 617–625.

39. Draft Guidance for Industry: Pediatric Rare Diseases – A Collaborative Approach for Drug Development Using Gaucher Disease as a Model. www.fda.gov/cder/guidance, posted 12/2017

40. Eichler HG, Baird LG, Barker R, et al. From Adaptive Licensing to Adaptive Pathways: Delivering a Flexible Life-Span Approach to Bring New Drugs to Patients. *Clinical Pharmacology and Therapeutics* 2015; 97: 234–246.

8

Multi-Arm, Multi-Drug Trials from a Reimbursement Perspective

Anja Schiel and Olivier Collignon

In Europe, regulatory decisions concerning approval of drugs are made centralized by the European Medicines Agency (EMA), while reimbursement decisions are made decentralised at the national level by all member states. Historically access to new drugs was dependent on the regulatory approval, but in recent years this has shifted towards reimbursement being the restricting factor. Main drivers of this development are the ever increasing costs of new drugs, the decline in quality and robustness of submitted data, and the increasing pressure to accelerate drug approval and reimbursement processes.

The traditional drug development focuses on a linear process where obtaining the regulatory approval is considered a first hurdle, with reimbursement decision often coming into consideration after important decisions about the development program have been made already. The observed shift in importance of the regulatory versus reimbursement decisions has also led to an understanding that acceptance of for example trial designs should not only be sought with regulators, but also with other downstream stakeholders.

Based on this understanding of shifting roles and need for closer interactions, EMA and the European network for health technology assessment (EUnetHTA) have facilitated interactions between drug developers, national health technology agencies (HTA), and EMA to provide consolidated advice on drug development programs.

One of the complicating factors in providing a HTA viewpoint is the huge diversity of methodology used to perform assessments at the national or even regional level. Historically, European member states have different preferences in techniques and philosophy based on their political and financial differences.[1] The field of HTA is also relatively young and still developing, something that makes reimbursement decision-making difficult to predict across the spectrum. As a consequence, the HTA landscape for medicines in Europe is currently fragmented; however in a recent legislative proposal by the EC (January 2018; https://ec.europa.eu/health/technology_assessment/eu) cooperation was adopted with the aim to establish a European system for health technology assessment, and harmonise health technology assessment criteria in order to assess the added therapeutic value of medicines. Such a network with mandatory uptake of relative effectiveness assessments can have a major impact on transparency and policy in the future, but will likely not be fully operational before 2024.

In December 2017, a workshop was organized by the EMA oncology working party on "Site and Histology – Independent Indications in Oncology." As a contribution to this workshop, EUnetHTA conducted an informal survey among national members of EUnetHTA as well as international HTA contacts. The results of this survey are not meant to be representative or provide a consolidated opinion, but rather reflect the current viewpoint of those HTAs that participated in it.

The survey focused on multi-arm, multi-drug trials such as 'Umbrella type' or 'Basket type' trials. Questions focused mainly on awareness, experience, and acceptability of these new trial designs. Five EUnetHTA members and two international HTAs contributed to the survey.

All HTAs were familiar with the concept of Basket/Umbrella trials, but the lack of a consolidated definition of such trials was pointed out as one of the major problems at the moment. Not all agencies had seen such trial designs in submissions, and those that had received submissions including such trials had seen them mainly in early development phases, not as pivotal source of evidence per se. While none of the agencies a priori disapproved these types of trial designs, a number of potential problems were identified across all agencies. Concerns were raised about the potential lack of statistical power, all agencies had concerns about the uncontrolled aspects of such trials, and the issue of independence of arms was raised. These concerns mirrored those already identified by regulators and methodologists (and discussed in earlier sections/chapters) and indicate that the acceptance of HTAs will not necessarily differ too much from that of regulators per se. One aspect that was specifically problematic from an HTA perspective was the lack of collection of Quality of life (QoL) data seen in some recent examples.

Umbrella-type trials, if defined as testing different drugs or drug combinations in identical populations, are less problematic from an HTA perspective. Such trials would potentially allow a direct comparison between arms (directly if populations are truly identical or possibly indirectly if not) and assessment of relative effectiveness is possible. Problems would arise if all drugs/drug combinations would represent non-approved, non-reimbursed substances, since anchoring results to existing treatments might not be possible.

Basket-type trials are perceived as more problematic, as they often resemble what can be perceived as a collection of single-arm trials, lacking the comparative context required to establish relative effectiveness. Since each arm/sub-study would be seen as a separate single-arm trial all problems connected to that approach would still apply, regardless whether the trial is conducted in a basket context (from a logistical perspective) or not. The only possible solution in absence of a comparative context is the attempt to establish relative effectiveness through comparison to historical or observational sources. Currently HTAs consider it problematic to use historical evidence to establish relative effectiveness; more progress has to be made in establishing common quality standards and criteria for such sources of real world evidence (RWE). Before such criteria have been established, the acceptance of use of RWE is largely dependent on the national HTAs regulations and is often determined case-by-case.

All HTAs acknowledged that multi-arm, multi-drug trial designs have certain advantages. Faster and more efficient drug development was mentioned by several HTAs, yet this is not considered a strong advantage from a reimbursement perspective if it does not result in lower prices and the guarantee that the provided evidence for decision-making has sufficient robustness. Seemingly, requirements for regulatory approval have been lowered, but this needs to be seen in light of the changing landscape of drug development in smaller, more targeted populations, and the accompanying ethical and logistic problems of conducting studies in such indications. Nonetheless, the changes in evidence robustness pose an increasing problem, in addition to the decreases seen in sample sizes and short follow-up times in standard randomized clinical trials. Increasing numbers of submissions based on single-arm trials will only further aggravate the methodological challenges for the HTAs.

In general, potential problems with statistical aspects such as lack of power, handling of missing data, randomisation, and independence when multiple assignment possibilities exist, as well as uncertainties around what other issues might be identified dependent on the chosen statistical analysis plan suggest that instead of a general acceptance of such trial designs a case-by-case approach will be required.

Answering multiple research questions in one trial has been mentioned as another advantage, as well as the possibility to conduct trials in relatively small populations in rare and ultra-rare diseases. It might be that acceptance of multi-arm, multi-drug trials in rare diseases is largest, in particular seen in light of guidance available by several HTAs on evidence requirements being different in such disease areas. This is based on a generally higher acceptance of uncertainty when plans to fill evidence gaps post-authorization are in place in rare diseases than in mainstream indications.

An important feedback from the HTA side was that reimbursement based on biomarker selection is not considered impossible. As long as both an identifiable population and a standard of care for such a population can be established, reimbursement could be granted based on a validated biomarker.

Only a few phase III studies with these types of designs have been conducted and submitted as pivotal evidence. It is therefore not surprising that such trials often lack information on QoL as this information is not necessarily considered of prime interest in the early phase drug development. HTA assessment often relies on the collection of generic instruments to collect QoL (such as EQ-5D of SF36), but some HTAs also require disease specific QoL data for their assessment. In absence of direct collection of information in a clinical study it is often considered acceptable to use historical/observational data, keeping in mind that this increases the uncertainty about the relative effectiveness assessment. In situations where very heterogeneous populations are investigated in the same studies, it is clear that collecting adequate and relevant QoL data is considered challenging.

In conclusion, it can be stated that acceptance of a multi-arm, multi-drug trial is dependent on the elements that make up such trials. The lack of a common definition complicates establishment of a consolidated guidance on the use and acceptability from an HTA perspective. The logistic advantages of Basket trials are acknowledged, but most HTAs expressed the view that the individual arms/sub-studies of such trials would be treated as independent trials and not seen as one large trial. While the advantages of the logistics might be most prominent and acceptable in early drug development, concerns are raised about their role in late phase/pivotal evidence generation. The lack of contextualization in absence of control arms for all included populations and potentially different comparators is a major shortcoming currently seen in published data. It should also be highlighted that QoL data need to be collected in order to enable HTAs to use such trial evidence to determine relative effectiveness. Another aspect often mentioned as an advantage is the potential time gain in drug development, providing faster access of new drugs to patients. This is achieved by the use of endpoints that reflect short-term effects with often little true clinical relevance for the patient. Those endpoints are not always acceptable from an HTA perspective and might rather delay or prohibit a positive reimbursement decision. The acceptance of certain endpoints is not necessarily connected to multi-arm, multi-drug studies per se, but is a general problem for HTA bodies.

All in all the role of multi-arm, multi-drug studies needs careful assessment. The advantages such designs provide need to outweigh potential methodological and statistical challenges. Advantages to only one stakeholder should not drive the motivation to utilize study designs that might not provide the required robustness of evidence for downstream stakeholders. Whether these trial designs can play a role in late-stage drug development remains to be seen, but at the moment from an HTA perspective too many concerns remain, and utilizing multi-arm, multi-drug designs should only be considered when other more conventional options have been assessed, and good arguments can be provided against their use. Drug developers are advised to discuss such plans with relevant stakeholders to reach agreement before embarking into such a program.

Reference

1. Allen N, Pichler F, Wang T, Patel S, and Salek S. (2013). Development of archetypes for non-ranking classification and comparison of European National Health Technology Assessment systems. *Health Policy* 113, 305–312.

9

Highly Efficient Clinical Trials

A Resource-Saving Solution for Global Health

Edward J. Mills, Jonas Häggström, and Kristian Thorlund

Introduction

Populations living in resource-limited settings are disproportionately affected by non-communicable and infectious diseases, experience shorter life expectancy, and have rates of child mortality that effect developmental and economic potential at national and regional levels.[1] The countries with the greatest burdens of disease are nearly consistently located in the global south, environments that have historically lacked adequate healthcare infrastructure.[2] While medicine and public health has always prided itself with caring for the disadvantaged, partnerships between well-resourced medical researchers and colleagues in resource limited settings has been hampered by a lack of interest, an assumption that poor uptake of medical interventions will occur, and the emergence of drug-resistant infections.[3,4] Within this belief, the prevalence of clinical trials among populations in resource limited settings were relatively rare, and typically poorly funded and planned.[5] A 2002 study found that 0.1% of trials conducted globally are done in sub-Saharan Africa even though 25% of the global burden of disease is there.[5]

The AIDS epidemic in southern Africa can likely be credited with bringing about a paradigm shift in assumptions about widespread public health interventions and the evaluation of interventions to reduce morbidity and mortality. Prior to the rollout of the U.S. President's Emergency Plan for AIDS Relief (PEPFAR), the provision of antiretroviral therapy (ART) for the largest infectious disease epidemic of the past 50 years, was rare. As roll-out of ART began, evaluations of the success of ART and implementation science revealed dramatic findings that challenged widespread assumptions of both drug effectiveness and the desire and behaviors of recipient patients and communities. Safe, effective, and adherent treatment led to dramatic decreases in mortality, morbidity, and transmission of the HIV virus.[3,6] The success of the PEPFAR program led to the expansion of services for other diseases, such as specific cancers, hepatitis C, and—more recently—non-communicable diseases.[7-9] Yet clinical trials to evaluate the effectiveness of interventions in these populations remain comparatively limited, and local infrastructure to successfully undertake clinical trials is typically limited.[10] Although there is often great enthusiasm at the local level for directly relevant evidence, funding and infrastructure needs often preclude clinical trials. Agencies such as the UK Medical Research Council (MRC), the U.S. Fogarty International Center, and the Bill & Melinda Gates Foundation aim to increase clinical trial prevalence and infrastructure. Yet achieving rapid improvements in the scale and infrastructure to conduct relevant trials presents challenges that are often embedded in the traditions of clinical trials and clinical investigator behaviors. Adaptive clinical trials offer a remarkable opportunity to improve the number and efficiency of clinical trials, but are typically poorly understood by funders and investigators. Platform trials, in particular, represent a long-term solution to infrastructure development, multiple evaluations, and long-term cost-savings.

Lesson Learned—Past Mistakes and Foregone Opportunities

Up to now, clinical trials in resource-limited settings have been, on average, relatively small, short duration, and often poorly conducted. For example, among 184 trials that we reviewed evaluating interventions to reduce childhood stunting from pregnancy to 2 years, the median duration was 26 weeks (interquartile range [IQR] 12–52) and the number of participants enrolled was 377 (IQR 135–1,213). Interventions chosen for evaluation have frequently compared established standards of care (e.g., nevirapine for prevention of HIV vertical transmission) versus inert controls (e.g., placebo), even when the standards of care have been established in other settings. Superiority trials dominate and relatively few head-to-head evaluations of current therapies are conducted. One of the reasons for this paucity in cutting-edge interventions has been the lack of involvement of pharmaceutical companies and thus the lack of funding. Clinical trials relying on peer-reviewed competitive funding are rare and many aid agencies have refused to conduct clinical trials to evaluate the effectiveness or harms of interventions or implementation of strategies. As a result, the majority of clinical trials documented in developing countries are two-arm superiority trials or cluster trials.[11,12] Cluster trials can present challenges in the conduct and interpretation of results, and examples exist of inappropriate interpretation of clustered interventions.[12] For example, in a mega-cluster randomized trial of mothers receiving antenatal corticosteroids for pediatric maturity in Argentina, Guatemala, India, Kenya, Pakistan, and Zambia (51 intervention clusters, 48,219 pregnant women, 47,394 livebirths, and 50 control clusters, 51,523 women, and 50,743 livebirths), the investigators found severe imbalance in cluster characteristics of ANC use (intervention clusters, most common in Pakistan [23.4%], Zambia and Argentina [14–17%], Guatemala and India [9–11%], and Kenya [2.9%]). Rates of C-sections were highest in Argentina (40%), then India and Guatemala (20%), Pakistan (12%), then Kenya and Zambia (≤2%). Rates of mortality were not different between the low birth weight groups (relative risk [RR] 0·96, 95% CI 0·87–1·06), but significantly increased among the overall population (RR 1·12, 1·02–1·22).[13] Interpretation of this study is difficult even when one has access to the individual participant data.

While much has been written about the past quality of trials conducted in low resource settings, studies of quality have almost exclusively examined pairwise clinical trials, and much less so cluster, pragmatic, and stepped wedge trials. The 2014 ebola virus disease (EVD) epidemic in West Africa was among the first circumstances where advocacy for adaptive clinical trials created thoughtful discussion about innovative trial designs in the global health arena.[14–16] This was a unique time in clinical trial history as no useful clinical trial infrastructure existed in Liberia, Guinea, or Sierra Leone. The local population was fearful of engaging with patients, while the outside investigators and agencies argued publicly about the best approach to treatment and investigations of experimental interventions.[17] Both private industry and, more often, investigator groups, supported by the UK Wellcome Trust and U.S. CDC, proposed haphazard designs that failed to provide useful information.[18,19] The only successfully completed trial in the ebola epidemic was the Bern vaccine trial using a ring-design demonstrating 100% effectiveness.[20,21] The Bill & Melinda Gates Foundation engaged numerous stakeholders, including Berry Consultants, to design an optimal clinical trial to efficiently answer questions of effectiveness of interventions. The proposed design for the trial was an adaptive platform design employing multiple agents and combinations.[22] The design permitted adding or dropping interventions arms according to interim examinations of the accumulating evidence. The trial recommends a response-adaptive randomization procedure. The study was approved by U.S. and Sierra Leone ethics committees, and reviewed by the U.S. FDA. In addition, data management, drug supplies, and local sites were prepared. However, because the ebola epidemic declined dramatically in incidence by the time the trial was designed, the trial was never initiated, although it remains ready if such an epidemic occurs again. This is, to our knowledge, the first example of a platform trial in a low-resourced environment.

The research agenda in global health (and specifically in clinical trials) has historically been uncoordinated.[23,24] For example, in 2012, a survey of all randomized trials for major neglected tropical diseases found 971 eligible randomised trials. The majority of studies were funded by NGOs and non-profit entities (hence possibly the neglected element). Either a single trial or trials with fewer than 100 participants comprised the randomized evidence for first or second line treatments for Buruli ulcer, human African trypanosomiasis, American trypanosomiasis, cysticercosis, rabies, echinococcosis, New World cutaneous leishmaniasis, and each of the foodborne trematode infections. Relative to its global burden of disease, lymphatic filariasis had the fewest trials and participants.[25] These findings make it challenging for health workers to interpret the evidence and make strong clinical recommendations. In all of these investigated neglected diseases, head-to-head comparisons were rare and trials funded by the pharmaceutical industry were sparse. The HIV community in 2007, recognized the need for a research agenda that established a coordinated approach to conducting trials in developing settings and called for the Sydney Declaration, a statement demanding that 10% of HIV/AIDS funding should be allocated to research; a demand that mostly landed on deaf ears.[26]

Creating a Functional Research Environment

Creating a research environment that meets the needs of the local medical communities requires five key elements: 1) Consultation with the local health staff about abilities and interest in clinical trials; 2) Interventions for research topics that are both available and of need in the local communities; 3) Funding for clinical trials that can provide definitive answers; 4) Human resource capacity to conduct high-quality trials; and 5) Dissemination of study findings back to the community to ensure the community is engaged and responsive to study findings. Box 9.1 elaborates on these key agenda setting elements.

Education in clinical trials is clearly a necessity for building future clinical trials. A 2017 survey of investigators working in low-income settings identified that local worker education on clinical trials was among the top concerns for agenda settings.[24] Efforts to build capacity for clinical trials have been led by organizations such as the Cochrane Collaboration or individuals and universities.[27,28] Clinical trial capacity building is frequently provided as short workshops by visiting investigators. A longer-term education on clinical research may involve students from low-income settings taking time out from their careers to reside in a wealthier environment for formal education that typically relies on a scholarship. These educational opportunities usually require the individual to spend a number of years away from their employment or family and often remove physicians from their clinical care—further contributing to inadequate health infrastructure. An irony of this form of education is that it is rarely provided to the lower cadres of health workers, those who actually conduct the day-to-day tasks of running medical research projects.[29,30] The clinical research community should be cautious about contributing to the brain drain of health workers by encouraging education afield. Efforts are needed to build capacity locally and to address long term local leadership.

BOX 9.1	
Key Components of Functional Global Health Trial Environments	
Component	**What to do?**
Consultation with the local health staff and the community about abilities and interest in clinical trials	The local community should be engaged and self-interested in assessing whether interventions can improve their health.[36] An absence of local buy-in from leaders can create tensions between the community and clinical trialists.[37]
Interventions for research topics that are both available and of need in the local communities	Interventions should be available to the local community upon convincing evidence from the clinical trial. The diseases researched should be of relevance to the community recruited for participation.[37]
Funding for clinical trials that can provide definitive answers	Funding is rarely available from host governments. Funding from wealthier settings should fund trials that are well designed and large enough to provide convincing evidence.
Cost-saving	The design of trials and the interventions evaluated should be considered when determining whether interventions are likely to be available post-trial.
Human resource capacity to conduct high-quality trials	Education and employment of staff is important to ensure that the trials are conducted correctly and that staff remain for future clinical trials that may be locally led or partnered.[36] A recent survey of African scientists found education of research staff was a chief concern, with a specific target of statistical expertise.[24]
Dissemination of study findings back to the community to ensure the community is engaged and responsive to study findings	Study findings should be provided to the local community representatives or community to ensure the population is aware of the study findings and the potential importance of the findings. This can lead to future engagement and update of findings.[38]

Of course, the paucity of clinical trials in most low resource settings also creates opportunities. Unlike more developed settings where research infrastructure has developed over decades, there is an opportunity to focus on innovative approaches to the conduct of clinical trials and do away with arduous elements of trial settings and infrastructure.[31] Bureaucratic elements of clinical trials are well established and include multiple differing ethics reviews, a one-size fits all approach to evaluating low risk interventions similarly as high-risk, excessive monitoring of drug safety,

---

BOX 9.2

Key Components of Highly Efficient Clinical Trials Infrastructure

Have staff been trained and planned for retention?	Building necessary human resource infrastructure for innovating clinical trial designs requires a knowledge of advanced statistical issues (often Bayesian) as well as trial methodology, all in the context of clinical questions. Staff that develop these skills should be retained for future trials to ensure the development of both local clinical trial infrastructure and leadership, but also the likelihood of increased funding and successful completion of trials
Is the clinical question of importance to the intended trial community?	Clinical questions should address topics of importance to the community where the trial is being undertaken. Questions should not be so nuanced that future trials are unlikely.
Have the investigators made efforts to compare and justify candidate designs?	Trial investigators considering a trial design are faced with a multitude of possible designs and adaptations (multiple allocation ratio adaptation schemes, criteria for dropping inferior/non-superior arms, sample size re-estimation, etc.). Investigators should demonstrate computer simulations that justify their choice of design.
Have the investigators planned *a priori* plan for changes in trial design?	Trials should pre-plan interim evaluations of accumulating evidence. Decisions about changes in design or analytics should be planned in advance or justified.
Have efforts been made to minimize costs associated with the trials?	Costs of clinical trials can be unwieldy if they are not closely monitored. Efforts to minimize the number of participants in a trial and the retention of staff should result in favorable cost savings.

---

and viable and outdated good clinical practice (GCP) guidelines.[31] Many low-resourced environments have the unique opportunity to develop clinical trial infrastructure by examining the higher functioning elements of more developed settings and rejecting arduous elements. This leap-frogging of clinical trial capacity can also be reflected in the clinical trial design. The adoption and development of education of elements of adaptive clinical trials and platform clinical trials is both cost-saving and advantageous to the local communities. We refer to the new archetype of clinical trials as *Highly Efficient Clinical Trials (HECT)* and it encompasses many elements of platform trials that assist in developing local infrastructure to arrive at strong inferences about interventions that can reduce suffering among populations in need. Box 9.2 illustrates key concepts of HECT infrastructure.

The Role of Highly Efficient Clinical Trials (HECT) and Perpetual Designs in Global Health

The proposed concept for highly efficient clinical trials in global health should be of no surprise to trialists working within the pharmaceutical industry, but would be a profound change from how trials are done within the predominantly academic-led field of global health. Key concepts of thinking beyond individual clinical questions are rare within global health and planning for long-term multiple trials would be relatively unheard of. Platform clinical trials address the majority of the issues we highlight as implicit to highly efficient clinical trials as they aim to build capacity, evaluate multiple interventions, are responsive to necessary changes, and plan for long-term answering of clinical questions. We use the term "perpetual platform trials" when thinking about optimal trial designs in global health, as trials that are planned for the long term can become increasingly more efficient over time. Our proposal for perpetual clinical trials represents a radical departure from traditional RCTs. However, it has the potential to build sustained infrastructure in low resourced environments, reduce human resource challenges and costs, and more efficiently partner with the local communities. Perpetual clinical trials are an opportunity to answer multiple questions of multiple interventions in the most efficient way we can imagine. Their uptake may be hindered by a lack of understanding of adaptive trial designs and local needs within the greater clinical trial community, as well as vested institutional interests. Building on successful examples of perpetual trials will allow educational opportunities and an openness by funders for innovative approaches to important clinical research questions.

Our suggestion that staff be adequately trained is focusing on the day-to-day conduct of staff involved with participant recruitment and interactions during clinical visits. Outside of South Africa, for example, (to our knowledge) there are no Clinical Research Associate (CRA) certifications available in Africa. Non-disruptive human resource utilization is key in facilitating perpetual trials. Investing in training staff is typically resource-intensive and takes staff outside of their usual routines (e.g., a clinical nurse). Many clinical trials hire select staff for the duration of the trial only to let them go after trial completion. For many, this results in unemployment and likely some reticence to participate in future clinical trials. Similarly, for trialists initiating a new trial, recruiting experienced staff is challenging and may delay the trial start date. If our long-term goal is to build local capacity for clinical research, then planning the long-term employment of staff is necessary. Perpetual trials encourage the retention and capacity building, thus avoiding common human resource challenges.

Access to relevant trial populations and their ongoing ownership and involvement of trial conduct is an equally important aspect. Perpetual clinical trials allow for the long-term involvement of the community and discourse with the community on the planning of future clinical trials. Examples of community involvement in clinical trials extend beyond recruitment of patients to networking with populations to introduce research teams to the patients and households and encouraging retention and patient follow-up. Key community members represent important knowledge translation agents of the trial conduct and study findings for the affected populations. Long-term trust can encourage patient enrollment, retention, and involvement of study findings dissemination.

Of course, clinical trials in the global context require oversight to ensure ethical conduct and quality infrastructure. Perpetual designs allow ongoing discussion with institutional bodies (e.g., ethics review boards), to permit dialogue for changes in the conduct or evaluation of trials. An example of institutional readiness is the perpetual platform efforts being piloted in Rwanda whereby investigators run mock institutional ethics submissions to address new designs, interventions, or harm outcomes, in an effort to achieve institutional approval within 72 hours. Rwanda has recently made a step to approve 10 hospital trial sites for conducting clinical research that meets the needs of the population. This will inevitably require establishing a regulatory framework to guide trial activities and building capacity to conduct clinical trials, primarily by educating healthcare professionals and identifying gaps in hospital infrastructure that are barriers to conducting clinical trials.

Highly efficient clinical trials can cover a wide spectrum of designs. Even for one particular category of designs, say platform trials, there are several possible modifications. Trial investigators considering any design are faced with a multitude of possible designs and adaptations (multiple allocation ratio adaptation schemes, criteria for dropping inferior/non-superior arms, sample size re-estimation, etc.). Unlike more traditional clinical trials that often only require an approximate sample size to elucidate the likelihood of trial success, or statistically, the risk of false positive or false negative finding, such measures are not immediately known for platform designs. Likewise, the likely gains (e.g., reduction in expected overall sample size) of conducting a platform trial versus a conventional trial are also not readily known. These properties nonetheless can be reasonably obtained with statistical simulations, and it is convention in adaptive trial planning to run several iterations of such simulations. This concept is foreign to the academic and global health arenas and will require both the support of clinical trial advocacy agents (e.g., Cochrane Collaboration, All trials, CONSORT) as well as concerted educational efforts to sensitize investigators to the techniques and benefits/risks of computer simulations.

Many trialists in global health will be unfamiliar with the concept of making changes to a trial design once the trial has begun. As with most adaptive trials, HECT and platform trials should be clear about what decisions exist for making changes during the conduct of the trial. Interim examinations of the accumulating data are the most likely strategy for informing a change. Having such a plan available typically also casts light on treatment or safety signals that may not be reported as final analyses (e.g., a treatment arm stopped for lack of efficacy may inform that this treatment should not be prioritized in clinical practice). It is important to assess whether the trial investigators followed the plan that was laid out a priori. While post-hoc changes are sometimes necessary due to unexpectedly pronounced signals (e.g., excessive harm), HECT are like other trial designs susceptible to bias from unplanned design modifications. For legitimacy of the trials going forward, it is important to assess how such adaptations may have influenced the ability of the trial to detect or refute clinically meaningful treatment effects.

Being considerate of the elements to improve efficiency of a clinical trial should result in cost savings of the trial. In the simplest form, reducing the number of participants required for a trial should decrease the overall cost of a trial or free up resources for further evaluations within a trial. Within the global health sphere, most clinical trials are insufficiently funded. A major inadequacy of clinical trials in resource-limited settings is that the funding is frequently managed by institutions in wealthier countries that take larger overheads than is typically permitted in the actual trial site countries. As a result, funds at the trial sites are typically stretched to employ as many staff as possible and enroll as many participants as possible. Applying HECT approaches to trials can save money, resources, and lives.

A recent high-profile clinical trial examining synbiotics for the prevention of sepsis among children in rural India illustrates potential time and cost savings well.[32] Here, the required sample size to demonstrate a 20% relative risk reduction assuming an 8% control risk with 80% power and 5% maximum type I error was 8,442 patients. The trial applied O'Brien-Fleming group sequential stopping boundaries (for superiority) with interim looks once per year (corresponding to over 1,000 patients enrolled per interim analysis).[33] Given a large observed relative risk reduction of 40% and control risk slightly larger than originally assumed (9%), the data safety monitoring board called for the trial to be terminated after the fourth interim analysis and 4,456 patients enrolled. While this signifies a substantial reduction in the required sample size, it is possible that the trial could have been stopped even earlier, thus reducing the number of participants exposed to the control and also costs associated with continuing the trial. Figure 9.1 illustrates a simple simulation with 1,000 replications of the trial applying O'Brien-Fleming group sequential stopping boundaries with equally spaced interim looks every 10% of the required sample size, which is more frequent than the yearly interim looks. In this simulation, about 1/3 of simulations has crossed the O'Brien-Fleming

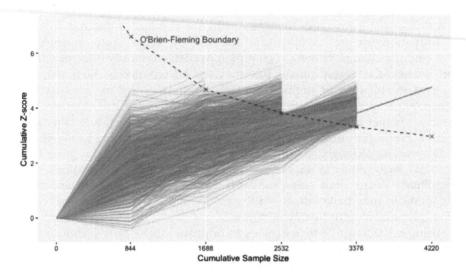

FIGURE 9.1
Distribution of 1,000 simulated Z-curves from Panigrahi, et al. synbiotic trial with two-sided 5%-alpha O'Brien-Fleming stopping,

stopping boundary after 2,582 patients enrolled, and all (except for 1/1,000) had crossed the boundary by 3,376 patients enrolled. This illustrates how multiple frequent looks at the data, particularly at the beginning of a global health trial, can be essential for trial success. While the trial by Panigrahi, et al. opted for conventional frequentist stopping rules, surely some adaptive design elements would have allowed for further optimization of the trial. The promising findings of the trial Panigrahi, et al. has stirred up controversy in the field of sepsis research and a platform trial applying HECT issues is now being planned.

Trials in resource-limited settings are both resource-intensive and lengthy. Applying HECT approaches to even complicated designs, such as cluster trials, can reduce costs, realize findings early, and permit the evaluation of novel interventions. Cluster trials can lend themselves well to HECT and platform designs. For example, in a published cluster randomized multi-arm trial enrolled 8,246 and 5,551 pregnant women in villages of rural Kenya and rural Bangladesh, respectively.[34,35] Clusters were randomized to either control (data collection only) or one of six WASH interventions: chlorinated water (water); upgraded sanitation (sanitation); promotion of hand washing with soap (hand washing); combined water, sanitation, and hand washing; counseling of appropriate child nutrition plus lipid-based nutrient supplement (nutrition); combined water, sanitation, hand washing, and nutrition. The randomization ratio was 2:1:1:1:1:1:1. The primary outcomes were prevalence of care-giver reported diarrhea in the past 7 days among children in utero or younger than 3 years at enrollment, and two year change in height-for-age Z-score (HAZ) among children born to enrolled pregnant women. In both Kenya and Bangladesh, the two intervention groups including nutrition significantly improved mean HAZ. All interventions including one or more WASH components significantly reduced diarrhea rates by 30–40% in Bangladesh, but no significant effects were observed in Kenya.

This trial represents a common trial scenario in global health, where a multitude of interventions and their potential combinations are of interest. Certainly, narrowing in on the final six active interventions during planning of this trial was no easy task. Although it is important to remember that the respective efficacies of the investigated interventions were unknown at the onset of the trial, substantial efficiencies could have been gained via use of a platform design. First, the assumed prevalence of diarrhea for the sample size calculations was 10%, whereas the realized prevalence was 27.1% in Kenya, and 5.7% in Bangladesh.[34,35] An early realization of this could have helped adapt the design, as power would be larger than expected in Kenya to either detect superiority or futility with approximately half of the originally estimated required sample size. In Bangladesh where diarrhea data was available from a total of 14,425 children (almost three eligible children per mother over the follow-up period of 2 years), the effects of any intervention versus control would also have been statistically apparent earlier than reaching the full sample size. Second, had a platform design with interim analysis on HAZ been incorporated, the four treatment arms that did not include a nutrition component would have been dropped for inferiority. For example, using a criterion of the posterior probability of superiority being less than 1% to drop an experimental treatment arm, the number of patients and clusters randomised to the non-nutrition arms could have been reduced by approximately 30–60%. Figure 9.2 illustrates a single simulation using the observed HAZ effects (and standard deviations) for each arm from the publications. In the simulation, water (alone) was dropped for inferiority after only 100 patients have been enrolled to each experimental arm (and 800 in total for the trial), sanitation (alone) and WASH were dropped after 200 patients had been enrolled to each arm (at a total of 1,500 patients), and hygiene alone was dropped after 300 patients (corresponding to a total of 2,000 patients). In 1,000 simulations of this trial based on the published effects, similarly allowing arms to be dropped by inferiority, over 96% of simulations enrolled a total of 2,000 to 3,000 patients, and the remaining 4% of simulations enrolled between 3,000 and 3,500 patients. Thus, rather than enrolling 5,551 pregnant women, the trial could have reached the same conclusion about comparative efficacy with respect to HAZ with 2,000 to 3,000 less participants. In addition, the trial could have allocated relatively more patients to the nutrition

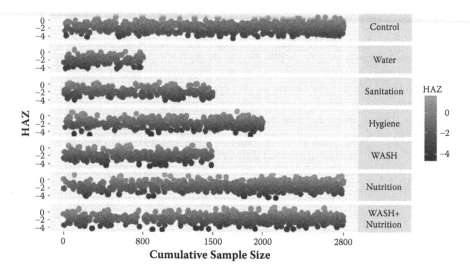

FIGURE 9.2
Illustrates an example of a simulated WASH-B trial, using the HAZ effect observed in the trial, where treatments are dropped for inferiority if the probability of being superior is less than 1%.

based interventions when non-nutrition arms were dropped and thereby reached a firm conclusion faster in addition to substantially reducing the number of patients.

These potential saving represent a large amount of funds that could have been allocated to other important research questions. With the above approximate estimates, it stands to reason that a platform trial incorporating well-established stopping rules for superiority and inferiority could have reduced the total cost by roughly one-third. As well, the time to completion could have been shortened importantly. This trial represents only one of many trials investigating interventions for preventing diarrhea and stunting. Several other promising "intervention bundles" have yet to be examined in large well-designed randomized trials. As such trials emerge, several costs and resources could likewise be saved by utilizing platform designs rather than non-adaptive multi-arm designs, or even less efficient, multiple two-arm trials. It is common in global health trials that investigators' guesstimates of baseline risks are highly inaccurate. In this trial, the estimated 10% risk of diarrhea in the control group was inaccurate. In reality, the observed risk was close to half of the guesstimate in Bangladesh and close to triple the guesstimate in Kenya. Sample size readjustment would have importantly changed both the sample enrolled and the costs associated with completing the trial.

Conclusion

Highly efficient clinical trials represent a radical departure from traditional RCTs in the global health context. Platform trials employing HECT efforts have the potential to build sustained infrastructure in low resourced environments, reduce human resource challenges and costs, answer questions quickly and reliably, and more efficiently partner with the local communities. Highly efficient platform trials are an opportunity to answer multiple questions of multiple interventions in the most efficient way we can imagine. Their uptake may be hindered by a lack of understanding of innovative trial designs and local needs within the greater clinical trial community, as well as vested institutional interests. Building on successful examples of highly efficient platform trials will allow educational opportunities and an openness by funders for innovative approaches to important clinical research questions of great global importance.

Acknowledgements

This work was supported by the Bill & Melinda Gates Foundation. The article contents are the sole responsibility of the authors and may not necessarily represent the official views of the Bill & Melinda Gates Foundation or other agencies that may have supported the primary data studies used in the present study.

References

1. GBD 2016 Disease and Injury Incidence and Prevalence Collaborators. Global, regional, and national incidence, prevalence, and years lived with disability for 328 diseases and injuries for 195 countries, 1990–2016: A systematic analysis for the Global Burden of Disease Study 2016. *Lancet* 2017; 390(10100): 1211–59.
2. GBD Mortality Collaborators. Global, regional, and national under-5 mortality, adult mortality, age-specific mortality, and life expectancy, 1970–2016: A systematic analysis for the Global Burden of Disease Study 2016. *Lancet* 2017; 390 (10100): 1084–50.
3. Ford N, Calmy A, Mills EJ. The first decade of antiretroviral therapy in Africa. *Globalization and Health* 2011; 7: 33.
4. Oxman AD, Bjorndal A, Becerra-Posada F, et al. A framework for mandatory impact evaluation to ensure well informed public policy decisions. *Lancet (London, England)* 2010; 375(9712): 427–31.
5. Isaakidis P, Swingler GH, Pienaar E, Volmink J, Ioannidis JP. Relation between burden of disease and randomised evidence in sub-Saharan Africa: Survey of research. *BMJ* 2002; 324(7339): 702.

6. Grinsztejn B, Hosseinipour MC, Ribaudo HJ, et al. Effects of early versus delayed initiation of antiretroviral treatment on clinical outcomes of HIV-1 infection: Results from the phase 3 HPTN 052 randomised controlled trial. *Lancet Infect Dis* 2014; 14(4): 281–90.

7. Oluwole D, Kraemer J. Innovative public-private partnership: a diagonal approach to combating women's cancers in Africa. *Bull World Health Organ* 2013; 91(9): 691–6.

8. Ford N, Singh K, Cooke GS, et al. Expanding access to treatment for hepatitis C in resource-limited settings: Lessons from HIV/AIDS. *Clin Infect Dis* 2012; 54 (10): 1465–72.

9. Mills EJ, Ford N. Political lessons from the global HIV/AIDS response to inform a rapid noncommunicable disease response. *AIDS (London, England)* 2012; 26(9): 1171–3.

10. Evans JA, Shim JM, Ioannidis JP. Attention to local health burden and the global disparity of health research. *PLoS One* 2014; 9(4): e90147.

11. Cohen ER, O'Neill JM, Joffres M, Upshur RE, Mills E. Reporting of informed consent, standard of care and post-trial obligations in global randomized intervention trials: A systematic survey of registered trials. *Dev World Bioeth* 2009; 9(2): 74–80.

12. Allanson ER, Tuncalp O, Vogel JP, et al. Implementation of effective practices in health facilities: A systematic review of cluster randomised trials. *BMJ Glob Health* 2017; 2(2): e000266.

13. Althabe F, Belizan JM, McClure EM, et al. A population-based, multifaceted strategy to implement antenatal corticosteroid treatment versus standard care for the reduction of neonatal mortality due to preterm birth in low-income and middle-income countries: The ACT cluster-randomised trial. *Lancet* 2015; 385 (9968): 629–39.

14. Kanters S. Evaluating Ebola interventions: Adaptive designs should be commonplace. *Lancet Glob Health Blog Lancet* October 10, 2014. http://globalhealth. thelancet.com/2014/10/10/evaluating-ebola-interventions-adaptive-designs-should-be-commonplace

15. Lanini S, Zumla A, Ioannidis JP, et al. Are adaptive randomised trials or non-randomised studies the best way to address the Ebola outbreak in west Africa? *Lancet Infect Dis* 2015; 15(6): 738–45.

16. Kanters S, Thorlund K, Mills EJ. Ethical testing of experimental Ebola treatments. *JAMA* 2015; 313(4): 421–2.

17. Fink S. Pattern of safety lapses where group worked to battle ebola outbreak. *The New York Times*, April 12, 2015. www.nytimes.com/2015/04/13/world/africa/pattern-of-safety-lapses-where-group-worked-to-battle-ebola-outbreak. html.

18. National Academies of Sciences Engineering, and Medicine. *Integrating Clinical Research into Epidemic Response: The Ebola Experience*. Washington, DC: The National Academies Press; 2017.

19. Rojek A, Horby P, Dunning J. Insights from clinical research completed during the West Africa Ebola virus disease epidemic. *Lancet Infect Dis* 2017; 17(9): e280–92.

20. Hossmann S, Haynes AG, Spoerri A, et al. Data management of clinical trials during an outbreak of Ebola virus disease. *Vaccine* 2017. doi:10.1016/j. vaccine.2017.09.094.

21. Henao-Restrepo AM, Camacho A, Longini IM, et al. Efficacy and effectiveness of an rVSV-vectored vaccine in preventing Ebola virus disease: Final results from the Guinea ring vaccination, open-label, cluster-randomised trial (Ebola Ca Suffit!). *Lancet* 2017; 389(10068): 505–18.

22. Berry SM, Petzold EA, Dull P, et al. A response adaptive randomization platform trial for efficient evaluation of Ebola virus treatments: a model for pandemic response. *Clin Trials* 2016; 13(1): 22–30.

23. Siegfried N, Volmink J, Dhansay A. Does South Africa need a national clinical trials support unit? *SAMJ S Afr Med J* 2010; 100(8): 521–4.

24. Rosala-Hallas A, Bhangu A, Blazeby J, et al. Global health trials methodological research agenda: Results from a priority setting exercise. *Trials* 2018; 19(1): 48.

25. Kappagoda S, Ioannidis JP. Neglected tropical diseases: Survey and geometry of randomised evidence. *BMJ* 2012; 345: e6512.

26. Cooper D, Cahn P, Lewin S, et al. The Sydney declaration: A call to scale up research. *Lancet* 2007; 370(9581): 7–8.

27. Machekano R, Young T, Rusakaniko S, et al. The Africa Center for Biostatistical Excellence: A proposal for enhancing biostatistics capacity for sub-Saharan Africa. *Stat Med* 2015; 34(27): 3481–9.

28. McGregor S, Henderson KJ, Kaldor JM. Capacity building in longitudinal HIV research. *Lancet Glob Health* 2015; 3(1): e18–19.

29. Mbuagbaw L, Thabane L, Ongolo-Zogo P. Training Cameroonian researchers on pragmatic knowledge translation trials: A workshop report. *Pan Afr Med J* 2014; 19: 190.

30. Scheffler RM, Campbell J, Cometto G, et al. Forecasting imbalances in the global health labor market and devising policy responses. *Hum Resour Health* 2018; 16 (1): 5.

31. Reith C, Landray M, Devereaux PJ, et al. Randomized clinical trials—Removing unnecessary obstacles. *N Engl J Med* 2013; 369(11): 1061–5.

32. Panigrahi P, Parida S, Nanda NC, et al. A randomized synbiotic trial to prevent sepsis among infants in rural India. *Nature* 2017; 548(7668): 407–12.

33. O'Brien PC, Fleming TR. A multiple testing procedure for clinical trials. *Biometrics* 1979; 35(3): 549–56.

34. Luby SP, Rahman M, Arnold BF, et al. Effects of water quality, sanitation, handwashing, and nutritional interventions on diarrhoea and child growth in rural Bangladesh: A cluster randomised controlled trial. *Lancet Glob Health* 2018; 6(3): e302–15.

35. Null C, Stewart CP, Pickering AJ, et al. Effects of water quality, sanitation, handwashing, and nutritional interventions on diarrhoea and child growth in rural Kenya: A cluster-randomised controlled trial. *Lancet Glob Health* 2018; 6(3): e316–29.

36. Rwandan Research and Implementation Writing Group. Building health research infrastructure in Rwanda. *Lancet Glob Health* 2014; 2(1): e9–10.

37. The trials of tenofovir trials. *Lancet* 2005; 365(9465): 1111.

38. Condo J, Kateera B, Mutimura E, et al. Building clinical trial priorities at the University of Rwanda. *Trials* 2014; 15: 467.

10

Decision Analysis from the Perspectives of Single and Multiple Stakeholders

Robert A. Beckman, Carl-Fredrik Burman, Cong Chen,

Sebastian Jobjörnsson, Franz König, Nigel Stallard, and Martin Posch

Decision analysis is a very useful tool that can be used to quantitatively and objectively optimize the benefit from individual conventional trials, individual master protocols, as well as systems of master protocols representing approval pathways (1). When making design choices, this is greatly preferable to relying on subjective impressions, arbitrary rules, or cherished customs of the field. While master protocols can deliver a range of benefits, increased planning and collaboration is needed (2). The ability of model-based decision analysis to facilitate communication (3), by clarifying assumptions, is therefore important.

The most important step in decision analysis is building a quantitative "utility function" by which the net benefit of any proposed strategy is quantitatively assessed. Net benefit takes both benefit and cost or risk into account, and all elements are weighted according to their respective probabilities of occurrence. Decisions are then guided by calculating the expected value of the utility function under different design choices and maximizing it. The utility function also provides a quantitative measure of the advantage of the optimal strategy compared to other possible designs. The development of a utility function requires an interdisciplinary team of drug developers, cancer biologists, and clinical oncologists who provide the qualitative guidance, which is then translated into quantitative terms and analyzed by mathematicians, statisticians, and/or computer scientists. Decision analysis can be utilized to optimize the design of a trial, to govern the adaptation in an adaptive design, to optimize groups or systems of trials, or to optimize decisions which may occur between phases of development. It may be applied to a single drug development program or to portfolios of drugs. We will present several examples of the application of decision analysis to conventional trials with and without biomarker defined subsets, and then discuss possible future applications to master protocols. There is a rich literature of decision analysis and the examples below are not meant to be comprehensive.

For example, Chen and Beckman (4–7) defined a utility function for randomized proof of concept (POC) trials based on a benefit to cost ratio (BCR). Benefit was defined as the expected number of true positive POCs (numerator in Equation 1), and cost was defined as the risk adjusted number of patients utilized in Phase 2 (first term in the denominator of Equation 1) and Phase 3 (second and third terms in the denominator of Equation 1), assuming that a Phase 3 trial was performed for every positive Phase 2 POC study (both true and false positives). A simplified version of the BCR is represented in Equation 1 where p represents the estimated probability that the therapy is effective in the true state of nature, and λ is the ratio of the patient numbers of Phase 2 to Phase 3 when both are designed with the same Type I (α) and Type II (β) errors, where Phase 2 usually involves a smaller sample size because it uses a more sensitive short-term (surrogate) endpoint. In order to evaluate the BCR for a portfolio of POC studies, one simply sums their expected benefits in the numerator and their risk adjusted costs (including downstream Phase 3 costs) in the denominator.

$$Benefit/cost\ ratio = \frac{p(1-\beta)}{\lambda + p(1-\beta) + (1-p)\alpha} \tag{1}$$

In the presence of a fixed POC budget which was insufficient to fund testing of all worthy POC hypotheses (a very common situation), this simple function was used to investigate the optimal size for individual POC trials and groups of POC trials performed in parallel. Surprisingly, it was discovered that smaller POC trials than traditional were optimal. The optimal trials had less power (i.e., a higher Type II error, or false negative rate) than the traditional trials, while having a similar Type I error or false positive rate. However, because these trials were smaller it was possible to fund more of them within the limited POC budget. The larger, traditional trials had lower Type II error but more opportunity cost because they were more expensive, causing other POC trials to fall below the funding line. Chen and Beckman later termed this opportunity cost Type III error (8).

A simple worked example is shown in Figures 10.1. Either one large POC trial (Figure 10.1A) with a Type II error of 0.15 (sample size of 120) or two small POC trials (Figure 10.1B) with Type II error of 0.4 (sample size of 60 each) are used to search for POC. Whenever an apparent POC is achieved in either trial, the corresponding Phase 3 trial will be executed with a sample size of 450. The POC hypothesis (involving a pairing of a therapy and a proposed application) is assumed to have a 30% chance of being actually positive and a 70% probability of actually being negative according to the true state of nature. All POC trials are executed with a one-sided Type I error of 0.05. A true positive POC is assigned a benefit one, all other outcomes zero. The figure illustrates the risk-adjusted benefit-cost ratio is higher in the case of two small POC trials conducted in

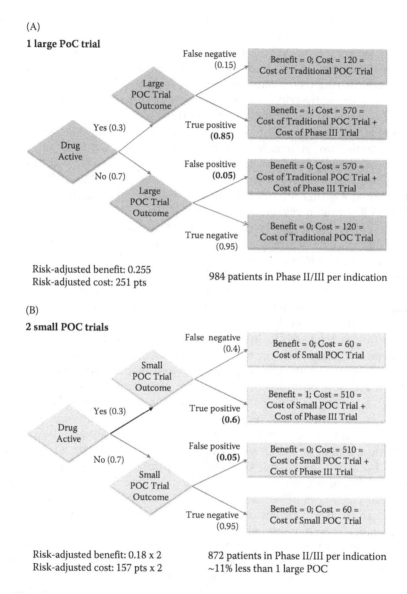

FIGURE 10.1

Illustration of advantage of two small POC trials compared to one traditionally sized POC trial at equivalent total POC cost. Either one large POC trial (Figure 10.1A) with a Type II error of 0.15 (sample size of 120) or two small POC trials (Figure 10.1B) with Type II error of 0.4 (sample size of 60 each) are used to search for POC. Whenever an apparent POC is achieved, a Phase 3 trial will be executed with a sample size of 450. The POC applications are assumed to have a 30% chance of being actually positive and a 70% probability of actually being negative according to the true state of nature. All POC trials are executed with a one-sided Type I error of 0.05. A true positive POC is assigned a benefit one, all other outcomes zero. The figure illustrates the risk adjusted benefit cost ratio is higher in the case of two small POC trials compared to one large POC trial with a lower Type II error. Reproduced from (5) with permission.

parallel compared to one traditional POC trial with a lower Type II error (7). It is straightforward to modify the analysis in case the prior probability, p, of efficacy is varying across candidate drugs. This is a simple but powerful example of where decision analysis altered a widely held and widely taught rule concerning the proper Type II error in a Phase II POC design. An alternative decision theoretic model for optimal sample size in Phase 2 is given by Miller and Burman (9).

The analysis defined optimal sizes for individual POC trials and groups of POC trials run in parallel under a fixed budget, as well as optimal criteria for moving from Phase 2 to Phase 3. Ongoing work is considering optimal sequential arrays of trials, where a smaller set of POC trials is used to determine whether a particular therapy will be subsequently funded for further POC trials in related settings (10,11). In another application, Antonijevic (12) has subsequently discovered that adaptive designs that adjust sample size may have suboptimal performance if the decision rules do not take Type III error into account.

Similar principles may be applied to clinical validation of predictive biomarkers, a key concern of current master protocols in oncology. For example, we can consider the possible results of a randomized Phase 2 POC trial stratified into biomarker positive and negative groups, and the decision about what to do in Phase 3, a problem which will be present whenever one trial hands off to another within any approval pathway. All possible Phase 2 results may be graphed two dimensionally in terms of the apparent efficacy, posterior probability for efficacy, or other efficacy measure in biomarker positive patients on one axis and in biomarker negative patients on the other axis (Figure 10.2) (8). Each of four regions of the graph may lead to a different optimal decision. Qualitatively, if efficacy is not demonstrated in either subgroup, the drug should be discarded. If efficacy is clearly demonstrated in both subgroups, the drug works, but the biomarker is not predictive, and a traditional Phase 3 trial should proceed in the full population. If efficacy is clearly demonstrated in the biomarker positive group only, an enriched Phase 3 trial in the biomarker positive only patients is recommended. Finally, if efficacy is clearly demonstrated in the biomarker positive population and there is an ambiguous positive "trend" in the biomarker negative population, indicating possible (if lesser) efficacy, an adaptive design is recommended in Phase 3 to gain further information. In this case, the question was how to optimally define the borders between regions on this graph, to deal with borderline results. This was accomplished using decision analysis. A team of experts was interviewed to assign quantitative positive or negative utilities to all possible outcomes resulting from any decision. For example, the decision to perform a traditional Phase 3 trial in the full population, if correct, could result in approval in a larger population; but if incorrect, could lead to a negative study in which benefit in the biomarker positive patients is diluted by the a lack of benefit in the biomarker

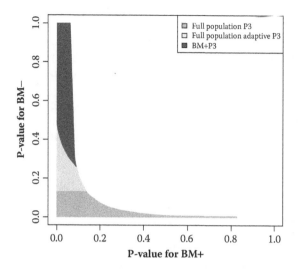

FIGURE 10.2

Two dimensional decision rule for deciding the Phase 3 design after a Phase 2 biomarker stratified POC study, according to a sponsor utility function. The x and y axes represent efficacy observed in the Phase 2 study for biomarker positive and negative subpopulations respectively. In the general case, any measure of efficacy may be used including posterior probabilities of efficacy. In this case, p values are used and therefore efficacy is greatest closer to the origin. The graph is divided into four regions. Near the origin (dark gray), the therapy is effective in both populations, and the optimal choice is to utilize a conventional Phase 3 trial in the full population without biomarker selection. In the upper left-hand corner (black), the therapy is clearly effective in the biomarker positive population but not the biomarker negative population, and the optimal strategy is a Phase 3 trial exclusively in the biomarker positive population. In the upper right hand corner (white), the therapy is ineffective in both populations, and no Phase 3 trial is recommended. In the middle left (light gray), the therapy is effective in the biomarker positive population, and there is lesser efficacy, or possibly an equivocal trend towards efficacy lacking statistical significance, in the biomarker negative population. In this setting, an adaptive Phase 3 study considering both full population and biomarker positive subpopulations in some fashion is recommended. Reproduced from (8) with permission.

negative patients. For each point in the graph, the corresponding Phase 2 data gave an estimate of the probability of different outcomes for each of the different decisions. The graph was then drawn in a way which maximized the overall expected utility subject to control of Type I error at a prespecified level (8).

The adaptive Phase 3 design in this example was a Phase 3 study in the full population, but where the Type I error permitted in Phase 3 was apportioned between the biomarker positive subgroup and the full population in a way that maximized the expected power of the study (a simple utility function), using data internal to the study as well as maturing data from the previous Phase 2 studies, according to pre-specified rules. This "adaptive alpha allocation" in effect prioritized the biomarker positive subgroup in proportion to the quality of the evidence supporting the predictive biomarker to that point (13). For confirmatory clinical trials involving predictive biomarkers, Bayesian decision theoretic methods have been proposed by several authors to optimize trial design and statistical testing procedures (13–17).

The above examples optimized utility functions from the perspective of the drug developer, a pharmaceutical or biotechnology company, assuming that the perspectives were generally aligned with the public health perspective, in that both of these stakeholders would prefer an efficient way to identify "true positives," or therapies that work. Antonijevic and Wang discuss in this volume the question of how a pharmaceutical sponsor can optimally design Phase 3 programs while taking into account the need to satisfy the requirements of two different stakeholders: national health authorities and payers (18).

Posch and colleagues have utilized decision analysis to optimize single Phase 3 study designs involving predictive biomarkers from the varying perspectives of a pharmaceutical sponsor, and from a public health perspective, with interesting results (19–21). For example, the net utility of studying a low prevalence biomarker positive subgroup was found to be negative in the public health perspective, and only weakly positive in the pharmaceutical perspective, and in the latter would still not be incentivized for development because more productive investments could be made in higher prevalence markets (this can change in cases where a very large benefit is anticipated in the small subgroup, but it is a matter of debate how common such cases will be). This finding exemplifies the need for master protocols. By combining many small indications with a common biomarker together in a single basket trial, for example, it is likely that efficiencies can be gained for these low prevalence biomarkers that would render development of the corresponding drugs cost effective from both the pharmaceutical and public health perspective. This is critical given the increasingly small molecular subsets which are being defined.

This work featured two subtle but important distinctions between the utility functions for the sponsor and public health perspectives. For the sponsor, the benefit was determined by the observed level of efficacy in the pivotal clinical trial, whereas from the public health perspective what mattered was the actual true level of efficacy, not the estimate. Further, the true net benefit for an individual patient (efficacy–toxicity) could be negative in the public health perspective, resulting in harm from a marketed product. For the sponsor, the price was assumed proportional to the estimated net benefit for an individual patient, but the drug would not be marketed if this quantity was negative, meaning a negative actual benefit was primarily a public health risk unless this negative actual benefit was detected (20). For both these reasons, a precise estimate of the true efficacy benefits the public health perspective more than the sponsor perspective. Indeed, these authors found that the public health perspective consistently recommended a larger Phase 3 sample size at optimum than the sponsor perspective (Figure 10.3) (20, 21).

Furthermore, in the context of an adaptive two stage Phase 3 study, where the second stage can be run in the full population, a fully enriched biomarker positive population, or a partially enriched biomarker positive population depending on the stage one results, the fully enriched biomarker positive population is less likely to be optimal for the sponsor. This is because the biomarker negative patients in the Phase 3 trial will potentially lead to a larger market for the sponsor even if they don't truly benefit (Figure 10.4) (21).

Master protocols represent an efficient way to generate precise efficacy data simultaneously for a variety of related therapies in multiple subgroups. Moreover, post-approval observational studies, possibly as parts of a linked system of master protocols (1), if coupled to adjustments in price based on the findings, might align the incentives affecting different stakeholders more closely.

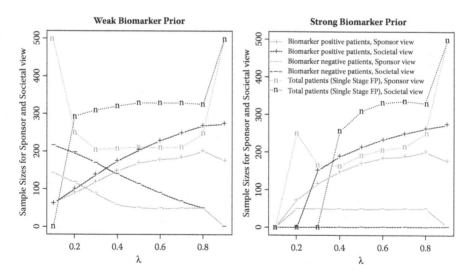

FIGURE 10.3

Recommended optimal sample size for a single stage biomarker stratified Phase 3 study using utility functions from the sponsor and societal (public health) perspectives, assuming the biomarker is weakly or strongly predictive of efficacy, for various values of the biomarker prevalence λ. The sponsor consistently prefers a smaller sample size than is optimal from a societal perspective, with the exception of the number of biomarker negative patients that are optimal in the case of a strongly predictive biomarker, where the public health perspective but not the sponsor perspective recommends a study in biomarker positive patients only. Reproduced from (14) with permission.

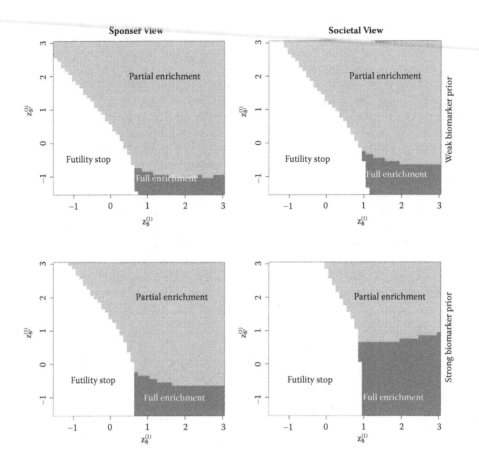

FIGURE 10.4

Two-dimensional decision rule for stage 2 of an adaptive Phase 3 study as a function of efficacy in the biomarker positive population S (*x* axis) and in the biomarker negative subpopulation S′ (*y* axis), from both sponsor and societal (public health) perspectives and in the case of strongly and weakly predictive priors about the biomarker hypothesis. Three options are available: stop for futility (white), proceed in the biomarker positive patients only (full enrichment, red), or proceed in the full population with some degree of enrichment of biomarker positive patients (partial enrichment, gray). Compared to the sponsor perspective, the public health perspective is more likely to be optimized with a full enrichment strategy if supported by evidence from stage 1 of the design. Reproduced from (14) with permission.

Decision analysis could also in principle be used to quantify the utility advantage of master protocols compared to individual trials. In order to quantify the benefits of master protocols, let's look at them in the context of a portfolio. A basket trial is a portfolio of indications with a common treatment and biomarker, while an umbrella trial is a portfolio of treatments and associated biomarkers in one broader indication. As we have seen in the context of POC trials, it may be more cost-effective to test more hypotheses within the portfolio if they are of approximately equal merit. One must consider the Type III error, or missed opportunity from not investing in trials (or arms of a master protocol) that might have identified good indications/treatments. It is possible, although still not investigated, that similar principles may apply to Phase 3 approval studies and to master protocols in both the Phase 2 and Phase 3 settings.

Let us now consider the comparison between master protocols and individual trials as development options. Proceeding with one individual trial is an extreme case of focusing on the minimum number of indications/treatments with maximum sample size. By investigating more possibilities within a portfolio, there is at least the potential that a master protocol may be more optimal.

Basket trials can result in a considerable efficiency gain from pooling indications (22). Basket trials also have a characteristic that overall pharmaceutical portfolios do not have, which is a potentially strong correlation among components, given that the same treatment is applied to all indications, which also share a common molecular characteristic. This correlation allows for "borrowing" of information among components, which results in a more efficient design, even in the absence of pooling. One way to account for this correlation is described in (23,24). In umbrella trials, additional savings may often be realized from using a common control arm (25) while each of a portfolio of individual trials would need their own control. In the light of recent data transparency initiatives (26,27) decision theoretic tools will provide an excellent tool to evaluate the role of historical data in drug development, e.g., by comparing single-arm threshold designs (28) to parallel group randomized controlled as pivotal trials.

Some platform trials, as I-SPY2 (29), involve several drugs which may be included and leave the trial at different points in time. Such innovations raise the question of whether previous control arm data can be borrowed to increase power. Decision analytic approaches may prove useful to optimize operating characteristics, as well as trading power vs. potential bias.

In quantifying these benefits of master protocols compared to individual trials, one would again need to define utility functions, perhaps from both the sponsor and the public health perspectives. From the sponsor perspective, optimization may be based on financial measures, whereas from the patient perspective optimization may involve the numbers of patients who benefit, the degree of benefit in terms of quantity and quality of life, and in some cases such factors as disease severity and the degree to which the medication is differentiated from other available options. While these incentives are generally aligned, we have seen exceptions using decision analysis. Systems of master protocols combined with post approval observational studies (1) may not only improve absolute benefit but also alignment between stakeholders. Finally, we note that decision analysis is also applicable for individual trial patients (30) and individual patients in clinical practice (31).

References

1. Trusheim M, Shrier AA, Antonijevic Z, Beckman RA, Campbell R, Chen C, Flaherty K, Loewy J, Lacombe D, Madhavan S, Selker H, and Esserman L. PIPELINEs: Creating comparable clinical knowledge efficiently by linking trial platforms. *Clinical Pharmacology and Therapeutics*, 100: 713–729 (2016).
2. Woodcock J and LaVange LM. Master protocols to study multiple therapies, multiple diseases, or both. *New England Journal of Medicine*, 377: 62–70 (2017).
3. Burman CF and Wiklund SJ. Modelling and simulation in the pharmaceutical industry – Some reflections. *Pharmaceutical Statistics*, 10: 508–516 (2011).
4. Chen C and Beckman RA. Optimal cost-effective designs of proof of concept trials and associated go-no go decisions, *Proceedings of the American Statistical Association, Biometrics Section*, pp. 394–399 (2007).
5. Chen C and Beckman RA. Optimal cost-effective designs of phase II proof of concept trials and associated Go-No Go decisions. *Journal of Biopharmaceutical Statistics*, 19: 424–436 (2009).
6. Chen C and Beckman RA. Optimal cost-effective Go-No Go decisions in late-stage oncology drug development. *Statistics in Biopharmaceutical Research*, 1: 159–169 (2009).
7. Chen C and Beckman RA. Maximizing return on socioeconomic investment in phase II proof-of-concept trials. *Clinical Cancer Research*, 20: 1730–1734 (2014).
8. Beckman RA, Clark J, and Chen C. Integrating predictive biomarkers and classifiers into oncology clinical development programmes. *Nature Reviews Drug Discovery*, 10: 735–749 (2011).
9. Miller F and Burman CF. A decision theoretic modeling for phase III investments and drug licensing. *Journal of Biopharmaceutical Statistics*, 28(4): 698–721 (2018).
10. Beckman RA and He L. Maximizing the efficiency of proof of concept studies and of arrays of proof of concept studies for multiple drugs or indications. *Proceedings of the Joint Statistical Meetings of the American Statistical Association, Biopharmaceutical Section*, pp. 2815–2838 (2016).
11. Chen C, Deng Q, He L, Mehrotra DV, Rubin EH, and Beckman RA. How many tumor indications should be initially studied in clinical development of next generation immunotherapies? *Contemporary Clinical Trials*, 59: 113–117 (2017).
12. Antonijevic Z. The impact of adaptive design on portfolio optimization. *Therapeutic Innovation and Regulatory Science*, 5: 615–619 (2016).
13. Chen C and Beckman RA. Hypothesis testing in a confirmatory phase III trial with a possible subset effect. *Statistics in Biopharmaceutical Research*, 1: 431–440 (2009).

14. Rosenblum M, Liu H, and Yen EH. Optimal tests of treatment effects for the overall population and two subpopulations in randomized trials, using sparse linear programming. *Journal of the American Statistical Association*, 109: 1216–1228 (2014).
15. Rosenblum M, Fang X, and Liu H. *Optimal, Two Stage, Adaptive Enrichment Designs for Randomized Trials Using Sparse Linear Programming*. Department of Biostatistics, Johns Hopkins University, Working Paper, 2014.
16. Krisam J and Kieser M. Decision rules for subgroup selection based on a predictive biomarker. *Journal of Biopharmaceutical Statistics*, 24: 188–202 (2014).
17. Krisam J and Kieser M. Performance of biomarker-based subgroup selection rules in adaptive enrichment designs. *Statistics in Biosciences*, 8: 8–27 (2015).
18. Antonijevic Z and Wang Z. Optimal approach for addressing multiple stakeholders' requirements in drug development. In *PlatormTrials:Umbrella Trials and Basket Trials*, Antonijevic Z and Beckman RA, eds. CRC Press, Boca Raton, FL, pp. XX–YY (2018).
19. Graf AC, Posch M, and König F. Adaptive designs for subpopulation analysis optimizing utility functions. *Biometrical Journal*, 57: 76–89 (2015).
20. Ondra T, Jobjörnsson S, Beckman RA, Burman CF, König F, Stallard N, and Posch M. Optimizing trial designs for targeted therapies. *PLoS One*, 11: e0163726 (2016).
21. Ondra T, Jobjörnsson S, Beckman RA, Burman CF, König F, Stallard N, and Posch M. Optimized adaptive enrichment designs. *Statistical Methods in Medical Research*, first published online. December 18, (2017),https://doi.org/10.1177/0962280217747312.
22. Beckman RA, Antonijevic Z, Kalamegham R, and Chen C. Adaptive design for a confirmatory basket trial in multiple tumor types based on a putative predictive biomarker. *Clinical Pharmacology and Therapeutics*, 100: 617–625 (2016).
23. Simon R, Geyer S, Subramanian J, and Roychowdhury S. The Bayesian basket design for genomic-variant driven phase II trials. *Seminars in Oncology*, 43: 13–18 (2016).
24. Berry DA. The brave new world of clinical cancer research: Adaptive biomarker-driven trials integrating clinical practice with clinical research. *Molecular Oncology*, 9: 951–959 (2015).
25. Hlavin G, Hampson LV, and Koenig F. Many-to-one comparisons after safety selection in multi-arm clinical trials. *PLoS One*, 12 (6): e0180131. (2017).
26. Bonini S, Eichler HG, Wathion N, and Rasi G. Transparency and the European Medicines Agency – Sharing of clinical trial data. *New England Journal of Medicine*, 371: 2452–2455 (2014).
27. Koenig F, Slattery J, Groves T, Lang T, BenjaminiY, Day S, Bauer P, and Posch M. Sharing clinical trial data on patient level: Opportunities and challenges. *Biometrical Journal*, 57: 8–26 (2015).
28. Eichler H, Bloechl-Daum B, Bauer P, Bretz F, Brown J, Hampson L, Honig P, Krams M, Leufkens H, Lim R, Lumpkin M, Murphy M. Pignatt F, Posch M, Schneeweiss S, Trusheim M, and Koenig F. Threshold-crossing: A useful way to establish the counterfactual in clinical trials? *Clinical Pharmacology & Therapeutics*, 100: 699–712 (2016).

29. Berry SM, Connor JT, and Lewis RJ. The platform trial: An efficient strategy for evaluating multiple treatments. *JAMA*, 313: 1619–1620 (2015).

30. Burman CF and Carlberg A. Future challenges in the design and ethics of clinical trials. In *Clinical Trial Handbook*, Gad SC, ed. Wiley, Hoboken, NJ, pp. 1173–1200 (2009).

31. Parmigiani G. *Modeling in Medical Decision Making: A Bayesian Approach*, Wiley, Hoboken, NJ, (2002).

11

Optimal Approach for Addressing Multiple Stakeholders' Requirements in Drug Development

Zoran Antonijevic and Zhongshen Wang

Introduction

In order to successfully market pharmaceutical products, sponsors need to pass several important hurdles. First and foremost, in order to get marketing approval, they need to pass regulatory requirements by demonstrating that the product is safe and effective. In the current environment, however, getting regulatory approval does not guarantee market success. Another critical factor is securing the payer's agreement to reimburse the product. What payers want to see in addition to safety and efficacy is demonstration of differentiation or value added. This generally requires collection of information beyond what is needed for regulatory approval. This additional information can range from collecting data on several additional endpoints, to conducting additional trials or adding active control arms. Therefore, a level of investment to address payers' expectations varies, but it can be substantial. The previous chapter of this book [1] discusses decision analysis from the perspective of multiple stakeholders. In this chapter we are proposing optimal criteria for addressing multiple stakeholders' requirements.

We are comparing two development approaches to address these requirements, sequential and parallel.

1) In the sequential approach sponsors are focused on addressing regulatory requirements first. Any additional payers' requirements are addressed if and when the regulatory approval is achieved. This approach can result in less than optimal rewards, since the peak will be achieved only after payers' expectations are satisfied.

2) In the parallel approach sponsors are addressing regulatory and payers' requirements simultaneously. This scenario results in much larger revenues due to extended time on the market, but it requires

sponsors to make larger investments at risk, prior to knowing whether the product would be approved by regulators.

Please note that intermediate scenarios for addressing payers' requirements are possible, but we are focusing on two distinct approaches to explain key principles more clearly. These two approaches are first compared at the program level. The optimal decision criteria are provided as a guideline for sponsors' development strategy by maximizing an expected reward function.

Investing at risk, however, has an impact not only on the development program itself, but on the company's portfolio as a whole. Given that budgets are set at the portfolio level, funds invested at risk in one program have to be taken away from other programs. Therefore, what is the best solution for one program in isolation may not be the best solution at the entire portfolio level. Because of this we are also providing an optimal solution at the portfolio level. The provided solution is subject to budget limits and considerations to proceed sequentially or in parallel in each of the programs.

Finally, we extend our methods onto basket designs to provide solution how to best address differing stakeholders' requirements for these types of trials. We are focusing on the approach described in Beckman, et al. [1] and Chen, et al. [2], because in the current environment this approach seems most likely to result in regulatory approval based on a basket design.

Development Options

Sequential Approach

In this approach, clinical trial outcomes are first submitted to regulators who evaluate safety and efficacy of a new drug and make the decision regarding approval. Pending regulatory approval, sponsors will then collect and submit additional information necessary for payers to decide if they will reimburse the product and at which price. In Figure 11.1 we use an outcomes tree to illustrate this process.

Here, C_R and C_P are the costs for addressing regulatory requirements and the additional payers' requirements respectively, T_R and T_P are corresponding time periods. P_OS_R and P_OS_P are the probabilities of success for regulatory approval and payers approval respectively, $R(T)$ is sponsor's reward measured as expected revenue. To keep it simple, we use a general form $R(T)$ as a measurement of interest and we assume that $R(T)$ is a linearly time-dependent cumulative function. $T_{SEQ} = T_{PATENT} - T_R - T_P$ is the remaining patent life after payers' decision under the

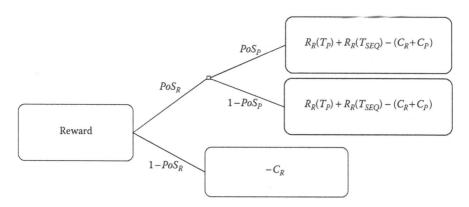

FIGURE 11.1
Outcomes Tree for Sequential Approach.

sequential approach. In reality, sponsors start accruing revenues once the marketing authorization is granted by regulators, but the reward increases much more rapidly when it also obtains payers approval of reimbursement. To distinguish the notations, we call the reward function when only regulatory approval is achieved as R_R (T) and we use R_P (T) to represent the reward when the new product is also approved by payers.

From the decision tree, the sponsor's expected reward (ER) under sequential approach can be calculated as:

$$ER_{SEQ} = P_OS_R \cdot R_R(T_P + T_{SEQ}) + P_OS_R \cdot P_OS_P[R_P(T_{SEQ}) - R_R(T_{SEQ})]$$
$$- (C_R + P_OS_R \cdot C_p) \tag{1}$$

Parallel Approach

As an alternative to sequential approach, we can also consider collecting information to address both requirements simultaneously. We call it the parallel approach, as shown in Figure 11.2.

Here we assume that the time addressing regulatory requirements is longer than the time addressing additional payers' requirements, i.e., $T_R > T_P$, and that remaining patent life under this parallel approach is $T_{PAR} = T_{PATENT} - T_R$.

We can then compute the expected reward under parallel approach:

$$ER_{PAR} = PoS_R \cdot R_R(T_{PAR}) + PoS_R \cdot PoS_P[R_P(T_{PAR}) - R_R(T_{PAR})] - (C_R + C_P) \tag{2}$$

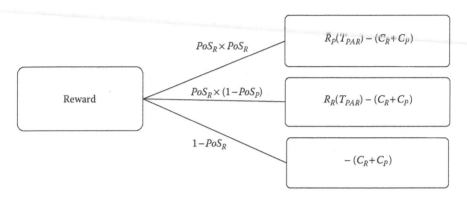

FIGURE 11.2
Outcomes Tree for Parallel Approach.

Now, the criteria for optimal approach selection can be summarized as follows: let

$$\Delta = ER_{SEQ} - ER_{PAR} = (1 - P_OS_R) \cdot C_p - P_OS_R \cdot P_OS_P \cdot (R_P - R_R)(T_P) \quad (3)$$

be the difference of the expected rewards between sequential and parallel approaches, then

- If $\Delta > 0$, choose sequential approach
- Otherwise, choose parallel approach

Note that the criterion (3) has a very intuitive explanation. The optimal design approach depends on a trade-off between C_P, the cost for addressing additional payers requirements and $(R_P - R_R)(T_P)$, the incremental gain during that period. If the cost C_P is playing a more important role, then it is very likely that Δ is positive, meaning that we should choose sequential approach for risk control. On the other hand, if the incremental gain $(R_P - R_R)(T_P)$ weights heavier, then there is a good chance that Δ is negative, suggesting the parallel approach might be more appropriate and the sponsor should take the risk for larger expected reward.

Case Study

Let's assume the following scenario: A new product is ready to enter phase 3, which will require two different trials. The first one (Study A) is a

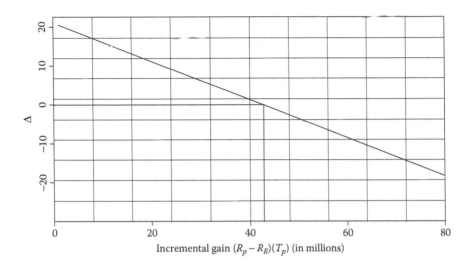

FIGURE 11.3
Sensitivity Plot for Incremental Gain.

placebo-controlled pivotal study to assess the effect of the new treatment compared with placebo is required for regulatory approval. The second one (Study B) is an active-controlled phase 3 study to compare the effect of the new product with a marketed drug is an additional payers' requirement if the product is to be reimbursed by them. At the time of planning, the estimated cost of Study B is $C_P = \$70M$, probabilities of success for Study A and B are both assumed to be 0.70, i.e., $P_OS_R = P_OS_P = 0.70$. We then apply Equation (3) to calculate the value of Δ as a function of the incremental gain $(R_p - R_R)(T_p)$.

As we can see from Figure 11.3, if the expected incremental gain is less than $43M, then Δ is positive, suggesting that under this scenario the sequential approach is a better option; otherwise, one should choose the parallel approach.

Portfolio-Level Optimization

So far we have been explaining how to select an optimal approach at the development program level. However, a decision to develop at risk, which is in this case the parallel approach, has an additional effect on company's portfolio. Investment C_P prior to regulatory approval competes with resources that could be allocated to other development programs. Given budget constraints, each program within the portfolio can have one of the following three possible designations; not executed, executed using sequential approach, or executed using parallel approach.

We then formulate portfolio optimization as a Knapsack Problem with budget constraints. For detailed discussions how this concept has been previously implemented see Martello and Toth [3] and Patel, Ankolekar, Antonijevic, and Rajicic [4].

Here we use subscript $i(i = 1,2,...n)$ for pharmaceutical products and $j(j = 1 \text{ or } 2)$ for development approach (sequential or parallel). For instance, let's assume that the drug in the previous program-level section is the first drug in the portfolio, then we can compute the expected reward (ER) and the expected cost (EC) for each development approach:

Sequential approach $(j = 1)$

$$ER_{11} = P_O S_R \cdot R_R(T_P + T_{SEQ}) + P_O S_R \cdot P_O S_P[R_P(T_{SEQ}) - R_R(T_{SEQ})] \\ - (C_R + P_O S_R \cdot C_P)$$

$$EC_{11} = C_R + P_O S_R \cdot C_P$$

Parallel approach $(j = 2)$

$$ER_{12} = P_O S_R \cdot R_R(T_{PAR}) + P_O S_R \cdot P_O S_P[R_P(T_{PAR}) - R_R(T_{PAR})] - (C_R + C_P)$$

$$EC_{12} = C_R + C_P$$

If we further define a decision variable as

$$z_{ij} = \begin{cases} 1, & \text{If Drug i uses strategy } j \\ 0, & \text{otherwise} \end{cases}$$

Then the optimal solution is the one that maximizes the following objective function:

$$\sum_j ER_{1j}Z_{1j} + \sum_j ER_{2j}Z_{2j} + \ldots + \sum_j ER_{nj}Z_{nj}$$

With the budget constraint

$$\sum_j EC_{1j}Z_{1j} + \sum_j EC_{2j}Z_{2j} + \ldots + \sum_j EC_{nj}Z_{nj} \leq B$$

and the approach constraint

$$\sum_j Z_{ij} \leq 1, \text{for all } i$$

where B is the total budget available over the entire portfolio.

Basket Designs with Accelerated Approval

In this section, we apply our program-level optimization results to basket designs. Such designs are not only useful for exploratory early-stage development, but also have the potential at confirmatory stage. We are addressing one such design, that was described in Beckman, et al. [5] and Chen, et al. [2]. We will first describe it at a very high level, such that a reader can follow the contents of this section.

This design has two stages: the "pruning" stage, and the "pooling" stage. In the pruning stage the trial starts with m indications. The outcome of the pruning stage is that a number (say k) of indications, satisfy the criteria, based on a faster interim endpoint, to advance into the second stage of this design. In oncology indications that pass the criteria may qualify for accelerated approval. In the second stage successful indications are pooled, and the final endpoint is tested on the combined indication. A successful outcome results in regulatory approval for all indications. This method is proposing a subsequent regulatory review by indication to ensure that there is at least a trend towards a positive risk/benefit. We are not addressing this part in order to provide a simpler algebraic solution.

Here a sponsor has three potential options when to generating payers information; (1) start at the beginning of the first stage of the basket trial, (2) start at the beginning of the second stage of the basket trial, or (3) start after both stages of the basket trial have been completed. In this chapter we will compare only options (2) and (3) above.

Since multiple indications are pooled in the basket trial, we modify our previous notations as follows: POS_r is the probability of success for regulatory approval. For each indication i, POS_{Pi} is the probability of success for payers' approval. C_{Ri} and C_{Pi} are the costs for addressing regulatory requirements and additional payers requirements. $R_{Ri}(T)$ is the cumulative reward function with regulatory approval only while $R_{Pi}(T)$ is the one which also has payers approval. For simplicity, we assume that the time for addressing payers' requirements is the same across all indications. In practice, however, they could vary. In that case the remaining patent time (also the cumulative reward) for each indication needs to be adjusted accordingly.

Assuming there are k out of m indications are qualified for accelerated approval. Without loss of generality, those k indications are numbered from 1 to k. Then following a similar method, we can obtain the decision trees for two approaches as shown in Figures 11.4 and 11.5:

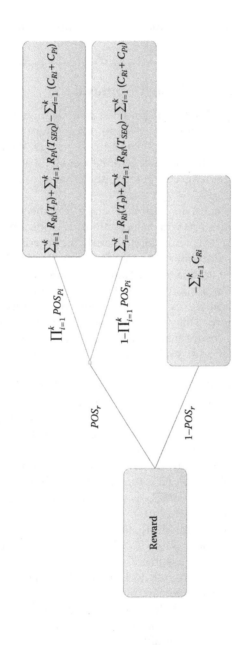

FIGURE 11.4
Sequential approach decision tree for basket designs.

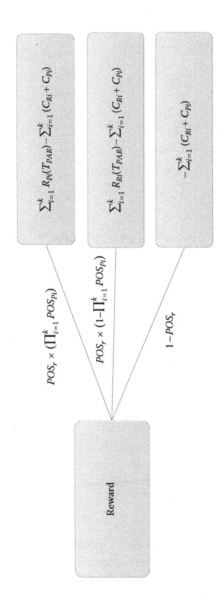

FIGURE 11.5
Parallel approach decision tree for basket designs.

The expected reward under each scenario can be computed as:

$$ER'_{SEQ} = POS_r \cdot \left(\sum_{i=1}^{k} R_{Ri}(T_P + T_{SEQ}) \right) + POS_r \cdot \left(\sum_{i=1}^{k} POS_{Pi}(R_{Pi} - R_{Ri})(T_{SEQ}) \right)$$
$$- \left(\sum_{i=1}^{k} C_{Ri} + POS_r \cdot \left(\sum_{i=1}^{k} C_{pi} \right) \right)$$

$$(4)$$

$$ER'_{PAR} = POS_r \cdot \left(\sum_{i=1}^{k} R_{Ri}(T_{PAR}) \right) + POS_r \cdot \left(\sum_{i=1}^{k} POS_{Pi}(R_{Pi} - R_{Ri})(T_{PAR}) \right)$$
$$- \sum_{i=1}^{k} (C_{Ri} - C_{Pi})$$

$$(5)$$

So for basket trials, the criteria for optimal approach selection is: let

$$\Delta' = ER'_{SEQ} - ER'_{PAR} = [1 - POS_r] \cdot \left(\sum_{i=1}^{k} C_{Pi} \right)$$
$$- POS_r \cdot \left(\sum_{i=1}^{k} POS_{Pi}(R_{Pi} - R_{Pi})(T_{SEQ} - T_{PAR}) \right)$$

$$(6)$$

be the difference of the expected rewards between sequential and parallel approaches, then

- If $\Delta' < 0$, choose sequential approach
- Otherwise, choose parallel approach

Summary

In this chapter, we compared two development approaches for addressing regulatory requirements and payers requirements at both program and portfolio level. For each individual program the sequential approach requires smaller up-front investment and generally smaller expected cost, but it also delays time for payers' approval, which is a crucial component for market success. The parallel approach, on the other hand, requires larger investment at risk at the development stage, but if successful it is faster to market approval, and it yields longer remaining patent life. To balance positive and negative impacts of these two approaches we provided the optimal decision criteria for traditional development as well as for basket designs with accelerated approval. The criteria can serve as a guideline for sponsors for development strategy and design of pharmaceutical programs.

Since budgets for individual programs are interdependent, it is preferable to optimize development decisions at the portfolio level. We provided an optimal solution for such problems by maximizing an objective function with budget and development approach constraints. This approach assures the optimal portfolio-level strategy.

References

1. Beckman RA, Burman CF, Chen C, Jobjörnsson S, König F, Stallard N and Posch M 2018. Decision analysis from the perspectives of single and multiple stakeholders. In *Platform Trial Designs in Modern Trial Development*, Antonijevic Z and Beckman RA (eds.), CRC Press, Boca Raton, Florida, pp XX–YY.
2. Chen C, Li N, Yuan S, Antonijevic Z, Kalamegham R Beckman RA 2016. Statistical design and considerations of a phase 3 basket trial for simultaneous investigation of multiple tumor types in one study. *Statistics in Biopharmaceutical Research* 8(3): 248–257.
3. Malrtello S Toth P 1990. *Knapsack Problems*. Wiley, Chichester.
4. Patel NR, Ankolekar SA, Antonijevic Z Rajicic N 2013. A mathematical model for maximizing the value of phase 3 drug development portfolios incorporating budget constraints and risk. *Statistics in Medicine* 32: 1763–1777.
5. Beckman RA, Antonijevic Z, Kalamegham R, Chen C 2016. Adaptive design for a confirmatory basket trial in multiple tumor types based on a putative predictive biomarker. *Clinical Pharmacology & Therapeutics* 100(6): 617–625.

Part III
Statistical Methodology

12

Primary Site Independent Clinical Trials in Oncology

Richard M. Simon

1. Introduction

Randomized clinical trials (RCTs) have been an important tool for evidence-based medicine. In oncology, RCTs historically involved a broadly defined population of patients who are representative of those with a specified primary site of disease and stage. Developments in tumor biology and genomics have indicated, however, that tumors of a primary site represent a heterogeneous collection of diseases that differ with regard to the oncogenic DNA alterations that drive their invasion. As genomic tools have become available to identify the driver DNA alterations in tumors, treatment has become increasingly based on molecular phenotypes. This movement has been called personalized or precision medicine. In oncology it is driven mainly by the somatic changes in tumor DNA, not the inherited germ-line changes, although both can be important.

The heterogeneous nature of tumors of the same primary site offers new challenges for therapeutics development and clinical trial design (1). Physicians have always known that cancers of the same primary site were different with regard to natural history and response to treatment. Today we have better tools for understanding these differences and using this knowledge to improve the development of drugs and the predictive biomarkers to guide their use. This approach provides the opportunity to tailor drugs to patients so that a greater portion of the treated population will benefit, the average benefit for the treated population will be larger, fewer patients will be exposed to the adverse effects of new regimens without benefit, clinical trials can be smaller, and payers more likely to reimburse since the cost-benefit is greater.

2. Phase II Basket Trials

Many of the cancer drugs being developed today are inhibitors of a signaling pathway that is driving tumor progression and is activated by mutation of a gene or amplification of a receptor. Drug discovery is based on screening for target inhibition. When the mechanism of action of the drug is well established and when the role of the relevant target in the pathophysiology of the disease is well understood, the drug is expected to be effective only in patients for whom the target is de-regulated by genomic alteration. In these cases, phase II clinical trials may be restricted to patients whose tumor carries the genomic alteration relevant for the test drug.

The increasing availability of affordable DNA sequencing of tumors has given rise to "basket" trials in which patient eligibility is based on a defined genomic alteration rather than on primary site. Basket trials are phase II trials. They can be non-randomized or randomized and include either a single drug or multiple individual drugs. If multiple drugs are involved, there is a separate specification of the genomic alteration determining eligibility for each of the drugs.

Single drug basket trials are generally non-randomized discovery trials (Figure 12.1). Eligibility depends on the presence in the tumor of a specified type of genomic alteration. For example, eligibility may require that the tumor contains a V600E mutation in the BRAF gene in a patient with any type of solid tumor other than melanoma and the drug being evaluated is a BRAF inhibitor (2). Basket trials often evaluate drugs which are approved for patients with a particular primary site of disease whose tumors bear a specific genomic alteration. The patients evaluated have tumors with the same alteration but with different primary sites. The primary site determines the cell of origin of the tumor and a given genomic alteration can have different biological effects depending on the cell type in which the alteration occurred.

For single treatment regimen studies, the eligible patients have had their tumor DNA sequenced and determined that their tumor contains a genomic alteration that indicates likelihood of benefit from the treatment regimen; that is, the genomic alteration is "actionable" for the specified regimen. The evidence that a drug is actionable for a given mutation varies and is often based on clinical evidence of effectiveness of the regimen in patients with the same genomic alteration but with a different primary site of tumor. Or the basis of actionability may just rest with the known importance of the drug target in pre-clinical tumor models.

A multi-drug non-randomized basket trial is like a collection of single drug basket trials with a common infrastructure for evaluating the patient's tumor for genomic alterations. Associated with each drug available in the multi-drug basket trial is a list of "actionable mutations" that make the patient eligible to receive that drug. The Molecular Analysis for Therapy Choice (MATCH) clinical trial recently launched by the National Cancer Institute, which opened with 400 clinical sites and10 drugs is an example of a large multi-drug basket design (3). Over 3,000 patients with

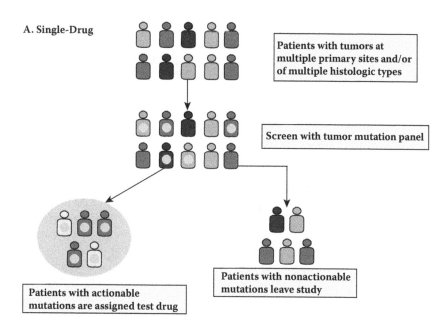

FIGURE 12.1
Single-drug Basket design

advanced metastatic cancer of many histologic types have been genomi-
cally tested with a common platform and triaged to a non-randomized
sub-study with an actionable drug; over 20 drugs are available. The
primary end-point for each of these sub-studies will be objective tumor
response or durable (> 6 months) disease stability.

Another large multi-drug non-randomized basket study is the Targeted
Agent and Profile Utilization Registry (TAPUR) of the American Society of
Clinical Oncology (4). That study is also for patients with advanced
metastatic cancer and a large number of approved drugs will be available
for investigating off-label use. This study differs from MATCH in that it
will not use a standard genomic screening platform and decisions about
which drug to use will be determined by the participating physicians, not
by a protocol.

The only endpoint clearly interpretable for the non-randomized basket
trials is objective tumor response or stable disease lasting longer than 6
months. Tumors generally do not shrink spontaneously, and so an objective tumor response can usually be attributed to the effect of the drug.
Whether stable disease is prolonged is more difficult to judge without a
control group because of the variability of tumor growth, but stable
disease durations in excess of 6 months for patients with advanced metastatic disease is unusual in the absence of treatment.

2.1. Statistical Designs for Basket Trials

The non-randomized drug basket trials are currently being planned similar to traditional phase II clinical trials. For MATCH, each drug-specific sub-study is designed to accrue 35 total patients with the same genomic alteration, but a range of primary sites in the expectation that data from 31 will be evaluable. The sub-studies are analyzed separately. If the observed response rate is at least 5/31, then the result will be considered positive and a subsequent expanded accrual study will be planned to better define how drug activity varies among the eligible histological types. A single stage accrual plan is used, instead of the usual two-stage accrual plan. This is because it was felt that a small first stage of accrual of patients heterogeneous with regard to primary site might lead to missing activity restricted to a single primary site. The BRAF inhibitor vemurafinib (2) was, for example, highly active for melanoma patients whose tumors contained the V600E BRAF mutation but not for patients with BRAF mutated colorectal cancer.

The TAPUR study is evaluating off-label use of drugs which have been approved by the Food and Drug Administration for patients with the genomic alteration in a specific primary site. Because these drugs have been approved for a given primary site, it uses an optimal two-stage design with activity level target of 35%, much larger than that used for MATCH. The two-stage designs for different drugs are analyzed separately. For planning phase II trials using an optimal two-stage design, extensive tables are available in reference (5) and an online design tool is available at http://brb.nci.nih.gov. For distinguishing a response rate $\geq$ 35% from a rate $\leq$ 15%, a design with power 90% and type I error 10% involves accruing 19 patients in the first stage. If fewer than 4 responses are seen, then the results are declared inconsistent with a 35% response rate and accrual ceases. If at least 4 responses are obtained, then accrual of that subtype continues to 33 total patients. If at that point 7 or fewer responses in 33 patients are observed, the results are declared inconsistent with a 35% response rate. Otherwise, results are considered inconsistent with a 15% response rate. The chance that a drug with a true 15% response probability will have 3 or fewer responses in the first 19 patients is 68%.

For each drug studied in a basket design, all of the patients generally share a common mutation, but have different primary disease sites. The standard phase II designs used for most basket clinical trials ignore this heterogeneity and pool all patients containing the same actionable mutations for analysis. To analyze separately the patients of each primary site would require much larger sample sizes. Jung et al. (6) described one and two stage designs for heterogeneous populations but the inference is on the average response rate for the population. Leblanc et al. (7) proposed a design similar to using separate optimal two-stage designs for the different histologic types, but it includes a futility test for the overall population.

They also proposed that histology specific futility tests be conducted after every 5–10 patients are accrued to the histology strata. Cunanan et al. (8) described a design in which the decision of whether to pool the primary sites or to accrue to them in a separate two-stage design for each is determined based on an interim test of treatment by primary site interaction.

Thall et al. (9) developed a design based on a Bayesian hierarchical model which could be used for making inferences about drug activity in primary type subsets of a basket clinical trial. The subset specific effects are viewed as random variables drawn from a "hyper-prior" distribution whose parameters are specified. This design was used prior to the Basket era in a trial of imatinib for multiple histologic subsets of sarcoma (10).

Berry et al. (11) have furthered the development of Bayesian hierarchical designs for Basket clinical trials. For distinguishing response probabilities of p_0 to p_1 they model the log odds ratio $\Theta_k = \log(p/(1-p)) - \log(p_1/(1-p_1))$ for each histologic site k. The prior for Θ_k is taken as normal with an almost non-informative hyper-prior mean distribution and an inverse Gamma distribution as hyper-prior variance distribution. The amount of "sharing" among histologic groups is determined by the inverse Gamma hyper prior. Unless the number of groups is large, the data contains very limited information about the variance of the Θ_k. Berry, et al. compared the design based on hierarchical modeling with frequent interim monitoring (i.e., every five patients) to performing a Simon two-stage design separately for each histology. They show that the design based on hierarchical modeling requires somewhat fewer patients per histology to conclude that $p < p_1$, when $p = p_0$ is true for all classes and that the probability of a false positive conclusion for some histology is reduced. This improved performance for the case where the drug is uniformly ineffective is achieved at the expense of greater false positive rates for cases where the drug is effective for some histologies and not for others.

2.2. Other Bayesian Basket Designs

Simon, et al. (12) have developed a different kind of Bayesian design for evaluating the response probabilities for the primary sites included in a basket trial of a drug. They assume that the response probability for histology stratum k (p_k) takes on either a low value p_{lo} of no therapeutic interest or a higher value p_{hi} of interest, as in previous phase II statistical models (5). Two hypotheses are considered for the ensemble $\{p_1, \ldots, p_K\}$; H_0 indicates that the stratum specific response probabilities are all equal. If H_0 is true, then the probability that the common value of the response probabilities is p_{hi} is taken as a specified value γ. The alternative hypothesis H_1 specifies that the response probabilities can be viewed as independent random variables drawn from a common two point prior distribution with $\Pr[p_k = p_{hi} | H_1] = \gamma$ independently for each k. The prior probability of H_0, denoted by λ.

At any interim analysis one can compute the posterior probability of activity (i.e., $p_j = p_{hi}$) for each of the stratum. If that posterior probability is too small, one may close accrual to that stratum. If that posterior probability is very large, one might wish to proceed with the next stage of development of the drug in that stratum.

An advantage of this model is that the posterior probabilities can be computed in closed form without the need for simulation. At the interim analysis assume that there are r_k responses among n_k patients treated in stratum k. The posterior probability for H_0 can be written

$$
\begin{aligned}
\Pr[H_0 | data] &= \frac{\Pr[data | H_0]\lambda}{\Pr[data]} \\
&= \frac{\Pr[data | H_0]\lambda}{\Pr[data | H_0]\lambda + \Pr[data | H_1](1 - \lambda)} \\
&= \left\{ 1 + \frac{\Pr[data | H_1](1 - \lambda)}{\Pr[data | H_0]\lambda} \right\}^{-1} \\
&= \left\{ 1 + \frac{(1 - \lambda) \prod\limits_{k=1}^{K} \{\gamma b(r_k; p_{hi}, n_k) + (1 - \gamma)b(r_k; p_{lo}, n_k)\}}{\lambda \left\{ \gamma \prod\limits_{k=1}^{K} b(r_k; p_{hi}, n_k) + (1 - \gamma) \prod\limits_{k=1}^{K} b(r_k; p_{lo}, n_k) \right\}} \right\}^{-1}
\end{aligned}
$$

$$(1)$$

where $b(r;p,n)$ denotes the binomial mass probability of r responses in n trials with propability p per trial.

The posterior probability that the drug is active in stratum k can be expressed

$$\Pr[p_k = p_{hi} | data] = \Pr[p_k = p_{hi} | data \ \& \ H_0]\Pr[H_0 | data]$$

$$+ \Pr[p_k = p_{hi} | data \ \& \ H_1]\Pr[H_1 | data] \quad (2)$$

The first factor of the first term on the right-hand-side can be written as

$$\Pr[p_k = p_{hi} | data \ \& \ H_0] = \left\{ 1 + \frac{(1 - \gamma) \prod\limits_{k=1}^{K} b(r_k; n_k, p_{lo})}{\gamma \prod\limits_{k=1}^{K} b(r_k; n_k, p_{hi})} \right\}^{-1} \quad (3)$$

and the first factor of the second term on the right-hand-side can be written as

$$\Pr[p_k = p_{hi}|\text{data \& } H_1] = \frac{\gamma b(r_k; n_k, p_{hi})}{\gamma b(r_k; n_k, p_{hi}) + (1 - \gamma)b(r_k; n_k, p_{lo})} \tag{4}$$

When the posterior probability of uniformity (H_0) is very small, there will be no sharing of information among strata and the stratum specific posterior activity probabilities can be computed from equation (4). When, however, the posterior probability of homogeneity is not negligible, then there will be sharing of information among strata and the stratum specific posterior activity probabilities are weighted combinations of expressions (3) and (4) with the weights determined by expression (1).

A website that performs the calculations for planning and analyzing Bayesian Basket Design is available at https://brpnci.shinyapps.io/main/.

The Bayesian Basket design described above requires specification of four parameters; p_{lo}, p_{hi}, the prior λ for H_0 and the prior γ for probability of activity in a stratum. For basket trials of drugs which have been approved for some primary site we have generally recommended parameter values $\lambda = 0.33$ and $\gamma = 0.5$. We like the need to specify these probabilities. You perform the basket trial because you believe that homogeneity across strata is credible and you are generally using a drug having a substantial response rate in another primary site of disease. Many statisticians are, however, uncomfortable with informative priors, even for phase II studies. We would point out, however, the assumption of a "non-informative" hyper-prior is itself informative.

The Bayesian Basket Design may be generalized by placing independent priors on λ and/or γ. If a prior $\pi(\lambda)$ is placed on λ but not γ, then expression (1) becomes

$$\Pr[H_0|\text{data}] =$$

$$\left\{ 1 + \frac{\prod_{k=1}^{K} \{\gamma b(r_k; p_{hi}, n_k) + (1 - \gamma)b(r_k; p_{lo}, n_k)\} \quad \int_0^1 (1 - \lambda)d\pi(\lambda)}{\left\{\gamma \prod_{k=1}^{K} b(r_k; p_{hi}, n_k) + (1 - \gamma) \prod_{k=1}^{K} b(r_k; p_{lo}, n_k)\right\} \quad \int_0^1 \lambda d\pi(\lambda)} \right\}^{-1}$$

and expressions (3) and (4) remain unchanged. Hence, results with the original model can be interpreted as results with a model having a prior $\pi(\lambda)$ with the ratio of $(1 - \lambda)/\lambda$ in (1) replaced by the ratio of expected values of the parameter λ.

If a prior is also placed on γ, then (1) becomes

$$\Pr[H_0|\text{data}] = \left\{1 + \frac{\int_0^1 \prod_{k=1}^{K} \left\{\gamma b(r_k; p_{hi}, n_k) + (1-\gamma)b(r_k; p_{lo}, n_k)\right\} d\pi(\gamma)}{\left\{\bar{\gamma} \prod_{k=1}^{K} b(r_k; p_{hi}, n_k) + (1-\bar{\gamma}) \prod_{k=1}^{K} b(r_k; p_{lo}, n_k)\right\}} \frac{1-\bar{\lambda}}{\bar{\lambda}}\right\}^{-1}$$

where the over-bar denotes the mean of the prior distributions. In expressions (3) and (4), the fixed parameters are replaced by the prior means.

3. Following a Basket Design

At the conclusion of the basket design, there may be some primary sites for which the activity level of the test drug is still uncertain. In these cases, extended phase II trials may be appropriate.

3.1. Separate Enrichment Phase III Trials for Prevalent Histologies

For the histologic types for which the drug was established as active in the basket trial, there are several options for further development. For those primary sites which are sufficiently prevalent, option one would be to conduct separate phase III enrichment trials, randomizing patients whose tumors contain the genomic alteration to a control regimen versus a regimen containing the test drug.

3.2. Histology Independent Phase III Confirmatory Trial

For active primary sites which are not sufficiently prevalent to support separate phase III trials, option two would be to conduct a histology independent phase III randomized trial as suggested by Beckman et al. (13) and illustrated in Figure 12.2. In such a trial, however, sample size would be established for testing whether the treatment group pooled across primary sites had better outcomes that a pooled control group. The control group may differ by primary site or be "physicians' choice" since for advanced disease patients who have failed standard treatment there may be no agreed upon control. Actually for the analysis of such a trial, a measure of treatment effect would be computed separately for each primary site and averaged across the primary sites. If the pooled analysis of the clinical trial were statistically significant, the sponsor would ask for approval of the drug for all of the primary sites included in the trial. The endpoint of the trial would most likely be either progression-free survival or overall survival.

Although the pooled design of Figure 12.2 would be conducted without sufficient statistical power to evaluate primary sites separately, some

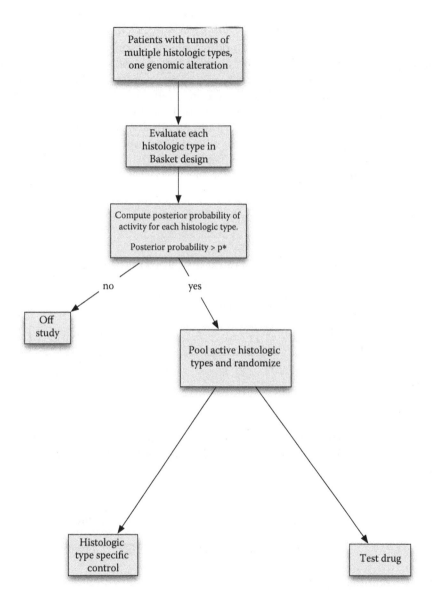

FIGURE 12.2
Phase III histology agnostic design

monitoring for large inter-histology differences could be monitored using a variant of the Bayesian basket method described as follows. Let β_k denote the log hazard ratio of the test treatment compared to control for primary site k. Ideally we would wish to determine whether the treatment is effective for primary site k (i.e., $\beta_k = \beta_{lo}$) or is not effective (i.e., $\beta_k = \beta_{hi}$) because a low value of the log hazard corresponds to effectiveness. Generally we would take $\beta_{hi} = 0$. As for the basket trial, the null hypothesis is that all the β_k are equal and the alternative is that they are independent selections from a two point distribution with probability γ that $\beta_k = \beta_{lo}$. The prior probability for the null hypothesis is specified as λ which would generally be taken as > 0.5 since all included primary sites showed activity in the basket design.

We will assume exponential distributions are are generally appropriate for DFS or OS data for patients with far advanced disease. For the randomized design, the posterior probability that the treatment effectiveness is uniform across primary sites is

$$
\begin{aligned}
\Pr[H_0 \mid \text{data}] &= \frac{\Pr[\text{data} \mid H_0]\lambda}{\Pr[\text{data}]} \\[2mm]
&= \frac{\Pr[\text{data} \mid H_0]\lambda}{\Pr[\text{data} \mid H_0]\lambda + \Pr[\text{data} \mid H_1](1-\lambda)} \\[2mm]
&= \left\{ 1 + \frac{\Pr[\text{data} \mid H_1](1-\lambda)}{\Pr[\text{data} \mid H_0]\lambda} \right\}^{-1} \\[2mm]
&= \left\{ 1 + \frac{(1-\lambda) \prod\limits_{k=1}^{K} \{\gamma\phi(\beta_k;\beta_{lo},\sigma_k) + (1-\gamma)\phi(\beta_k;\beta_{hi},\sigma_k)\}}{\lambda\left\{ \gamma \prod\limits_{k=1}^{K} \phi(\beta_k;\beta_{lo},\sigma_k) + (1-\gamma) \prod\limits_{k=1}^{K} \phi(\beta_k;\beta_{hi},\sigma_k) \right\}} \right\}^{-1}
\end{aligned}
$$

(5)

Where β_k is the maximum likelihood estimation (mle) of the log hazard ratio in stratum k, σ_k equals 2 divided by the number of events in stratum k and ϕ denotes the normal density function.

The analog of expression (2) is

$$
\Pr[\beta_k = \beta_{lo}|\text{data}] = \Pr[\beta_k = \beta_{lo}|\text{data \& } H_0]\Pr[H_0|\text{data}]
$$

$$
+ \Pr[\beta_k = \beta_{lo}|\text{data \& } H_1]\Pr[H_1|\text{data}].
$$

The analog of expression (3) is

$$
\Pr[\beta_1 = \cdots = \beta_K = \beta_{lo}|\text{data \& } H_0] = \left\{ 1 + \frac{(1-\gamma) \prod\limits_{k=1}^{K} \phi(\beta_k;\beta_{hi},\sigma_k)}{\gamma \prod\limits_{k=1}^{K} \phi(\beta_k;\beta_{lo},\sigma_k)} \right\}^{-1}
$$

and the analog of expression (4) is

$$\Pr[\beta_k = \beta_{lo}|\text{data \& H}_1] = \frac{\gamma\phi(\beta_k;\beta_{lo},\sigma_k)}{\gamma\phi(\beta_k;\beta_{lo},\sigma_k) + (1-\gamma)\phi(\beta_k;\beta_{hi},\sigma_k)}$$

One can monitor the posterior probability of H_0 in the phase III trial to try to detect heterogeneity of effect. But if the trial is designed to detect a uniform treatment effect across histologies, then this may not provide a sensitive indicator of heterogeneity. Nevertheless, under these conditions, the power for rejecting the hypothesis of no average treatment effect will be low and so approval of the drug for ineffective histologies will be unlikely.

3.3. Extended Indications for Low Prevalence Histologies Based Solely on the Basket Trial Results

For the rare sites of disease in which the posterior probability of activity of the drug is substantial in the basket design and the drug has already been approved for some primary site, the best course of action may be regulatory approval without further clinical trial. This approach might be justified if the basket trial established that the drug provided substantial rates of durable responses in patients with advanced disease for whom no other effective treatment was available. One would, of course, have to consider the safety profile in these new disease site patients and that can be difficult to evaluate in non-randomized studies. Generally for basket trials, however, the disease is life threatening in all primary sites of disease and the patients have exceeded all available therapy. The histology independent randomized trial described previously might be difficult to recruit patients or physicians to because for patients with such advanced disease there is no treatment of established value and because the test drug will have already demonstrated activity in such patients.

---

4. Randomized Basket Trials

Several multi-drug basket trials have been conducted which involve randomization to either a test drug which targets a mutation in the patient's tumor or to a control drug. For example, in the Molecular Profiling-Based Assignment of Cancer Therapy (MPACT) clinical trial five different treatment regimens were used in the experimental arm, each targeted to patients with a specified type of genomic alteration (14). Patients are randomized to either receive the drug actionable for a genomic alteration in their tumor or to receive a non-matched control drug. This design was also used for the French SHIVA clinical trial (15).

With randomization the trial may test the general policy of trying to match the drug to the genomics of the tumor. The null hypothesis here relates to a matching policy for a given set of drugs and genomic alterations used in the study. This policy is also determined by the type of genomic characterization performed and by the "rules" for matching drug to tumor. Rejection of the null hypothesis provides a proof of principle that matching can be useful overall but that null hypothesis is specific for the genomic alterations and the drugs on which the study is based (16). This type of trial is sized like a phase III trial for testing the null hypothesis that mutation matching does not lead to improved outcome overall for the full set of drugs.

Randomization makes it more feasible to use progression-free survival as endpoint rather than objective tumor response for evaluating the component single drug basket trials. Time until progression and survival can in some cases be quite variable and a randomized control arm facilitates their use as endpoint. One can compare the patients who received a matched drug to those who did not, stratified by the genomic alterations. This involves pooling all of the patients regardless of their genomic alterations and primary sites of disease. Separate analysis of the genomic alteration subsets using the corresponding randomized control group is possible but the statistical power of the comparison is generally limited by the small sample size. The relative merits of several types of basket designs has also been discussed by Trippa and Alexander (17).

5. Discussion

Recognition of the molecular heterogeneity of human diseases and availability of tools for characterizing this heterogeneity presents new opportunities for the development of more effective treatments and challenges for the design of new kinds of clinical trials (18). This paper has attempted to review some of these newer designs.

Initially, there was some reluctance of cancer drug developers to target molecularly defined sub-populations of patients. The many examples in which drugs were developed to target specific genomic alterations in oncogenes resulting in enrichment studies that demonstrated much larger treatment effects than used to be obtained in more heterogeneous populations has convinced most investigators and sponsors however. These larger treatment effects facilitate both regulatory approval and payer approval. The new generation of phase 2/3 umbrella studies represent an attempt to increase the efficiency of enrichment designs by linking them together in a common infrastructure for screening and triaging patients to the appropriate study.

The successes seen with molecularly targeted drugs have stimulated basket trials to evaluate off-label use of such drugs in patients with the same genomic alterations for which the drug was approved.

Identifying the right patient population for a drug regimen can dramatically improve the efficiency of clinical development and avoid treatment of patients with regimens that do not benefit them. It can also play an important role in controlling societal costs of medical care. Shankaran et al. (19) estimated that restricting use of the anti-EGFR antibody Cetuximab to patients without KRAS mutations in advanced colorectal cancer reduced the health care costs in the U.S. alone by 740 million dollars per year. Developing drugs with candidate predictive biomarkers is, however, more complex than the traditional practice of developing drugs for broad heterogeneous populations (20). Larger phase II studies with much more extensive biological characterization of the participating patients are often needed to adequately understand the role of candidate biomarkers in the disease.

References

1. Simon RM. (2013). *Genomic Clinical Trials and Predictive Medicine*. Cambridge, Cambridge University Press.
2. Hyman DM, Puzanov I, Subbiah V, Faris JE, Chau I, et al. (2015). Vemurafenib in multiple nonmelanoma cancers with BRAF V600 Mutations. *The New England Journal of Medicine* 373: 726–736.
3. Conley BA, Doroshow JH. (2014). Molecular analysis for therapy choice: NCI MATCH. *Seminars in Oncology* 41: 297–299.
4. Chakradhar S. (2016). Group mentality: Determining whether targeted treatments really work for cancer. *Nature Medicine* 22: 222–224.
5. Simon R. (1989). Optimal two-stage designs for phase II clinical trials. *Controlled Clinical Trials* 10: 1–10.
6. Jung SH, Chang MN, Kang SJ. (2012). Phase II cancer clinical trials with heterogeneous populations. *Journal of Biopharmaceutical Statistics* 22: 312–328.
7. LeBlanc M, Rankin C, Crowley J. (2009). Multiple histology phase II trials. *Clinical Cancer Research* 15: 4256–4262.
8. Cunanan KM, Iasonos A, Shen R, Begg CB, Gonen M. (2017). An efficient basket trial design. *Statistics in Medicine* 36: 1568–1579.
9. Thall PF, Bekele BN, Champlin RE, Baker LH, Benjamin RS. (2003). Hierarchical Bayesian approaches to phase II trials in diseases with multiple subtypes. *Statistics in Medicine* 22: 27–36.
10. Chugh R, Wathen JK, Maki RG, Benjamin RS, Patel SR, et al. (2009). Phase II multicenter trial of imatinib in 10 histological subtypes of sarcoma using a Bayesian hierarchical statistical model. *Journal of Clinical Oncology* 27: 3148–3315.
11. Berry SM, Broglio KR, Groshen S, Berry DA. (2013). Bayesian hierarchical modeling of patient subpopulations: Efficient designs of phase II oncology clinical trials. *Clinical Trials* 10: 720–734.

12. Simon R, Geyer S, Subramanian J, Roychowdhury S. (2016). The Bayesian basket design for genomic alteration driven phase II clinical trials. *Seminars in Oncology* 43: 13–18.

13. Beckman RA, Antonijevic Z, Kalamegham R, Chen C. (2016). Adaptive design for a confirmatory basket trial in multiple tumor types based on a predictive biomarker. *Clinical Pharmacology and Therapeutics* 100: 617–625.

14. Kummar S, Williams M, Lih CJ, Polley EC, Chen AP, et al. (2015). Application of molecular profiling in clinical trials for advanced metastatic cancers. *Journal of the National Cancer Institute* 107(4). doi:10.1093/jnci/djv003.

15. Le Tourneau C, Delord JP, Goncalves A, Gavoille C, Dubot C, et al. (2015). Molecularly targeted therapy based on tumour molecular profiling versus conventional therapy for advanced cancer (SHIVA): A multicentre open-label, proof-of-concept randomised, controlled phase 2 trial. *The Lancet Oncology* 16: 1324-1334.

16. Simon R, Polley E. (2013). Clinical trials for precision oncology using next generation sequencing. *Personalized Medicine* 10: 485–495.

17. Trippa L, Alexander BM. (2017). Bayesian baskets: A novel design for biomarker-based clinical trials. *Journal of Clinical Oncology* 35: 1–16.

18. Mandrekar SJ, Dahlberg SE, Simon R. (2015). Improving clinical trial efficiency: Thinking outside the box. *American Society of Clinical Oncology Education Proceedings*, ASCO.

19. Shankaran V, Bentrem DJ, Mulcahy MF, Bennett CL, Benson AB, III. (2009). Economic implications of Kras testing in metastatic colorectal cancer. American Society of Clinical Oncology 2009 Gastrointestinal Cancers Symposium, *Abstracty 298*, San Francisco, CA.

20. Simon R, Roychowdhury S. (2013). Implementing personalized cancer genomics in clinical trials. *Nature Reviews Drug Discovery* 12: 358–369.

13

Platform Trials

Ben Saville and Scott Berry

1. Introduction

Traditionally, clinical trials have been designed to evaluate a single treatment in a homogeneous group of patients. Such trials have proven useful for answering the following question: "Does a single treatment offer a benefit on average to a study population?" However, the answer to this question does not provide the physician with the necessary information to make decisions regarding the best treatment for an individual patient, especially when the patient may differ from patients in the study population and there are multiple treatment options to consider.

In addition, medical research is quickly moving beyond the simplistic view of an average treatment benefit in a homogenous group of patients. Biomarker development and personalized medicine are leading to a future in which the many diseases will be rare diseases. This will make slow, large scale clinical trials with a single hypothesis within a single disease impractical to conduct, and the speed of medical discovery will outpace the planned completion of such trials. Advances in personalized medicine are also leading to increasingly complex treatment regimens. This is forcing researchers to address a different question: "Which treatment or combination of treatments is best for each type of patient?" The answer to this question will provide the practicing physician with the information needed to make informed decisions on individual patient care.

To efficiently answer the latter (and more relevant) question, we advocate the use of adaptive platform trial designs. We define a platform trial as a clinical trial with a master protocol that has the broad goal of determining the best treatment for a disease by simultaneously and sequentially investigating multiple treatments, using specialized statistical tools for allocating patients and analyzing results [1–3]. Platform trials are inherently adaptive, and offer flexible features such as dropping treatments for futility, graduating treatments to confirmatory trials, or adding new treatments to be tested during the course of a trial. A platform trial is often intended to investigate treatment combinations, to quantify differences in treatment effects in subgroups, and to treat patients as effectively as possible within the trial. The focus is on the disease and the population of potential therapies rather than any specific experimental therapy.

2. Key Statistical Tools

Each platform trial is unique and will have objectives specific to the context of the disease and available treatments. Hence there is no "one-size-fits-all" approach to platform trial design, and there are a number of features and statistical tools that can be combined and incorporated into any one master protocol. Below we summarize some common statistical tools used in platform trial designs.

2.1. Adaptive Patient Allocation

Adaptive patient allocation is a key feature that allows platform trial designs to efficiently explore multiple treatments in multiple patient subgroups. Given the potentially large number of treatment by sub-group combinations in such trials, a fixed patient allocation would be inefficient and even infeasible in many contexts. Response adaptive randomization (RAR) [4] allows patients to be allocated with greater probability to the treatments that are performing best for a given type of patient. Less effective therapies will receive fewer randomization assignments and may be dropped from the study in one or all sub-groups according to the master protocol decision rules. Frequent interim analyses are required to update the randomization probabilities to maximize the efficiency of patient allocation. In addition to statistical efficiencies gained by response adaptive randomization compared to fixed allocation, RAR will generally provide better patient outcomes for patients in the trial, as patients are being allocated to the treatments that are performing best [2,5]. This is particularly helpful in diseases with severe or life-threatening symptoms, such as Ebola, where inefficient patient randomization to ineffective therapies can lead to unnecessary patient burden or death. Depending on the goals of the study, some treatments may be dropped early for futility from a platform trial with relatively small sample sizes, thus lacking precision for an estimated treatment response. But in many disease areas such as Ebola, the estimation of each possible treatment response is secondary relative to the goal of finding the best therapy or combination of therapies for each type of patient.

2.2. Hierarchical Modeling

The exploration of multiple treatments and multiple patient subgroups within a single platform trial can dramatically increase the dimensions required for estimation. For example, instead of estimating a single treatment effect within a single homogenous group of patients as in a traditional trial, a platform trial may investigate five treatment arms in five subgroups of patients, requiring a total of 25 cells requiring estimation of patient response. It would be extremely inefficient to independently estimate a treatment response within each of the 25 cells; hence more sophisticated methods of modeling are required to navigate the more complex space. Bayesian hierarchical modeling allows sharing of information across the respective cells in a measurable and pragmatic manner. In fact, Stein [6] showed in 1956 that shrinkage estimators that leverage information from multiple groups provide better estimators than maximum likelihood methods that estimate each group independently. In the context of clinical trials, if a treatment is beneficial to a particular subgroup, it is more likely to be beneficial to other related subgroups, which can be modeled via hierarchical modeling. Bayesian prior distributions can be calibrated to control the amount of sharing and to limit false positives. For example, tighter prior distributions around the null value (i.e., greater shrinkage) can be used for modeling the interactions of treatments with patient subgroups, thereby requiring greater evidence to convince investigators of heterogeneity in patient response. This would assume fairly homogenous treatment response until the sample size is sufficient to convince otherwise.

2.3. Predictive Modeling

Bayesian predictive probabilities [7,8] are extremely useful tools on which to base decision rules within the master protocol. For example, I-SPY2 [9] is a phase 2 trial in neoadjuvant breast cancer for the screening of multiple treatments within multiple biomarker subgroups. Based on a pre-specified master protocol, investigational treatments may "graduate" to a phase 3 trial within a specific patient biomarker group if the phase 3 predictive probability of success (given phase 2 data) is greater than 0.85. Predictive probabilities are also helpful as futility metrics on which to drop treatments from a study, and also for sample size adaptations for an arm in the presence of delayed outcomes, i.e., a delay between the time of randomization and the collection of the primary outcome such as is found with a 6-month or 12-month endpoint. Longitudinal models using auxiliary outcomes (e.g., using intermediate 6-month outcomes to predict 12-month outcomes for incomplete patients) [10] allow decision rules to harness all available information on patients with incomplete primary outcomes.

2.4. Perpetual Trial Design

In contrast to a traditional clinical trial with a fixed sample size, a platform trial may not have a fixed number of patients but may intend to enroll patients perpetually. Provided there is funding and continued need to explore the population of treatments within a disease, the treatments available in a platform trial may evolve over time, with ineffective therapies dropped from the study, and effective therapies remain to be compared to new investigational therapies. A master protocol dictates the decision rules that allow arm dropping, as well as the procedure for adding additional treatments to the ongoing study. Hence, when new treatments are available, there is no need to re-design the trial or start a new trial; the treatments are simply inserted into the existing platform trial given a pre-specified algorithm as described in the master protocol.

2.5. Leveraging Control Data

A key concept of platform trial designs is the ability to efficiently leverage data across multiple experimental interventions, often done through the management of a common control arm. For example, consider a disease in which there are five potential interventions to assess. A more traditional strategy may involve five independent trials, each with 100 active and 100 control patients, resulting in 1,000 total patients to evaluate all interventions. A platform trial design could randomize 100 patients to control and 500 patients to experimental arms to address the same questions with identical power but only requiring 600 patients.

An important issue in many of these trials will involve analyses of an arm compared to combined controls, some of which may not overlap the enrollment period of the experimental arm. Sections 2.6 and 4.3 address modeling the effects of time, allowing the borrowing of information from all controls for understanding the treatment effect of each experimental intervention.

In addition, control data from historical databases can be leveraged with platform trial designs to provide a natural history of the disease. Such data can be used to build disease progression models, enabling more innovative and relevant primary outcome analyses, and ultimately greater statistical power for the comparison of interventions. Control subjects from the platform trial can be combined with this natural history for model building. For example, the Dominantly Inherited Alzheimer Network [11,12] has launched a phase II/III platform trial in which a long-term observational control cohort is used for disease progression modeling and learning about the variations in the natural progression of cognitive decline. The design gains tremendous efficiency and power from the natural history modeling and creation of the primary endpoint. In addition, the long-term observational cohort data is used to set simulation parameters that enable exploration of design performance (e.g., power, Type I error, etc.). In another Alzheimer's platform trial, EPAD, a longitudinal observational cohort is used in a similar manner to build a disease progression model, but also forms the population of subjects for the randomized trial. This allows for a greatly reduced screen failure rates as well as longer exposure of natural history before the interventional trial.

2.6. Population-Drift Modeling

Because of the ability of platform trials to be sustained over long time periods (in particular for perpetual trials) with adaptive allocation of patients to treatments across time, there is a risk that population drift in patient characteristics may impact the interpretation of results. This could be due to either internal factors, such as adding additional study sites, or external factors, such as the availability of related external trials. To alleviate this risk when present, we recommend statistical modeling that specifically accounts for changes in the response of the patient population over time. This is typically done via Bayesian hierarchical modeling and can provide a trajectory of population drift over time. Proper adjustment for this drift in the primary outcome modeling enables the comparison of treatments with staggered entry (i.e., treatments in which patients are not enrolled concurrently), and also avoids bias that can result from adaptive allocation in the presence of a changing population.

2.7. Simulation Studies

Because of the complexity of platform trial designs, there is no simple formula from which to calculate frequentist operating characteristics such as power and Type I error. Hence, simulation studies are essential in the design stage to both (1) understand the operating characteristics of the design (e.g., power, Type I error, patient allocation, bias, etc.); and (2) iteratively calibrate the master protocol decision rules to align with the goals of the study. In the design stage, thousands of virtual trials are simulated over a wide range of plausible assumptions, and summaries are calculated across the simulated trials to ensure the master protocol provides desirable performance over a wide range of plausible truths. In addition, individual example trials are simulated to investigate the adaptive decisions of the master protocol given specific observed results. This is an opportunity for investigators to "see the trial in action before they run the trial," which helps all collaborators better understand the adaptive platform design as well as propose modifications or refinements that improve the design.

3. Applications of Platform Trials

Platform trial designs have been used or are planning to be used in many different disease areas, including various types of cancer (breast, brain, pancreatic), Alzheimer's disease, infectious diseases (flu, pneumonia, Ebola), antibiotics, and cystic fibrosis. In this section we provide a general summary of several key platform trials. In addition, Table 13.1 summarizes some of the features incorporated into these various trials, including the following: phase (2,3,4); multiple arms (Y/N); staggered entry of arms (Y/N), perpetual enrollment (Y/N), embedded within clinical care (Y/N); multifactorial combinations of treatments (Y/N); type of controls used (common controls shared among arms, Y/N indicating that some arms have controls while others do not); blinding of randomized treatment (Y/N); enrichment of the study population (Y/N); frequency of interim analyses (weeks, months, years, or "n" if based on sample size), primary Bayesian analysis (Y/N); adaptive sample size (Y/N), RAR for patient allocation (Y/N), longitudinal modeling of primary endpoint (Y/N); population drift modeling over time (Y/N); subgroup differential treatment effects (Y/N); and the use of Bayesian predictive probabilities (Y/N).

3.1. Breast Cancer

As noted previously, I-SPY2 is a platform trial in neoadjuvant breast cancer [3,9]. The objective of this phase 2 trial is to screen experimental agents (initially five plus standard therapy) within 10 genetic signature groups, with the goal of graduating promising agents to a focused phase 3 trial within the specified genetic subgroup (randomized 1:1 versus standard therapy). Traditional drug development typically involves a small to moderate number of patients in phase 2, followed by a much larger and expensive phase 3 clinical trial. I-SPY2 takes an inverted approach, as it involves a large phase 2 trial spanning multiple agents and multiple subgroups (up to 120 patients for each drug), followed by smaller focused phase 3 trials (300 patients) for the promising agent/subgroup combinations. The hope is that this paradigm will shorten the time and cost required to obtain regulatory approval.

The primary endpoint of I-SPY2 is pathological complete response (pCR), and incorporates longitudinal modeling of MRI volume as an auxiliary endpoint for decision making. As the trial progresses, the longitudinal model learns about the correlation between MRI volume and pCR, and this information is harnessed for patients with incomplete primary outcome data (pCR) in the calculation of predictive probabilities. An experimental treatment will graduate to a smaller focused phase 3 trial (randomized 1:1 vs. standard care) operationally seamless if the predictive

TABLE 13.1

Summary of Platform Trial Features

Features	ISPY-2	REMAP-CAP	GBM-AGILE	EPAD	DIAN-TU	Precision Promise	ADAPT	Ebola	PREPARE-ALICE	Cystic Fibrosis
Phase	2	4	2/3	2	3	2/3	3	3+4	4	4
Multiple Arms	Y	Y	Y	Y	Y	Y	Y	Y	Y	Y
Staggered Arms	Y	Y	Y	Y	Y	Y	Y	Y	N/Y	Y
Perpetual	Y	Y	Y	Y	Y	Y	Y	Y	N	Y
Embedded	N	Y	N	N	N/?	N/?	N	Y	Y	Y
Multifactorial	N	Y	N	N	N	N	N	Y	N	Y
Control?	Com	Y/N	Com	Com	Com	Com	Com	Either	Y	Y/N
Blinding	N	N	N	Y	Y	N	?	N	N	?
Enrichment	Y	Y	Y	Y	N	Y	Y	N	N	?
Interims	2w	1m	1m	3m	2y	1m	1m	1w	1y	?
Primary Time	6m	2m	TTE	Var/4y	4y+	TTE	<1m	2w	<1M	<1m
Prim. Bayesian	Y	Y	Y	Y	Y	Y	Y	Y	Y	Y
Adapt N	Y	Emb	Y	Flex/U	N	Y	Y	Emb	N	Emb
RAR	Y	Y	Y	N	N	Y	N	Y	N/Y	Y
Long. Model	Y	N/?	Exp	Y	Y	Exp	N	N	N	N
Drift Model	Y	Y	Y	N	N	Y	N	Y	Y	Y
Subgroups	Y	Y	Y	Y	N	Y	Y	N	Y	Y
Pred. Prob.	Y	N	Y	N	N	Y	N	N	N	?

Y = Yes, N = No, Com = Common, TTE = Time to Event, Var = variable, w = weeks, M = months, y = years
Emb = Embedded sample size, Flex/U = flexible sample size that is user(sponsor)-defined
Exp = Expected, ? = unknown

probability of success in the future phase 3 given current phase 2 data exceeds 0.85. In addition, I-SPY2 incorporates response adaptive randomization within subgroups in which allocation is proportional to the probability of being superior to control. The trial can drop or add treatment arms during the course of the trial, and includes modeling of the population-drift over time in the estimation of treatment effects. Additionally, a treatment arm can be restricted to a subset of the biomarker subgroups based on clinical data prior to entering the study.

3.2. Community Acquired Pneumonia

REMAP-CAP [13] is a large European platform trial funded by the European Commission for preparing against emerging epidemics. The objective of the trial is to determine the best care for community acquired pneumonia (CAP). The trial has distinct domains of treatment corresponding to antibiotic treatment (five choices), steroid treatment (yes vs. no), and the use of mechanical ventilation (yes vs. no). The impact of each of these treatment domains (and factors within a domain) is assessed within four distinct strata defined by the presence of shock and degree of hypoxemia. The primary outcome is mortality. Response adaptive randomization is driven by a statistical model with a full factorial design, including two-way and three-way interactions between the treatment domains. Prior distributions are calibrated to allow for the possibility of interaction effects, but only if there are sufficient data. The trial can add treatment domains or factors within a domain during the course of the trial.

REMAP-CAP currently has funding to enroll over 7,000 patients, and is intended to be perpetual in nature. One of the primary goals of the trial is to embed the study into routine care as a "Randomized Embedded, Multifactorial, Adaptive Platform (REMAP) trial" [14]. For every patient who presents with severe CAP, the clinical teams calls the interactive voice response system (IVRS) to collect the patient's randomized order set. This approach is a cost-effective strategy for simultaneously treating patients with best known care while simultaneously learning about effective therapies for various types of patients, and may be a glimpse of the future of randomized clinical trials.

3.3. Ebola

Based on recent outbreaks of the deadly Ebola virus, academics and industry have partnered to pre-emptively plan a platform trial design that can be used in the next Ebola epidemic [5]. Ebola is unique in that the outcome of interest is relatively short (14-day mortality) and there is no known effective therapy. For a number of reasons unique to the disease and third-world location, it is impractical to conduct traditional clinical trials with one or two experimental treatments per trial. Rather, a platform trial that focuses on the best treatment of the disease is ideal in this setting. Response adaptive randomization is critical in this context, as we want to quickly move away from ineffective therapies and allocate patients to the more promising arms. The trial has primary and secondary agents, as well as combinations of primary agents plus secondary agents. Controversially, a standard of care arm can also be included, which receives a minimum of 20% of patients until it is replaced by a more effective agent. 50% of the remaining patients are allocated to single-agent arms and the other 50% are allocated to combination arms. However, the master protocol allows the exclusion of a control arm depending on available therapies at the time of the epidemic. The design incorporates Bayesian RAR and modeling for population drift.

A notable feature of this design is that the treatment labels in the master protocol are completely generic, and when the time comes to implement this trial, these specific drugs/agents are simply inserted into the trial based on the master protocol, with simulations updated depending on the number of available treatments, and the trial design is ready for implementation. Speed is of the essence in this setting, as the trial must begin enrolling patients before the epidemic peaks.

3.4. Alzheimer's Disease

DIAN-TU is a phase II/III platform trial in Dominantly Inherited Alzheimer's Disease [11,12], which is a rare form of Alzheimer's caused by a gene mutation. It has an early age of onset and provides rare opportunity to enroll preclinical patients that are certain to progress. The DIAN platform trial design employs an innovative disease progression model for the modeling of the primary endpoint (based a long term observational cohort). The model estimates a proportional treatment effect in the randomized study to assess slowing in the rate of cognitive progression. The trial incorporates multiple treatments, in which the placebo group for a given treatment includes all patients that would have been eligible to be randomized to that treatment. Early biomarker analyses are used to demonstrate target modulation or to stop an arm early for futility.

The European Prevention of Alzheimer's Dementia Consortium (EPAD) [15] has launched a phase II platform trial in Alzheimer's disease with the goal of understanding the early stages of the disease and preventing dementia before symptoms occur. The trial randomizes patients to multiple interventions within multiple groups' biomarker-driven subgroups. The primary analysis uses an innovative Bayesian model to compare the rate of disease progression for a given treatment versus placebo. The trial design includes regular master protocol evolution analyses, and monitors interventions for early futility or success based on measured cognitive effect.

3.5. Antibiotics

ADAPT [16] is a platform trial design in antibiotics with the goal of providing an efficient pathway to evaluate multiple potential novel agents in multiple body sites, in a unique context where a successful treatment for a resistant pathogen should be used minimally to preserve its effectiveness. The trial design includes the sharing of a control arm across multiple agents; adaptive starting and stopping of novel agents with a potentially perpetual time frame, and hierarchical borrowing of information across body sites. This design does not use response adaptive randomization because finding the second and third best drugs are highly valued objectives, as opposed to single goal of finding the best drug. Hence power for comparing each treatment versus control is preserved for all arms by using a fixed randomization scheme.

3.6. Brain Cancer

GBM-AGILE (Glioblastoma Multiforme Adaptive Global Innovative Learning Environment) [17] is a phase 2/3 platform trial in glioblastoma multiforme and is similar conceptually to I-SPY2. Its design features therapies that enter and exit the trial at different times, and it combines the inferential tasks of screening new therapies for efficacy, identifying populations who benefit from therapies, and confirming treatment effects. Drugs may enter a trial with targeted biomarker subgroups. Response adaptive randomization is used to allocate patients within biomarker subgroups to more effective treatments (maximum of 150 patients per arm in phase 2), with overall survival as the primary outcome. A longitudinal model is used to harness the correlation between MRI and performance status with overall survival. Extensive simulations are used to show appropriate power and Type I error in order to support registration. The trial is privately funded and is the collaborative effort of academics, industry (drug makers), and the FDA.

3.7. Cystic Fibrosis

A platform trial design is also currently being planned in Australia to investigate treatment of patients with Cystic Fibrosis (CF), which is a genetic disorder characterized by persistent respiratory infections. Similar to REMAP-CAP conceptually, the trial design incorporates multiple domains for the treatment of CF-induced pulmonary exacerbations, such as primary antibiotic, adjunct antibiotic, muco-active therapy, immunomodulation therapy, and airway clearance; in which each domain has multiple factors of treatment. In addition, the trial recognizes the hetero-geneity of patient response with subgroups defined by age, CF mutation type, and bacterial colonization. The trial is expected to enroll up to 5,000 patients. Response adaptive randomization is used to efficiently navigate the large dimensional space from treatment by subgroup interactions, and treatments may be added or dropped throughout the trial.

3.8. Influenza

PREPARE-ALICE [18] is a sister trial to REMAP-CAP funded by the European Commission, but with a focus on influenza. The platform trial is a pragmatic trial designed to evaluate the benefits of antiviral medica-tions versus usual care in the treatment of patients presenting with influenza-like symptoms. The trial has 36 pre-specified subpopulations defined by combinations of age, severity of illness, duration of symptoms at time of initial visit, and the presence of comorbidities, with a primary outcome of time to return to usual activities with only minor presence of flu-like symptoms. The design incorporate Bayesian modeling for the estimation of treatment effects within the 36 subpopulations. Although the trial currently only has two treatment arms (one antiviral versus usual care), the master protocol allows for additional antiviral medications to be added during the course of the trial, in which case RAR will be used for patient allocation.

3.9. Pancreatic Cancer

Precision Promise [19] is a platform trial in pancreatic cancer. Therapies may enter the trial at different times and are evaluated within multiple patient sub-populations. A therapy may graduate from an exploratory stage to a confirmatory stage within a targeted population. The design incorporates response adaptive randomization, and allows patients to be re-randomized to a new treatment if the first treatment is ineffective.

---

4. Other Considerations

4.1. Statistical Efficiencies of Platform Trials

Recall the traditional drug development paradigm of evaluating a single treatment versus a control in a homogenous group of patients. In addition to the conceptual advantage of addressing the relevant question pertaining to the practicing clinician, platform trial designs can also have substantial statistical advantages relative to this traditional paradigm (e.g., power, sample size, etc.). The most obvious statistical efficiency is savings in sample size due to the sharing of a common control arms between multiple experimental treatments. For example, a fixed (non-adaptive) trial with two experimental therapies versus a common control would require 25% fewer patients total than two independent two-arm trials in order to maintain power for evaluating the same hypotheses.

Saville and Berry [2] conducted a simulation study to quantify the statistical efficiencies of a platform trial strategy versus the traditional two-arm paradigm of drug development. They considered a relatively simple setting with a binary outcome in a disease with severe morbidity and for which many experimental treatments exist, of which only a small proportion are effective (e.g., cancer). They compare two general strategies for drug development:

1. A sequence of traditional two-arm trials comparing a single treatment versus a control, which is repeated until a beneficial treatment is found
2. A perpetual platform trial comparing five active treatments versus a control, in which treatments are dropped and new ones added per a master protocol, which continues until a beneficial treatment is found

The authors considered variations of the above designs which incorporated adaptive features such as response adaptive randomization, adaptive stopping, and arm dropping/adding. The platform trial design was superior to the traditional paradigm on every evaluated metric. The platform trial design required fewer patients, had better overall patient outcomes, required less time, and had a greater probability of finding a beneficial treatment that the traditional strategy. In fact, the perpetual platform trial design could result in as much as 70% savings in sample size compared to the traditional strategy!

4.2. Embedding within Health Care Systems

Unlike most traditional trials, platform trial designs are uniquely suited to be embedded within existing clinical care systems. This is because 1) the focus of platform trials is on the disease with many options for treatment; 2) platform trials can account for heterogeneity of patient response; and 3) a primary goal is often to treat patients better during the course of a platform trial. In addition, the goals of platform trial designs typically align with the task of the practicing physician (i.e., to determine the best treatment for a single unique patient). Hence, it is natural and cost-effective to embed such trials within existing health care systems. This concept is summarized nicely by Angus [14] and is referred to as a "Randomized Embedded, Multifactorial, Adaptive Platform (REMAP) trial." Electronic health records and interactive response systems (IRS) enable the enrollment and randomization of patients in real time. Frequent analyses can be automated to update the randomization probabilities and evaluate treatments according to the master protocol. As platform trials become more prevalent and understood by patients and the health care industry, we anticipate a significant number of future randomized trials will be embedded within health care systems.

4.3. Concurrent Comparisons

One of the challenges associated with platform trials in which treatments can have staggered entry is how to manage comparisons between treatments (e.g., test vs. control) if patients between treatments are not randomized concurrently. For example, suppose an experimental treatment is added 2 years into a platform trial in which a control arm has been enrolling patients since the start of the trial. Should patients with the new treatment be compared to all control patients, or compared only to control patients who are enrolled during the same window of time as the new treatment? It seems wasteful and grossly inefficient to ignore the control data collected prior to the time of the new treatment entering the trial, yet there is a risk of bias in the comparison of the new treatment versus control if there is a population drift over time. Furthermore, how does one compare the new treatment versus a treatment that was previously dropped or graduated from the study? The solution is to provide a comparison between treatments that explicitly models and accounts for the population drift over time. This harnesses all available information in the comparison arms, yet avoids the issue of bias and confounding across time. This is possible mathematically because there is overlap among the treatments over the course of the trial. Such modeling is currently being implemented in I-SPY2 (mathematical details and papers are forthcoming), and is helpful in any trial with response adaptive randomization in which population drift may effect patient response over the course of the trial.

4.4. Operational Bias

Operational bias in in clinical trials is often minimized through the blinding of treatment assignments to both patients and investigators, as well as limiting investigator access to aggregate outcome data. In traditional two-arm clinical trials, the blinding of treatment assignment are relatively straightforward in many disease areas. However, in platform trial designs there may be additional complexity, in which there is blinding to active or control, but also to which possible experimental arm. As an example, suppose there are three experimental agents; A, B, and C, each with a control matching their experimental agent, A0, B0, and C0. Subjects could be blinded to active vs control, but aware of which experimental cohort (A,

B, C). Full blinding may require many "masking" therapies (A0, B0, and C0) to blind a subject on A0. This can be incredibly onerous and even impossible when there are arms with staggered enrollment. Such is the setting in the DIAN Alzheimer's trial, in which patients know the cohort (A/B) but not whether they are randomized to active or control. In such settings, investigators must carefully consider the different aspects of treatment blinding relative to the risks of operational bias.

Relatedly, investigators must also consider whether operational bias could occur due to unintentional unblinding of trial outcome results. With response adaptive randomization and potentially unblinded experimental cohorts, it may become obvious to investigators which intervention is performing best. Moreover, in trials with staggered entries and potential graduation such as I-SPY2, sponsors of the failed or graduated therapies may desire to see full outcome data pertaining to their particular intervention; but the disclosure of shared control data may potentially disclose information pertaining to the ongoing trial.

For these issues, there is no single remedy that will alleviate the concern of operational bias within a platform trial design. Rather, each platform trial is unique and all pertinent factors must be carefully considered and addressed prior to running the trial.

4.5. Regulatory Interactions

Many of the trials discussed above have involved substantial regulatory interaction with the FDA, and have benefitted tremendously from the collaboration of regulatory personnel. In general, representatives of the FDA (including CDER) have been very supportive and proponents of platform trials. High level leaders, most notably Woodock and LaVange [20], have been quoted in various settings emphasizing the key role that such trials will play in the future of drug development. Because of the complexity in planning platform trials, and the large number of simulations required to evaluate statistical properties of such designs, it is imperative to involve regulatory agencies in the initial stages of planning.

5. Conclusion

Adaptive platform trial designs provide a path for evaluating medical treatments in a future with increasingly complex science and solutions. Such designs can improve statistical efficiency and address the research questions most pertinent to the practicing physician. Advancing technology with real-time patient data collection, randomization, and analyses will help overcome logistical challenges of platform trial implementation.

Extensive simulation studies are essential in the trial design process by enabling investigators and regulatory agencies to understand and calibrate design performance. When properly implemented, platform trial designs will provide tremendous benefit to science, physicians, and most importantly patients.

References

1. Berry SM, Connor JT, Lewis RJ. The platform trial: An efficient strategy for evaluating multiple treatments. *Journal of the American Medical Association*. doi: 10.1001/jama.2015.2316, 2015.
2. Saville BR,, Berry SM. Efficiencies of platform clinical trials: A vision of the future. *Clinical Trials*, 13(3): 358–366, 2016.
3. Berry DA. Emerging innovations in clinical trial design. *Clinical Pharmacology & Therapeutics*, 99(1): 82–91, 2016.
4. Berry DA. Adaptive clinical trials: The promise and the caution. *Journal of Clinical Oncology*, 29(6): 606–609, 2011. PMID: 21172875.
5. Berry SM, Petzold EA, Dull P, Thielman NM, Cunningham CK, Corey GR, McClain MT, Hoover DL, Russell J, Griffiss JM, et al. A response adaptive randomization platform trial for efficient evaluation of Ebola virus treatments: A model for pandemic response. *Clinical Trials*, 13(1): 22–30, 2016.
6. SteinC. Inadmissibility of the usual estimator for the mean of a multivariate normal distribution. *Proceedings of the Third Berkeley Symposium on Mathematical Statistics and Probability*, 1: 197–206, 1956.
7. Berry DA. Bayesian clinical trials. *Nature Reviews Drug Discovery*, 5(1): 27–36, 2006.
8. Saville BR, Connor JT, Ayers GD, Alvarez J. The utility of Bayesian predictive probabilities for interim monitoring of clinical trials. *Clinical Trials*, 11(4): 485–493, 2014.
9. Barker AD, Sigman CC, Kelloff GJ, Hylton NM, Berry DA, Esserman LJ. I-SPY2: An adaptive breast cancer trial design in the setting of neoadjuvant chemotherapy. *Clinical Pharmacology & Therapeutics*, 86(1): 97–100, 2009.
10. Berry SM, Carlin BP, Lee JJ, Muller P. *Bayesian adaptive methods for clinical trials.* CRC Press Taylor & Francis Group, Boca Raton, FL.
11. The Dominantly Inherited Alzheimer Network. https://dian.wustl.edu/, 2018.
12. Dominantly inherited Alzheimer Network Trial: An opportunity to prevent dementia. A study of potential disease modifying treatments in individuals at risk for or with a type of early onset Alzheimer's disease caused by a genetic mutation. (DIAN-TU), https://clinicaltrials.gov/ct2/show/NCT01760005, 2013.
13. Randomized, embedded, multifactorial adaptive platform trial for community-acquired pneumonia (REMAP-CAP). https://clinicaltrials.gov/ct2/show/NCT01760005, 2017.
14. Angus DC. Fusing randomized trials with big data: The key to self-learning health care systems? *JAMA*, 314(8): 767–768, 2015.
15. European Prevention of Alzheimer's Dementia Consortium, http://ep-ad.org/, 2018.

16. Antibiotic Platform Design, www.berryconsultants.com/antibiotic-platform-design/, 2017.

17. Alexander BM, Sujuan B, Berger MS, Berry DA, Cavenee WK, Chang SM, Cloughesy TF, Jiang T, Khasraw M, Wenbin L, et al. Adaptive global innovative learning environment for glioblastoma: GBM AGILE. *Clinical Cancer Research*, http://clincancerres.aacrjournals.org/content/early/2017/09/20/1078-0432. CCR-17-0764, 2017.

18. Platform for European Preparedness Against (Re-)emerging Epidemics, https://www.prepare-europe.eu/About-us/Workpackages/Workpackage-4, 2015.

19. Precision Promise, www.pancan.org/research/precision-promise/, 2017.

20. Woodcock J, La VangeLM. Master protocols to study multiple therapies, multiple diseases, or both. *New England Journal of Medicine*, 377(1): 62–70, 2017.

14

Efficiencies of Platform Trials

Satrajit Roychoudhury and Ohad Amit

1. Introduction

Platform trials have the potential to drive tremendous efficiencies in the development of new therapeutics. These efficiencies can be operational or statistical in nature. Statistical efficiencies are derived from many sources including the use of a shared control arm and adaptive randomization. In rare or difficult to enroll populations, platform trials offer the opportunity to steer important new therapies into a standing clinical trials infrastructure, potentially expediting the availability of badly needed new therapies. Efficiency can also be gained from statistical modeling to formally leverage both historical information and concurrent information in related populations. In this chapter, the various sources of efficiency will be described in more detail and examples will be provided to demonstrate their relative contribution to a more economical paradigm for clinical trials.

The majority of this chapter will be focused on statistical efficiencies offered by platform trials. It is worth reviewing and documenting many operational efficiencies.

2. Operational Efficiencies

Significant up-front investment is often required for platform trials. This has created a perception that platform trials are innately complex and difficult to execute. After up-front investment, there are many operational efficiencies to be realized once the trial is initiated. The benefits of platform trials include:

- Pooling of resources
- Decreased trial costs for sponsors

- Standardization of medical practice
- Standardization of data collection

To date, most platform trials have been designed as public-private and inter-company collaborations. When designed as such, there are clear benefits that arise from pooling of resources. For example, a public or non-profit group may sponsor a platform trial with multiple companies contributing drugs into the platform, thus sharing the cost across multiple organizations and requiring less investment from individual companies. This framework may be particularly useful in rare diseases or difficult to enroll populations where both resources and patients are scarce.

An important advantage of platform trials is the ability to bring new treatments into the trial without writing a new protocol. This is typically accomplished through a master protocol which provides details of the trial in a treatment agnostic fashion. Details of individual treatments and associated requirements are provided separately as new treatments are ready to enter the platform. Typically, this is achieved through appendices that can be bolted on to the master protocol. The advantages of this approach are apparent given the time and resources required to create separate protocols for each treatment one wishes to study.

Platform trials are at times referred to as standing trials. This is an appropriate reference to the fact that such trials offer a standing platform by which to evaluate interventions in one or even multiple disease states. This provides an immediate and obvious operational benefit to researchers. Rather than writing, reviewing, and implementing multiple protocols to evaluate multiple treatments a single infrastructure can be used instead. This offers considerable savings in terms of up-front investment that is typically required to initiate a study. These savings should offset any additional logistical costs associated with initiating platform trials relative to a traditional clinical trial.

Standardization of data collection and medical practice are additional operational efficiencies offered by platform trials. Standardization of medical practice is particularly relevant in rare disease settings, where a platform trial may represent one of the few treatment options for patients. Standardization of data collection is desirable regardless of disease state. Such standardization offers researchers and regulators an efficient way to analyze and interpret data.

3. Statistical Efficiencies

There are many statistical efficiencies to be gained from platform trials. The most notable is the use of a shared control arm. Historically, not all platform trials have used a shared control. Several recent examples are useful to document. The I-SPY2 trial does allows for a shared control arm within the various biomarker defined strata [1]. The new GBM-AGILE trial also allows for a shared control [2]. The Lung-MAP trial does not use a shared control [3]. ADAPT, a proposed platform trial in multi-drug resistant bacterial infections also uses a shared control within the different sites of infection [4]. Subjects in this trial are stratified into cohorts based on a biomarker profile. Each cohort has a unique control arm.

The efficiencies of a shared control arm, manifested by a reduction in sample size are great. Complex statistical methodology is not required to elucidate them. A simple example is used to illustrate. Suppose one were designing a platform trial to evaluate four experimental treatments concurrently in a disease state of interest. The required sample size to run a phase 2 study for each experimental treatment is 120 subjects randomized equally between the experimental and control arms. If separate phase 2 studies are initiated for each of the four treatments, 480 subjects would be required with a total of 240 patients randomized to control. Now consider if we studied all these four experimental treatments concurrently in a platform trial. A total of 300 subjects would be needed with 60 subjects randomized to the control arm. This amounts to a 37.5% reduction in total sample size and 75% reduction in the number needed to be treated on a control arm. The reduction in sample size of 180 patients allows for three additional arms to potentially join the platform trial. The savings are illustrated in a figure that looks at percent savings in total sample size and in control as a function of the number of arms concurrently studied (Figure 14.1).

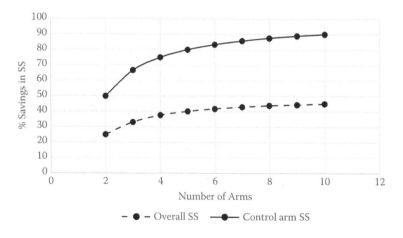

FIGURE 14.1
Savings in Overall and Control Arm Sample Size.

In practice, all treatments will not be studied concurrently and this will lead to some loss in efficiency. Using the same example as above, suppose that we now study two treatments versus control in the platform trial initially followed by two additional treatments versus control. The total sample size now becomes 360 with a total of 120 subjects treated on control, a 25% and 50% savings respectively. This loss in efficiency can be mitigated by further minimizing randomization to the control and augmenting the control arm with the non-contemporaneous control arm data collected earlier in the trial. Statistical methods to augment the control arm will be described later in this chapter. Continuing further with our example, now suppose we only randomized 20 patients to the control arm for the second set of two experimental treatments that come into the trial. the trial size is now 320 with 80 subjects randomized to control, a respective savings of 33% and 67% in total number of subjects and subjects randomized to control. We have provided an illustrative and simple example with the aim of elucidating the extremes (maximum and minimum in savings) of what can be accomplished by using a shared control within a platform trial. It is important to again acknowledge that in practice there will be overlap between when treatments leave and enter a platform trial.

Another consideration when using a common control to evaluate multiple treatments is control of the overall type 1 error. Coming back to our example of four experimental treatments, if four independent trials are run the overall type 1 error (i.e., the chance of at rejecting the null hypothesis for at least one treatment) is $1 - (0.95)^4$ or 0.19. We contrast this with a worst-case scenario for the platform trial of 0.25 which assumes almost perfect correlation in the comparisons. For two experimental treatments, the overall type 1 error approximates to 0.0975 as compared to 0.1. There is minimal inflation in the overall type 1 error when studying interventions in a platform trial with a common control versus independent trials. This does not suggest that type 1 error should not be a consideration in platform trials as it should in the development of any therapeutic intervention, but rather suggests there is only a minimal amount of additional likelihood that we would carry ineffective treatment by studying them in a platform trial versus studying them in independent trials.

We noted previously that there are several statistical methods that allow for borrowing of information from historical sources. There are several sources of external data that can be leveraged into a platform trial, and several mechanisms by which that data can be leveraged. We will restrict our discussion here to leveraging additional data into the control arm. There are predominantly two sources of historical that could be leveraged into a platform trial. Often there are multiple trials in the same disease state with the same control arm as the platform trial. This is a potential important source of historical data external to the platform trial. A second is the non-contemporaneous data generated on the control arm within the platform trial itself. Some platform trials have been designed such that an experimental arm is only compared to the control arm data generated contemporaneously with the enrollment of the former [5]. While this offers the most robust comparison in terms exchangeability of the data, it also ignores a large amount of data generated on the control arm under identical experimental conditions. At the other extreme is a straight pooling of the contemporaneous and non-contemporaneous control-arm data. This is approach seems reasonable when a platform trial is open for a short time. When there a significant time-lag in collection of the data on the control arm in a platform trial spanning many years, pooling may not be appropriate. To further drive the efficiency of platform trials, it is important to leverage this data. In the next part of this chapter we provide statistical methods for incorporating both historical and non-contemporaneous control arm data.

4. Statistical Methodology to Incorporate Historical Information for a Control Arm in Platform Trial

In this section, we describe a statistical methodology to incorporate historical control data in a platform trial. Figure 14.2 shows two design strategies of platform trial with multiple treatments. Strategy 1 in Figure 14.2 allows *concurrent control* to each treatment arm. This is a sequence of traditional two-arm trials comparing a single treatment versus control. This design is appropriate when the target populations are treatment specific, e.g., biomarker driven treatment (BATTLE trial) [6]. The success or failure of a treatment depends on the pairwise comparison of each treatment with corresponding control. In contrast; strategy 2 is a platform trial design with *shared control* [5]. In this design, a fixed proportion of subjects will be always allocated to a shared control arm. If the patient population is wide, design strategy 2 is appropriate. In this strategy, each treatment will be compared with the shared control arm. Both strategies are dynamic in nature as in practice not all treatments are available at the beginning of the trial. Therefore, each treatment arm (and corresponding control) can start at different times during trial.

Each strategy has certain advantages and disadvantages. Strategy 2 is appealing to practitioners as less number of patients are exposed to control (or standard of care [SOC]). However, if clinical efficacy is heterogeneous among different disease characteristics the study results will be questionable and require larger sample size for appropriate comparison. Moreover, if the trial recruitment is slow, the shared control group may not be homogeneous enough due to a change in clinical practice. Strategy 1 typically requires higher sample size for the control group, but allows a formal comparison when target patient population varies among experimental treatments. The sample size under strategy 1 can

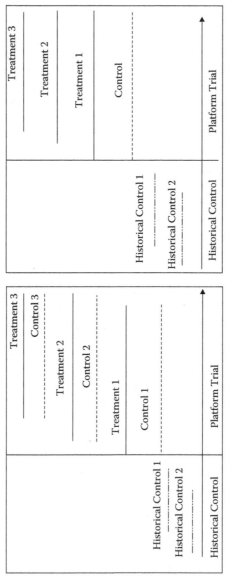

FIGURE 14.2
Platform Trial Designs with Historical Data.

be reduced by combining information across different control arms. In certain scenarios it is acceptable, as the underlying disease is the same. However, this poses an additional statistical challenge. A robust statistical methodology is required to combine information from different sources in the analysis.

Several statistical methodologies are available in the literature for borrowing information from historical sources. The notable ones include the *bias model* [7], *power prior* [8], *commensurate prior* [9] and the *meta-analytic predictive prior* [10,11]. However, modifications are required to incorporate these methods in a *co-data* setting. In the next section, we have described a meta-analytic framework for a platform trial with concurrent and shared control. The proposed methodology is in a Bayesian framework and adopted from [12]. Similar techniques can be applied to other types of platform trials [5]. This methodology is further illustrated using a simulated example of a platform trial in Non-small cell lung cancer (NSCLC).

4.1. Meta-Analytic Combined (MAC) Approach for Platform Trial with Concurrent Control

We consider a platform trial comparing M test treatments with concurrent control (strategy 1). Furthermore, relevant historical data on the control group is available. The aim is to borrow across historical and concurrent control for efficient design (e.g., smaller sample size). We assume Y_1, Y_2, ..., Y_H are data of control arm from H historical trials and Y_{*1}, Y_{*2}, ..., Y_{*M}, are the contemporaneous control data generated within the platform trial. The structure of the data suggests a hierarchical model to model Y_h's (h = 1, 2, ..., H) and Y_{*l}'s together.

$$Y_h \sim F(\theta_h); Y_{*l} \sim F(\theta_{*l})$$
$$\theta_h, \theta_{*l}|\tau \sim G(\omega, \tau); \quad h = 1, 2, \ldots, H \, and \, 1 = 1, 2, \ldots, M \qquad (1)$$
$$\omega, \tau \sim P_1, P_2$$

Where θ_h and θ_{*l} are the control parameters associated with historical and current study. F, G, P_i (i = 1, 2) are the likelihood, parameter model and priors for hyper-parameters respectively. The simplest parameter model (G) to link the parameters in historical and current study assumes "*exchangeability*" when no study level predictors are available. This assumption can be extended to "*partial exchangeability*" if clinically important predictors are present. Especially, for non-contemporaneous control arm data, a time effect needs to be the part of the model. For example, if the endpoint is binary (e.g., the number of responders) then under exchangeability the equation (1) is reduced to

$$Y_h \sim Bin(n_h, p_h); \; Y_{*l} \sim Bin(n_{*l}, p_{*l})$$
$$\theta_h, \theta_{*l} \mid \mu, \tau \sim N(\mu, \tau^2); \quad h = 1, 2, \ldots, H, \tag{2}$$
$$\theta_h = logit(p_h), \; \theta_* = logit(p_*)$$

n_h and n_{*l} are the sizes of historical and control arms of new platform trial respectively. Note that the weight of historical data depends on the *between trial heterogeneity* parameter τ. One way to quantify the amount of borrowing is *effective sample size (ESS)*. We calculated the ESS using ratio of variance approach [10].

$$ESS_{*l} = ESS_0 \frac{Var_0}{Var_{*l}}$$

where ESS_0 and Var_0 are the ESS and posterior variance respectively under complete pooling. Var_{*l} is the posterior variance under MAC model.

However, for platform a trial the model (2) requires some additional flexibility. We propose two extensions of model (2) to incorporate historical control and concurrent control data simultaneously in the analysis.

1. We extend the parameter model in (2) from one to K between-trial standard deviations. Since the quality of *co-data* can vary across historical and contemporaneous control, introducing different between-trial standard deviations can be useful. For the platform trial in Figure 14.1, two standard deviations ($K = 2$) are advised. In case of more complex setting $K > 2$ can be used.

2. The second extension allows each parameter θ_h and θ_{*l} to deviate from parameter model in (2). That is, it may be nonexchangeable with any of the other parameters. On the one hand, this adds robustness to the model for mis-alignment between data from different sources, but on the other hand implies less borrowing from the *co-data* (lower ESS). Non-exchangeability is introduced by the mixture model.

The extended model can be expressed as

$$y_h \sim Bin(n_h, p_h); \; Y_{*l} \sim Bin(n_{*l}, p_{*l})$$
$$\theta_h = logit(p_h), \; \theta_* = \log it(p_*)$$
$$\theta_h = p_h \theta_h' + (1 - p_h)\theta_h''; \quad h = 1, 2, \ldots H$$
$$\theta_{*l} = p_l \theta_{*l}' + (1 - p_l)\theta_l''; \quad l = 1, 2, \ldots \ldots M \tag{3}$$
$$\theta_h' \mid \mu, \tau_1 \sim N(\mu, \tau_1^2), \theta_h'' \sim N(m_h, v_h^2)$$
$$\theta_{*l}' \mid \mu, \tau_2 \sim N(\mu, \tau_2^2), \theta_{*l}'' \sim N(mm_l, vv_l^2)$$

Weakly informative priors can be used for μ and θ''_{*l}. For example, we suggest the use of unit information prior [13]. The mixture weights p_h and p_l represents the degree of confidence on the historical control and concurrent control data. Below are the few characteristics of model parameter in (3)

- $p_h = p_l = 0$ and $\tau_1 = \tau_2 = 0$: complete pooling of the historical and concurrent control data
- $p_l = 0$ and $\tau_2 = 0$: complete pooling of concurrent control data evolved during platform trial
- $p_h = 0$ and $\tau_1 = 0$: complete pooling of historical control data

Mixture parameters are fixed *a-priori* in the model (3). Standard Bayesian calculus for mixture models [14,15] implies that the mixture weights for the posterior distributions will be updated. The latter depend on the a-priori weights and on how likely the data are under the mixture components.

For platform trial with a shared control (strategy 2 in Figure 14.2), the MAC approach described above is still applicable. For a shared control, equation (3) can still be applied with M = 1 and $\tau_1 = \tau_2$. Alternatively, the Meta-analytic predictive (MAP) approach can be used to derive an informative prior for a shared control arm using available historical data. MAC and MAP approaches are theoretically equivalent.

Finally, in practice τ_1 and τ_2 are often unknown. Especially when H is small, it is not feasible to estimate τ_1 and τ_2 from small number of estimates of trial parameters. Therefore, prior judgements are required for τ_1 and τ_2. We suggest a weakly informative prior for τ_1 and τ_2 that covers a wide range of plausible values of between trial heterogeneity. Typically half-normal, half-t, half-Cauchy, and log-normal priors have been used [10,11]. For example, in the binary case a half-normal prior with scale parameter 0.5 implies a prior median of 0.34 and 95% prior interval (0.016, 1.12). This covers small to large between trial heterogeneity. A larger value of the scale parameter for a half-normal distribution allows larger between trial heterogeneity and higher discounting of the data. However, in practice the historical data is chosen under stringent conditions [7]. Therefore, it is reasonable to use priors that allow non-negligible weights to historical data.

Analytical forms of the posterior distribution of θ_{*l} from model (3) are not tractable except in some simple cases. Closed form expressions are provided in [10] for simple normal-normal hierarchical model (NNHM) with fixed values of $\tau(\tau_1 = \tau_2)$ and $p_h = p_l = 0$. For (3), MCMC sampling is required for estimating the trial specific parameters. This can be achieved using the modern computation tools, e.g., WinBUGS, JAGS, STAN, etc.

5. Application

We now introduce a phase II platform study to compare four experimental treatments with Docetaxel in second line NSCLC. Docetaxel is an approved treatment for locally advanced or metastatic NSCLC. Patients will be randomized either in one of the four experimental treatments arm or the concurrent Docetaxel arm. Experimental drugs with considerable advantage over Docetaxel will be considered for further development. The ORR data for Docetaxel in second line NSCLC is available from four historical studies (Table 14.1). There is substantial variability present in the historical ORR of Docetaxel (2.5%–8.8%) [16].

To expedite the overall development, the trial will start with two experimental treatments. The remaining two experimental drugs will be introduced 2 months after the trial starts. Therefore, the response data for concurrent Docetaxel arms will be available at later time points during the trial. For simplicity, we assume one final analysis after all data is available. The final analysis will be performed in the Bayesian method in order to utilize all the available data. However, the proposed methodology is flexible enough to incorporate intermediate analysis.

The number of responders for the i-th treatment and Docetaxel arms are denoted by $r_T^{(i)}$ and $r_C^{(i)}$ (i = 1, 2, 3, 4). The likelihood is given by

$$r_T^{(i)} \sim Bin(n_T^{(i)}, \pi_T^{(i)}) \text{ and } r_c^{(i)} \sim Bin(n_c^{(i)}, \pi_c^{(i)})$$

The measure of interest is the difference in ORR $\delta^{(i)} = \pi_T^{(i)} - \pi_c^{(i)}$. An experimental treatment is declared promising if the posterior probability of experimental arm better than Docetaxel is at least 95%, i.e., $P(\delta^{(i)} > 0|data) > 0.95$.

Under the alternative hypothesis $\delta^{(i)} = 0.3$, each comparison will require 80 patients (40 per arm) for 90% power and 2.5% Type-I error. Since historical and concurrent information for other Docetaxel arms are available at the time of analysis, we'll reduce the sample size in each Docetaxel arm. In addition, we'll also look into shared control platform design.

TABLE 14.1

Historical Data of Docetaxel in Second Line NSCLC

Study	Treatment	N	ORR (%) and 95% CI
TAX317 [17]	Docetaxel 75 mg/m^2 q21	55	5.5 (1.1–15.1)
TAX320 [18]	Docetaxel 75 mg/m^2 q21	120	6.7 (3.1–13.1)
DISTAL-01 [19]	Docetaxel 75 mg/m^2 q21	110	2.7 (0.5–7.8)
JMEI [20]	Docetaxel 75 mg/m^2 q21	288	8.8 (5.7–12.5)

6. Hypothetic Case Study

Below are the two hypothetic trial scenarios to illustrate the statistical inference. For this analysis we have assumed $\tau_1 \sim$ HalfNormal(0.5) and $\tau_2 \sim$ HalfNormal(0.25). The heterogeneity between different control arms may be driven by the biomarker or other patients characteristics. This allows higher discounting of the historical data compare to concurrent or shared control data. We have used three models for the analysis;

1. **MAC:** This assumes $p_h = p_l = 1$. This model assumes complete exchangeability of the historical and on-study control data.
2. **rMAC:** This assumes $p_h = p_l = 0.5$. This model allows non-exchangeability between historical data and current data in order to handle prior-data conflict.
3. **Stratified:** This model allows no borrowing. A weakly informative beta prior (centered at 10%) is used to analyze the on study control data.

Finally, a weakly informative beta prior (centered at 10%) is used to analyze the data from treatment arms.

Table 14.2 shows two data analysis for concurrent control and shared control cases. Both MAC and rMAC models increase precision of the estimate by borrowing information across arms and helps to make a sensible decision. The MAC model often borrows aggressively, however, both of them provide better precision than the stratified model.

7. Operating Characteristics

Finally, we have done a small simulation study to understand the long term operating characteristics of the MAC and rMAC designs. The simulations are performed for a concurrent control setting. It assumes

1. 5:1 randomization between treatment and concurrent control: 40 patients for each treatment arm and eight patients for concurrent control
2. Success criteria: $P(\delta^{(i)} > 0 | data) > 0.95$
3. We assume one final analysis after all data is collected.

We assume two scenarios: a) the true control rates of the platform trial are aligned with the historical control data from four Docetaxel trials, b) it is not aligned. 1,000 simulations are performed using MAC and rMAC models. Overall rMAC provides a better control of Type-I error and

TABLE 14.2

Hypothetic Data and On-trial Decisions

Control Arms$(r_c^{(i)}/n_c^{(i)})$	Experimental Arms$(r_T^{(i)}/n_T^{(i)})$	Analysis Method	Posterior Summary$(\delta^{(i)})$	$P(\delta^{(i)} > 0\|data)$
Concurrent Control (Strategy 1)				
1/8, 1/8, 2/8, 2/8	10/40, 5/40, 16/40, 9/40	MAC	0.15 (–0.01, 0,30)	0.9701
			0.03 (–0.11, 0.16)	0.6641
			0.29 (0.11, 0.46)	0.9985
			0.12 (–0.04, 0.27)	0.9372
		rMAC	0.14 (–0.10, 0.31)	0.9117
			0.02 (–0.22, 0.16)	0.6021
			0.24 (–0.15, 0.44)	0.9097
			0.07 (–0.31, 0.25)	0.7103
		Stratified	0.14 (–0.16, 0.33)	0.8504
			0.02 (0.18, 0.58)	0.5827
			0.17 (–0.18, 0.42)	0.8477
			0.00 (–0.34, 0.24)	0.5131
Shared Control (Strategy 2)				
4/20	10/40, 5/40, 16/40, 9/40	MAC	0.15 (0.02, 0.31)	0.9848
			0.03 (–0.08, 0.16)	0.7267
			0.30 (0.14, 0.46)	0.9996
			0.13 (–0.00, 0.28)	0.9716
		rMAC	0.14 (–0.05, 0.30)	0.8232
			0.02 (–0.16, 0.15)	0.4511
			0.27 (–0.03, 0.44)	0.9696
			0.10 (–0.19, 0.26)	0.7771
		Stratified	0.06 (–0.17, 0.25)	0.6922
			–0.07 (–0.17, 0.11)	0.2387
			0.20 (–0.03, 0.40)	0.9525
			0.03 (–0.19, 0.22)	0.6151

reasonable power under both alignment and conflict case (Table 14.3). For MAC the Type-I error is significantly inflated under co-data conflicts (almost 10%).

The purpose of this simulation study is to provide a general idea about the design behavior. Further extensions are possible by allowing heterogeneity among different control arms and using shared control. Another interesting feature will be adding the interim analysis into a simulation.

8. Discussion

In the preceding pages the various sources of efficiency arising from platform trials have been documented. Numerous operational efficiencies have been

TABLE 14.3

Frequentist Operating Characteristics

True Control Rate (%)	MAC	rMAC
Null:		
$\delta^{(i)} = 0$	0.024, 0.024, 0.048, 0.036	0.004, 0.020, 0.016, 0.008
7 (aligned)		
10	0.076, 0.084, 0.092, 0,092	0.032, 0.036, 0.056, 0.056
Alternative:		
$\delta^{(i)} = 0.3$	0.996, 0.996, 0.992, 1.000	0.872, 0.860, 0.848, 0.872
7 (aligned)		
10	0.996, 0.992, 0.996, 1.000	0.832, 0.816, 0.776, 0.836

noted accounting for the initial investment in resource and difficulties in setting up the platform. The majority of operational efficiencies result from a platform trial's ability to provide a standing infrastructure into which new interventions can be quickly evaluated and either discarded or progressed. The most important scientific efficiency offered by platform trials is the ability to use a shared control when evaluating multiple interventions. Statistically this is a very simple yet powerful concept. The reduction in sample size is notable and increases as the number of concurrent arms in a platform trial increase. Efficiency of the trial and control arm can be further increased by incorporating historical data on the control arm external to the trial and non-contemporaneous control arm data internal to the trial. There is opportunity to further increase efficiency by pooling the non-contemporaneous control data. Statistical methods need to be developed to evaluate the exchangeability of the contemporaneous and non-contemporaneous control arm data prior to performing such a step.

References

1. Barker AD, Sigman CC, Kelloff GJ, Hylton NM, Berry DA, Esserman LJ. (2009). I-SPY2: An adaptive breast cancer trial design in the setting of neoadjuvant chemotherapy. *Clinical Pharmacology & Therapeutics* 86, 97–100.
2. Alexander B, Berger MS, Berry DA, Cavenee WK, Chang SM, Cloughesy TF, et al. (2018). Adaptive global innovative learning environment for glioblastoma: GBM AGILE. *Clinical Cancer Research*, 24(4), 737–743.
3. Herbst RS, Gandara DR, Hirsch FR, Redman MW, LeBlanc M, Mack PC, et al. (2015). Papadimitrakopoulou VA. Lung master protocol (Lung-MAP)–A biomarker-driven protocol for accelerating development of therapies for squamous cell lung cancer: SWOG S1400. *Clinical Cancer Research* 21(7), 1514–1524.
4. Viele K. (2016) Adapt platform trial, ADAPT Public Meeting, December 7.
5. Saville B, Berry S. (2016). Efficiencies of platform clinical trials: a vision of the future. *Clinical Trials* 13(3), 358–366.

6. Kim ES, Herbst RS, Wistuba II, Lee JJ, Blumenschein GR Jr, Tsao A, et al. (2011). The BATTLE trial: personalizing therapy for lung cancer. *Cancer Discov* 1, 44-53.

7. Pocock SJ. (1976). The combination of randomized and historical controls in clinical trials. *Journal of Chronic Diseases* 29, 175–188.

8. Chen MH, Ibrahim JG. (2006). The relationship between the power prior and hierarchical models. *Bayesian Analysis* 1, 551–574.

9. Hobbs BP, Carlin BP, Mandrekar SJ, Sargent DJ. (2011). Hierarchical commensurate and power prior models for adaptive incorporation of historical information in clinical trials. *Biometrics* 67, 1047–1056.

10. Neuenschwander B, Capkun-Niggli G, Branson M, Spiegelhalter DJ. (2010). Summarizing historical information on controls in clinical trials. *Clinical Trials* 7, 5–18.

11. Schmidli H, Gsteiger S, Roychoudhury S, O'Hagan A, Spiegelhalter D, Neuenschwander B. (2014). RobustMeta-analytic-predictive priors in clinical trials with historical control information. *Biometrics* 70, 1023–1032.

12. Neuenschwander B, Roychoudhury S, Schmidli H. (2016). On the use of co-data in clinical trials. *Statistics in Biopharmaceutical Research* 8(3), 345–354.

13. Kass RE, Wasserman L. (1995). A reference Bayesian test for nested hypotheses and its relationship to the Schwarz criterion. *Journal of the American Statistical Association* 90, 928–934.

14. O'Hagan A, Forster J. (2004). *Bayesian Inference, Kendall's Advanced Theory of Statistics*, Volume 2B. Chichester: Wiley.

15. Spiegelhalter DJ, Abrams KR, Myles JP. (2004). *Bayesian Approaches to Clinical Trials and Health-Care Evaluation*. Chichester: Wiley.

16. Lazzari C, Bulotta A, Ducceschi M, Vigano MG, Brioschi E, Corti F, Gianni L, Gregorc V. (2017). Historical evolution of second-line therapy in non-small cell lung cancer. *Frontiers in Medicine*, 4, 4.

17. Shepherd FA, Dancey J, Ramlau R, Mattson K, Gralla R, O'Rourke M, et al. (2002). Prospective randomized trial of docetaxel versus best supportive care in patients with non-small-cell lung cancer previously treated with platinum-based chemotherapy. *Journal of Clinical Oncology* 18(10), 2095–2103.

18. Fossella FV, DeVore R, Kerr RN, Crawford J, Natale RR, Dunphy F, et al. (2000). Randomized phase III trial of docetaxel versus vinorelbine or ifosfamide in patients with advanced non-small-cell lung cancer previously treated with platinum-containing chemotherapy regimens. The TAX 320 non-small cell lung cancer study group. *Journal of Clinical Oncology* 18(12), 2354–2362.

19. Gridelli C, Gallo C, Di Maio M, Barletta E, Illiano A, Maione P, et al. (2004). A randomised clinical trial of two docetaxel regimens (weekly vs 3 week) in the second-line treatment of non-small-cell lung cancer. The DISTAL 01 study. *British Journal of Cancer* 91(12), 1996–2004.

20. Hanna N, Shepherd FA, Fossella FV, Pereira JR, De Marinis F, Von Pawel J, et al. (2004). Randomized phase III trial of pemetrexed versus docetaxel in patients with non-small-cell lung cancer previously treated with chemotherapy. *Journal of Clinical Oncology* 22(9), 1589–1597.

15

Control of Type I Error for Confirmatory Basket Trials

Cong Chen and Robert A. Beckman

1. Introduction

Increasing biological understanding is changing cancer classification and treatment. Cancer is largely becoming a collection of diseases defined by specific molecular subtype(s) with low prevalence for each individual subtype. This shift to a molecular basis of diagnosing and treating cancer requires a corresponding shift in our drug development paradigm. Conventional approaches to drug development (i.e., one tumor indication at a time), if used exclusively, will not be sustainable due to small patient populations and are deemed inefficient.

A viable alternative approach is to study patients with a common biomarker signature in a "basket" trial across multiple histologies. "Basket" or "bucket" trials study an experimental treatment across multiple histologic tumor indications with a common biomarker signature under the assumption that the fundamental etiology of cancer is molecular (1–5). Basket trials have been used primarily in exploratory settings or proposed for therapies with potentially transformative effect(s) (6).

We sought to develop a general method for confirmatory basket trials that would be applicable to any effective therapy, whether or not it was transformative. Such a method would have many benefits. Patients with different tumor types ("rare" or not) will potentially have access to effective drugs for which a cost-effective development approach might not have been available. For sponsors, development of biomarker-driven drugs would be facilitated and overall costs would be lowered by pooling indications. Health authorities may have more robust data for risk and benefit evaluation across tumor indications. To reap the benefit of a confirmatory basket trial, a general design which is broadly applicable to any effective therapy (transformative or not) in patients with or without other therapy options is proposed in (7,8). In the early stage of a basket trial, there is uncertainty about which tumor types/indications will be active and which will not. Prior Phase 2 study reduces but does not eliminate this risk. A key clinical and statistical strategy proposed in (7,8) is to use an interim analysis to prune inactive tumor indications and only pool active ones in the final analysis. The uncertainty about drug activities in a tumor indication is often under-estimated. For example, the imatinib basket trial studied 186 patients in 40 different malignancies with known genomic mechanisms of activation of imatinib target kinases (9). However, only four tumor indications were deemed active by FDA for regulatory approval (after pooling with other trials and case reports). Vemurafenib is a highly effective therapy for patients with BRAF V600E mutated melanoma (10), but is ineffective as a single agent in patients with BRAF V600E mutated colorectal cancer due to subsequently discovered tissue specific feedback loops (11). In an exploratory basket trial in BRAF V600E mutated non-melanoma patients, it was found to have some activity in non–small-cell lung cancer, Erdheim–Chester disease and Langerhans'-cell histiocytosis but not in other tumor types studied (12). A Phase 3 basket trial of vemurafenib in BRAF V600E mutated patients without careful tumor selection and pruning could have resulted in a negative outcome.

Given that not all experimental therapies are transformative, unless the clinical benefit clearly outweighs the risk and/or a standard of care (SOC) doesn't exist, a randomized controlled trial should be the norm. Biases within a development team that developed the predictive biomarker hypothesis may cause them to underestimate clinical equipoise. By default, in a randomized controlled basket trial, each individual tumor indication has its own control group. A shared control group may be used for indications with a common SOC as appropriate. Single arm trials must rely on objective response rate (ORR) as the primary endpoint for assessment of anti-tumor activity where a high rate of durable response may provide evidence for drug approvals as seen from studies of PD-1/PD-L1 immune checkpoint inhibitors. A critical statistical issue within a confirmatory basket design, randomized or not, is Type I error (alpha) control for the pooled analysis after pruning. Ideally, pruning is based on external data so that no penalty needs to be paid for Type I error control. However, in practice, pruning often has to rely on trial data which is our focus in this chapter. While pruning may be seen as cherry-picking and tends to inflate the Type I error, it also shares similarity with a binding futility analysis in a Phase 3 study which tends to deflate the Type I error if all indications are pruned. Thus, the net impact of pruning on the pooled analysis is complicated. The use of different endpoints for pruning and pooling further complicates the issue. Sample size is subject to adjustment after pruning. This chapter will provide statistical details on Type I error control for the general basket design under three sample size adjustment strategies when same or different endpoints are used for pruning and pooling.

Not all tumor indications "pruned" at the interim analysis are deemed failures. For example, a tumor indication that barely misses the bar for pooling in a third line setting may be considered in an earlier line setting with or without combination with SOC. It has to be also understood that not all tumor indications pooled into the final analysis will necessarily yield clinically meaningful benefit in the final analysis. Each individual indication is subject to regulatory review of benefit-risk prior to label inclusion. Further, a basket trial may not be the only confirmatory study for a particular tumor indication. Parallel studies may be conducted in a different line of therapy and they will have an impact on the decision for pruning and pooling. For simplicity, we treat a basket trial as an isolated study in this chapter without considering program level clinical and regulatory strategies.

2. Statistical Designs of a Phase 3 Basket Trial

Consider a basket trial of an experimental therapy that consists of k tumor indications, each with same planned sample size N. We assume that for all tumor indications the drug has the same standardized effect size Δ (treatment effect divided by standard deviation) and the estimator is normally distributed. When a time-to-event variable is the primary endpoint of interest in a controlled trial, Δ refers to negative logarithm of hazard ratio (experimental arm vs. control arm) and N refers to number of events. When a continuous or categorical variable is the primary endpoint of interest, N refers to number of patients. Denote by (α, β) the doublet of one-sided Type I error rate and Type II error rate for hypothesis testing in the pooled population. When a controlled study with 1:1 randomization (experimental arm and control arm) is used for each indication, the Type I error, Type II error and total sample size in the pooled population (kN) satisfy the following equation:

$$kN = 4(Z_{1-\alpha} + Z_{1-\beta})^2/\Delta^2 \qquad (1)$$

where $Z_{(.)}$ denotes the respective quantile of the standard normal distribution. With such sample size, an observed effect of $\Delta Z_{1-\alpha}/(Z_{1-\alpha} + Z_{1-\beta})$ or greater would approximately consist of a positive outcome. The corresponding sample size in the pooled population to a non-randomized single-arm study is $kN/4$. We call a design with fixed sample size that includes all tumor indications in the pooled analysis without any pruning "Design zero" or "D0" in short for later reference.

An alternative design strategy to D0 is to conduct an interim analysis independently for each tumor indication. For ease of presentation, we assume that the interim analysis is conducted at a common information time t for all tumor indications (i.e., the interim analysis is based on Nt events or Nt patients depending on type of endpoint), although in reality it can differ by tumor indication. A tumor indication will be pruned from the pooled analysis if it does not meet the bar for pooling, and only the ones that cross above the bar will be included in the pooled analysis. We also assume a common bar (α_t in terms of one-sided nominal Type I error rate) for all tumor indications for simplicity.

The endpoints for pruning and pooling may be the same (the primary endpoint), or different (an intermediate for pruning and the primary endpoint for pooling). Let Y_{i1} be the standardized test statistics based on the endpoint used for pruning at the interim analysis, and Y_{i2} be the standardized test statistics based on the endpoint for pooling for the i-th tumor indication at the final analysis ($i = 1, \ldots, k$). We assume that they are respectively independent of each other across tumor indications in this chapter. This assumption holds in single arm designs or when each indication has its own control group. However, it does not hold when a shared control group is used, which represents an extension beyond the scope of this chapter. The i-th tumor indication will be excluded in the pooled analysis if the p-value based on Y_{i1} is $> \alpha_t$. Suppose that m tumor indications are included in the pooled analysis ($m \geq 1$). Let V_m be the corresponding standardized test statistics pooled from Y_{i2}, which can be written as the sum of Y_{i2} ($i = 1, \ldots, m$) divided by $\sqrt{m}$. An immediate question is which alpha level (denoted by α^*) should be used at the final analysis (pooled analysis) to keep the overall Type I error rate of the basket trial controlled at α (2.5% one-sided by default), understanding that m is unknown in advance. We will investigate this problem in the next section. Just as in a related problem to biomarker subgroup selection (13), throughout the chapter, Type I error rate is controlled under the null hypothesis that there is no treatment effect in terms of the primary endpoint in any tumor indication studied. We will discuss Type I error control under the same endpoint first, followed with the discussion under different endpoints in the following subsections.

2.1. Pruning and Pooling Based on the Same Endpoint

Interim analysis provides an opportunity to adjust sample size for remaining tumor indications. In this subsection, we investigate how pruning and pooling impacts Type I error rate under three different sample size adjustment strategies, and compare operating characteristics when number of active tumor indications varies.

Type I Error Rate

The null hypothesis that there is no treatment effect in any of the tumor indications is denoted as H_0. The probability of V_m being statistically significant at the α^* level is

$$Q_0(\alpha^*|\alpha_t, m) - \Pr_{H_0}(\cap\{Y_{i1} > Z_{1-\alpha_t} \text{ for } i = 1, ..., m\},$$
$$\cap\{Y_{j1} < Z_{1-\alpha_t} \text{ for } j = m+1, ...k\}, V_m > Z_{1-\alpha^*}) \tag{2}$$

Since Y_{i1}'s ($i = 1, ...,$ k) have independent and identical standard normal distribution under the null hypothesis, equation (2) can be rewritten as

$$Q_0(\alpha^*|\alpha_t, m) = \Pr_{H_0}(\cap\{Y_{i1} > Z_{1-\alpha_t} \text{ for } i = 1, ..., m\}, V_m > Z_{1-\alpha^*})(1 - \alpha_t)^{(k-m)} \tag{2'}$$

Each tumor indication has the same probability of being selected under the null hypothesis. Let c(k, m) be the number of choices to select m tumor indications from k, or $k!/((k - m)!m!)$, the overall Type I error rate is then $\sum_{m=1}^{k} c(k\,m)Q_0(\alpha^*|\alpha_t, m)$. The adjusted Type I error rate α^* is obtained from the following equation:

$$\sum_{m=1}^{k} c(k\,m)Q_0(\alpha^*|\alpha_t, m) = \alpha \tag{3}$$

To solve for α^* from equation (3), we need the correlation between Y_{i1} and V_m. Since V_m can be written as the sum of Y_{i2} ($i = 1, ..., m$) divided by $\sqrt{m}$, all we need is the correlation between Y_{i1} and Y_{i2} as the correlation between Y_{i1} and V_m is $\text{corr}(Y_{i1}, V_m) = \text{corr}(Y_{i1}, Y_{i2})/\sqrt{m}$. Intuitively speaking, the higher the correlation, the lower the α^* (or the greater the penalty on Type I error control). The correlation between Y_{i1} and Y_{i2} is driven by the overlap between Y_{i1} and Y_{i2}, and it differs by sample size adjustment strategy after pruning. We consider the following three sample size adjustment strategies:

1) Sample size for each tumor indication is fixed upfront at N as planned. There is no sample size increase for those included in the pooled analysis. The total sample size for the overall study will be less than kN if not all tumor indications are included in pooled analysis. We call it "Design one" or "D1" in short for later reference. Under D1, the correlation between Y_{i1} and Y_{i2} is $\sqrt{t}$ and correlation between Y_{i1} and V_m is $\sqrt{t/m}(i = 1, ..., m)$. Notice that D1 degenerates to D0 when $\alpha_t = 1$.

2) Sample size for each tumor indication will increase after the interim analysis so that the total sample size in the pooled analysis remains at kN. The sample size in the overall study is greater if not all tumor indications are included in pooled analysis. We call it "Design two" or "D2" in short for later reference. Under D2, each tumor indication

that has passed the interim analysis will have a sample size of kN/m in the end. The correlation between Y_{i1} and Y_{i2} is $\sqrt{tm/k}$ and the correlation between Y_{i1} and V_m is $\sqrt{t/k}$ $(i = 1, ..., m)$.

3) Sample size for each tumor indication will increase after the interim analysis so that the total sample size in the overall study remains at kN. The sample size in the pooled analysis is smaller if not all tumor indications are included in pooled analysis. We call it "Design three" or "D3" in short for later reference. Under D3, the remaining sample size of $kN(1 - t)$ will be equally distributed to the m remaining tumor indications after pruning so that the sample size is $Nt + kN(1 - t)/m$ for each. The correlation between Y_{i1} and Y_{i2} is $\sqrt{t/(t + k(1 - t)/m)}$ and the correlation between Y_{i1} and V_m is $(1 - (1 - \alpha_t)^k)\sqrt{t/(mt + k(1 - t))}$ $(i = 1, ..., m)$ in this case.

Except when all indications are pooled (i.e., $m = k$), the correlation between Y_{i1} and Y_{i2} is the largest under D1 and the smallest under D2. With the correlation between Y_{i1} and V_m defined for each strategy, α^* can be readily solved from (3) [see R codes in (8)]. The above three strategies keep the sample sizes around the planned sample size for fair comparison with D0. In practice, depending on the desired operating characteristics, a different sample size adjustment strategy may be used. The corresponding correlation will be different but the derivation will be similar.

Figure 15.1 provides α^* under different k (4 or 8) and α_t (0.3 or 0.5) when the information time t ranges from 0 to 100%. As expected, the penalty on Type I error increases with information time. The α^* takes the largest value under D2 and the smallest value under D1 for a given t. It decreases slightly when k increases from 4 to 8. When the bar increases (i.e., when α_t decreases from 0.5 to 0.3), α^* has greater value when t is small (impact of binding futility) and smaller value when t is large (impact of cherry-picking). Mathematically, since the probability of pruning all indication is $(1 - \alpha_t)^k$, the left hand side of equation (3) approaches $(1 - (1 - \alpha_t)^k)\alpha^*$ when t approaches 0. Because $(1 - (1 - \alpha_t)^k)$ is less than one, this explains why α^* tends to be greater than 2.5% when t is small as seen in Figure 15.1.

Power and Sample Size Calculations

The pruning and pooling strategy is devised to mitigate the risk when not all the tumor indications are active. For the purpose of planning a hypothetical basket trial, we assume that g out of the k tumor indications are active with a common treatment effect Δ (> 0) and the remaining ones do not have any effect (i.e., $\Delta = 0$). We call this alternative hypothesis H_{1g}. Again, we assume that m tumor indications are selected at the interim analysis. When j of the m chosen indications are truly active, the probability of V_m being statistically significant at the α^* level is

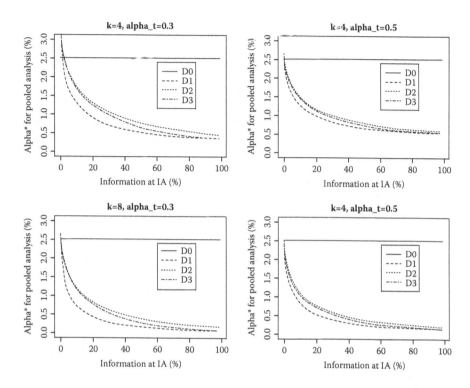

FIGURE 15.1

Adjusted alpha (α^*) under different pruning and pooling strategies when k = 4 or 8 and α_t = 0.3 or 0.5.

$$Q_1(\alpha*|\alpha_t, j, m) = \Pr_{H_{1g}}\{\cap_{i=1}^{m}(Y_{i1} > Z_{1-\alpha_t}), V_{mj} > Z_{1-\alpha^*}\}\Pr_{H_{1g}}\{\cap_{i=m+1}^{k}(Y_{i1} < Z_{1-\alpha_t})\} \tag{4}$$

where Y_{i1} has a $N(\Delta\sqrt{Nt/4}, 1)$ distribution for active indications including g-j pruned and j selected, and a $N(0,1)$ distribution for inactive indications. The probability of pruning k-m indications is $\Pr_{H_{1g}}\{\cap_{i=m+1}^{k}(Y_{i1} < Z_{1-\alpha_t})\} = \left(\Phi(Z_{1-\alpha_t} - \Delta\sqrt{Nt/4})\right)^{g-j}(1-\alpha_t)^{k-g-m+j}$ Since j out of m indications are truly active, the distribution of V_{mj} is $N((\Delta j/m)\sqrt{mN/4}, 1)$ under D1, $N((\Delta j/m)\sqrt{kN/4}, 1)$ under D2 and $N(\Delta j/m)\sqrt{(mt + k(1-t))N/4}, 1)$ under D3.

For a basket trial powered at $1 - \beta$, where β is the Type II error rate, the sample size N for each tumor indication is solved from the following equation by noticing that $m - j$ cannot be greater than k - g [see R codes in (8)]:

$$\sum_{m=1}^{k} \sum_{j=\max(0,m+g-k)}^{\min(m,g)} \binom{g}{j}\binom{k-g}{m-j} Q_1(a*|\alpha_t, j, m) = 1 - \beta \qquad (5)$$

where $Q_1(a*|\alpha_t, j, m)$ is given in equation (4).

While pruning will reduce the chance of including inactive indications in pooled analysis, it will also inadvertently exclude active ones. The probability of including an active tumor indication in the pooled analysis is $1 - \Phi(Z_{1-\alpha_t} - \Delta\sqrt{Nt/4})$, and the probability of including an inactive tumor indication is α_t. The expected number of tumor indications in the pooled population is $S = g\left(1 - \Phi(Z_{1-\alpha_t} - \Delta\sqrt{Nt/4})\right) + (k - g)\alpha_t$, of which $g\left(1 - \Phi(Z_{1-\alpha_t} - \Delta\sqrt{Nt/4})\right)$ are expected to be active. The proportion of expected tumor indications in the pooled population that are active measures the expected true treatment effect in the pooled population relative to Δ.

The expected sample size of the pruned tumor indications at the interim analysis is $(k-S)Nt$. When the sample size for each tumor indication is fixed at N (D1), the expected sample size in the pooled population is NS and the expected total sample size in the overall study is $NS + (k - S)Nt$. When the sample size for the pooled population is fixed at kN (D2), the expected total sample size for the overall study is $kN + (k - S)Nt$. When the total sample size for the overall study is fixed at kN (D3), the expected sample size in the pooled population is $kN - (k - S)Nt$, which is coincidentally equal to $NS + (k - S)Nt$ (the expected total sample size in the overall study under D1) when $t = 0.5$.

Comparison of Operating Characteristics among D0, D1, D2 and D3

Figure 15.2 provides study power under different pruning and pooling strategies in a basket trial when the number of tumor indications is 6, the midpoint for numbers of tumor indications considered in Figure 15.1. The total planned sample size (kN) ranges from 150 to 350 (i.e., sample size per indication ranges from 25 to approximately 58) and the number of active indications (g) varies from three to six. The true treatment effect is assumed to be $-\log(0.6)$. This corresponds to a hazard ratio of 0.6 for a time-to-event endpoint. The interim analysis is conducted at 50% information for each indication with α_t fixed at 0.4 (the midpoint considered for α_t in Figure 15.1). The bar for pruning corresponds to an observed hazard ratio of approximately 0.87 to 0.91 with respect to a time-to-event endpoint, which is a reasonable choice that is consistent with the proposed futility bar for a Phase 3 trial based on the benefit-cost ratio standpoint (14).

Table 15.1 provides study power and sample sizes under different pruning and pooling strategies for selected kN (200 and 300). Table 15.2 provides the number of tumors and the expected true treatment effect in

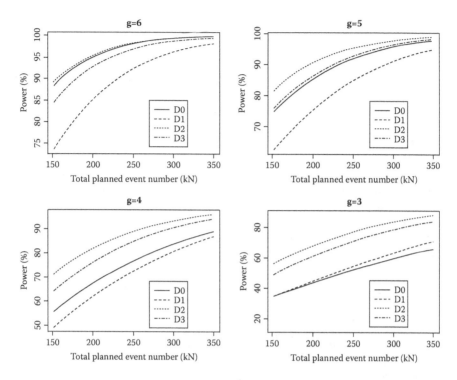

FIGURE 15.2
Study power under different pruning and pooling strategies when number of active indications (g) varies from 3 to 6 in a basket trial with 6 tumor indications. The true treatment effect is assumed to be $-\log(0.6)$ (or a hazard ratio of 0.6 for a time-to-event endpoint). The interim analysis is conducted at 50% information for each indication with $\alpha_t = 0.4$.

the pooled population with pruning (D1, D2, and D3) or without pruning (D0) under the same setting as that in Figure 15.2. Solved from equation (3), α^* for the pooled analysis is 0.32% under D1, 0.50% under D2, and 0.42% under D3. After paying the penalty for pruning, they are all considerably smaller than 2.5% which is used under D0.

As expected, the study power in Figure 15.2 decreases with decreasing g and increases with increasing kN. Among the three sample size adjustment strategies, D2 is always the most powerful followed with D3 and D1, consistent with the ordering of sample size in the pooled population. The relative performance to D0 depends on g. When all indications are active ($g = 6$), D2 has similar if not slightly higher power than D0, in spite of the fact that they have the same sample size in the pooled population. However, the overall study under D2 will need approximately 20 to 40 more samples when $kN = 200$ and approximately 20 to 60 more samples when $kN = 300$ (Table 15.1). D0 has higher power than D1 and D3 when all indications are active. As g decreases, the power of D0 decreases much faster than the pruning-based designs so that D0 has the lowest power when half of the indications are inactive (i.e., $g = 3$). This is not surprising because the true treatment effect in the pooled population decreases much faster without pruning than with pruning (Table 15.2). While pruning-based designs will miss a fraction of active indications in the pooled population, many more inactive indications are excluded (Table 15.2).

The above comparisons are for illustration purposes. The timing of interim analysis or the bar for pruning is not optimized. More investigation is needed when the true and target treatment effects are different across tumor types. Nevertheless, the illustration above has confirmed the potential benefit of the pruning-based strategies as expected. When designing a basket trial in practice, the project team should come up with an objective prior assumption about treatment effect and the probability of success in each indication based on preclinical and clinical data prior to the study design. The project statistician can then generate the design properties under different design options based on the prior assumptions.

TABLE 15.1

Study power and sample sizes under different pruning and pooling strategies when number of active indications varies from 3 to 6 in a basket trial with six tumor indications. The true treatment effect is assumed to be $\Delta = -\log(0.6)$ (or a hazard ratio of 0.6 for a time-to-event endpoint) for an active indication. The interim analysis is conducted at 50% information for each indication with $\alpha_t = 0.4$. The hypothesis on pooled population is tested at 2.5% under D0, 0.32% under D1, 0.50% under D2 and 0.42% under D3.

Planned events	Number of active tumors	Power (%) for a positive study				Exp. number of events for pooled population			Exp. number of events for overall study		
		D0	D1	D2	D3	D0/D2	D1	D3	D0/D3	D1	D2
200	6	95	85	95	93	200	157	179	200	179	221
200	5	85	75	91	86	200	144	172	200	172	228
200	4	67	62	82	76	200	131	166	200	166	234
200	3	44	45	68	61	200	119	159	200	159	240
300	6	99	96	99	99	300	254	277	300	277	323
300	5	96	81	98	96	300	232	266	300	266	334
300	4	84	81	94	91	300	209	255	300	255	345
300	3	60	64	84	79	300	187	244	300	244	356

TABLE 15.2

Numbers of tumor indications and expected true treatment effect in pooled population with pruning (D1, D2 and D3) or without pruning (D0) when number of active indications varies from 3 to 6 in a basket trial with six tumor indications. The true treatment effect is assumed to be $\Delta = -\log(0.6)$ (or a hazard ratio of 0.6 for a time-to-event endpoint) for an active indication. The interim analysis is conducted at 50% information for each indication with $\alpha_t = 0.4$.

Planned events	Number of active tumor indications	Exp. number of active tumor indications in pooled population		Exp. total number of tumor indications in pooled population		Exp. true effect in pooled population relative to Δ (%)	
		No pruning	With pruning	No pruning	With pruning	No pruning	With pruning
200	6	6	4.7	6	4.7	100	100
200	5	5	3.9	6	4.3	83	91
200	4	4	3.1	6	3.9	67	80
200	3	3	2.4	6	3.6	50	66
300	6	6	5.1	6	5.1	100	100
300	5	5	4.2	6	4.6	83	91
300	4	4	3.4	6	4.2	67	81
300	3	3	2.5	6	3.7	50	68

A Hypothetical Example of a Single-Arm Basket Trial

We now consider an example in the refractory disease setting where ORR is an acceptable endpoint for approval and single arm studies are advisable. We apply the Simon optimal two-stage design to each tumor cohort included in the basket, which optimizes the expected number of patients utilized per indication when ORR is the primary outcome (15). We will assume in this example a true ORR of greater than or equal to 30% is of interest, whereas a true ORR of less than 10% is not of interest. (In real applications, the ORR of interest will depend on a variety of factors, such as the duration and depth of responses and the tradeoff between the safety risk posed by the therapy and potential benefits of the therapy. Prediscussion with health authorities would be highly advisable in designing such a study.) Each indication will be powered at 90% with a 10% one-sided alpha per the Simon approach.

We will study ten tumor indications at once. The individual indications are evaluated according to the optimal two-stage approach. After the first stage, in which 12 patients are enrolled, any indication with fewer than two responses is dropped. The remaining indications are expanded to 35 patients each. Only indications which achieve at least five responses are pooled in the final analysis. In this example, $a^* = 0.29\%$ based on the exact binomial distribution instead of an asymptotic normal distribution. The fewer indications remain in the pool, the higher pooled response rate is required for demonstrating a positive outcome. For example, if only one indication remains in the pool, a 30% ORR must be observed, whereas if four indications remain, an observed ORR of 20% is sufficient.

In summary, in this non-randomized example, a confirmatory study of 120–350 patients has the potential to result in approval of up to 10 indications based on ORR.

2.2. Pruning and Pooling Based on Different Endpoints

Type I Error Rate

While the pooled analysis is usually based on a clinical endpoint (e.g., OS), pruning can be based on an intermediate endpoint. The intermediate endpoint, which may be used for accelerated approval, can be progression-free-survival (PFS) or ORR, based on prior discussions with national health authorities. The use of an intermediate endpoint at interim analysis for accelerated approval and the use of a clinical endpoint in a pooled analysis for full approval is a distinctive feature of the proposed general design (7,8). It represents a more efficient registration strategy than a basket design strategy that only aims for full approval or accelerated approval, but not both. An intermediate endpoint can also be any efficacy endpoint sensitive to the experimental treatment (e.g., tumor size change at a landmark time point as a continuous variable) which may be used to terminate inactive tumor indications early to save the time and cost of the trial and to reduce patient exposure. The choice of endpoint in this case is mainly at the sponsor's risk, and careful assessment of the statistical properties of the intermediate endpoint is required (16). Regardless of the objective, the bar for pruning based on an intermediate endpoint will be higher than in the previous section. For illustration purposes, the pruning bar at the interim analysis is assumed to be $a_t = 0.05$.

Let ρ be the correlation between the test-statistics for the two endpoints based on the same patient population. Let t be the proportion of patients included in the interim analysis (i.e., Nt patients in interim analysis population). Let Y_{i1} be the test statistics based on the interim patients using the intermediate endpoint and Y_{i2} be the test statistics based on all patients using the clinical endpoint in the i-th tumor cohort ($i = 1, \ldots, k$). For illustration purpose, without loss of generality, we assume that all endpoints are either binary or continuous. With the above set-up, the correlation between Y_{i1} and Y_{i2} is $\rho\sqrt{t}$ under D1, $\rho\sqrt{tm/k}$ under D2, and $\rho\sqrt{t/(t + k(1 - t)/m)}$ under D3. Clearly, ρ has a multiplicative effect on the correlation that is similar to $\sqrt{t}$. Notice that the correlation would be more complicated when t is defined as the information fraction with respect to a time-to-event endpoint, since the multiplicative property does not necessarily hold for time-to-event endpoints.

With two endpoints, the parameter space for the hypotheses becomes more complicated. While the null hypothesis for the clinical endpoint in the pooled analysis may remain the same as in the previous section, which is of our primary interest, there is no restriction of the treatment effect for the intermediate endpoint under the null hypothesis. It can vary from no effect to large treatment effect purely from a statistical standpoint. A conservative approach for multiplicity control would pick the smallest α^* over the entire parameter space for the intermediate endpoint (8,17). A less conservative approach is to conduct a meta-analysis of historical data (18–20) to find a more restrictive parameter space for the intermediate endpoint. In order to gauge the maximum penalty, we apply the conservative approach in this chapter. Let δ_i be the hypothetical treatment effect on the intermediate endpoint for the i-th tumor indication ($i = 1,\ldots, k$). The parameter space formed by δ_i ($i = 1,\ldots, k$) is less tractable under the conservative approach. We will try to simplify it first. To be consistent with the definition of t, we assume that Y_{i1} is a continuous or a categorical variable so that the test statistics Y_{i1} have standard normal distribution with mean $\delta_i\sqrt{Nt/4}$ ($i = 1, \ldots, k$). Notice that, from equation (2), α^* is determined by the joint distribution of $\{Y_{i1}, i = 1,\ldots, k\}$ and V_m. Since for any set of δ_i ($i = 1,\ldots, k$), there is a common δ which yields the same value for the joint distribution function, a natural parameter space for consideration is formed under the assumption that the treatment effect can take any value but remains the same for all tumor indications. We call the overall null hypothesis formed this way $H_{0\delta}$ whereas the first term in subscript refers to the endpoint for pooled analysis and the second term refers to the endpoint for pruning. Under this assumption, the adjusted Type I error for the pooled analysis (α^*) for each δ satisfies the following equation and the smallest α^* is chosen to be the final adjusted Type I error.

$$\sum_{m=1}^{k} c(k,m) \mathrm{Pr}_{H_{0\delta}}\left(\bigcap_{i=1}^{m}(Y_{i1} > Z_{1-\alpha_t}), V_m > Z_{1-\alpha^*}\right)\left(\Phi(Z_{1-\alpha_t} - \delta\sqrt{Nt/4})\right)^{k-m} = \alpha$$

(6)

R codes for solving α^* from the above equation are provided in (8). Notice that, unlike in equation (3) in the previous section, α^* also depends on N. More specifically, it is driven by δ and N via $\delta\sqrt{N}$ for a given t. In order to find the smallest α^*, all we need to do is to conduct a grid search of $\delta\sqrt{N}$ by treating it as an entity (or alternatively conduct a grid search of δ while keeping N fixed).

To get some insight about how α^* is impacted by δ, consider ρ to be small (or equivalently $\sqrt{t}$ be small). When there is no effect in any tumor indication, the chance of terminating the study is high because α_t is small. As a result, α^* would be greater than 2.5% following the same discussion after Figure 15.1. However, when δ is large, no indication will be pruned and α^* degenerates to 2.5%. In general, δ should be chosen to properly balance the probability of inclusion and exclusion of an indication in order to minimize α^*. Based on our calculations, δ does not degenerate to infinity (or zero) in general at the point when minimum α^* is reached. To illustrate, Figure 15.3 provides adjusted alpha (α^*) under different δ for selected ρ when k = 6 and t = 0.5 or 0.8. All analyses are conducted under D1. As shown in Figure 15.3, the shape of α^* is convex with minimum reached at non-trivial values for δ. (N is set at 30 in the calculation. When N is set at a different value, the value of minimal α^* will not change. However, it will be reached at a different δ but at the same $\delta\sqrt{N}$.)

Figure 15.4 provides the minimized α^* for different k (4 or 8) when ρ ranges from 0 to 1 under D1, D2 and D3 (compare minimized α^* to Figure 15.3 at same ρ). A reference line corresponding to α^* = 2.5% is also

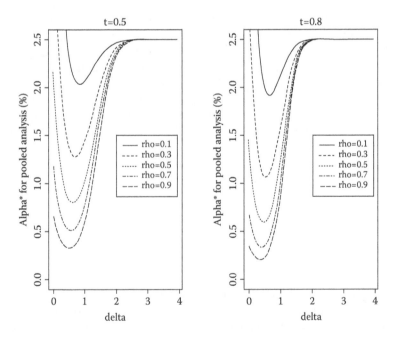

FIGURE 15.3
Adjusted alpha (α^*) under different δ for select correlations between the endpoint for pruning (α_t = 0.05) and the endpoint for pooling when k = 6 and t = 0.5 or 0.8. All analyses are conducted under D1, and N is set at 30 in the calculation.

provided. As expected, the minimized α^* is always less than or equal to 2.5% and decreases as ρ increases. The bar for pruning is set at $\alpha_t = 0.05$. It is misleading to compare Figures 15.1 and 15.4 directly because α_t is different between the two, and even when α_t is the same a comparison between Figures 15.1 and 15.4 can only be made when the correlations are the same.

In practice, we need an estimate of ρ (or the correlation between Y_{i1} and Y_{i2} in general) based on historical data prior to study start for planning purposes. For example, a reasonable starting point for the correlation between PFS and OS is around 0.5 based on our experience with various oncology studies. Once the study is finished, we can estimate ρ from the trial data to retrospectively calculate the minimized α^*. There are many ways to estimate the correlation. For example, when both are time-to-event endpoints (e.g., PFS and OS), the WLW option from the SAS procedure PROC PHREG may be considered (21). Pearson's correlation may be considered when neither one is a time-to-event

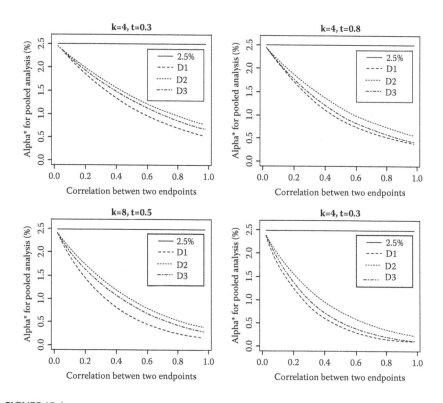

FIGURE 15.4

Adjusted alpha (α^*) under different correlations between the endpoint for pruning ($\alpha_t = 0.05$) and the endpoint for pooling when k = 4 or 8, and t = 0.5 or 0.8. The adjusted alpha is minimized over a common treatment for all tumor indications.

variable. In the case of concern that the correlation may differ with the underlying treatment effect, the allocation schedule for treatment assignment may be scrambled to facilitate the estimation of the correlation under null. The bootstrap method may be used to assist with the estimation as needed. Type I error rate is asymptotically controlled as long as a consistent estimator of ρ is used for calculation of α^*.

A Hypothetical Example of Special Interest

Once a minimized α^* is determined, the same analyses as presented in the previous section can be applied to the sample size and power calculation for the pooled analysis. We will not repeat them in this section. Instead, we will present an example when a key objective of the basket trial is to file for accelerated approval at an interim analysis (following existing regulatory paradigm) and full approval at the final analysis. PFS and OS are the respective endpoints considered in this hypothetical example. Different endpoints (e.g., ORR and OS for immunotherapies) may be considered in practice upon discussion with regulatory agencies.

Consider a randomized controlled basket trial with 1:1 randomization in six tumor indications. Each targets a hazard ratio of 0.5 in PFS at the interim analysis with 90% power. The hypothesis on PFS will be tested at 2.5% alpha each. The target number of PFS event size for each tumor indication at the interim analysis is approximately 88 based on equation (1). An observed hazard ratio of 0.66 will approximately meet the bar for a positive PFS outcome.

It is assumed that 80% of the patients will have a PFS event at the data cut-off date for the interim analysis if enrolling approximately 110 patients for each tumor indication. The D2 design will be used for sample size adjustment after the interim analysis so that the final sample size of patients in the pooled population is fixed at approximately 660 (i.e., 110 multiplied by 6). The interim analysis for each tumor indication will be conducted separately unless they reach the target number of PFS events at approximately same time. Whenever an indication has a negative PFS outcome, a total of 110 patients will be equally distributed to the remaining indications. Notice that, t = 1 based on the above set-up and the minimized α^* is 0.8% when ρ is 0.5. Assuming that 65% of the patients in the pooled population will die by the cut-off date for the final analysis, with a total of 430 events, the study has approximately 90% power to detect a hazard ratio of 0.7 in OS at the 0.8% alpha (after adjusting for the penalty). An observed hazard ratio of 0.79 will approximately meet the bar for a positive OS outcome. As a comparison to a design without an interim analysis for accelerated approval, the observed hazard ratio in OS would be approximately 0.83 for the trial to be positive at 2.5% alpha (no penalty). The chance of observing a hazard ratio of 0.83 would be higher than observing a hazard ratio of 0.79 when all tumor indications are equally active, but it could be much lower otherwise as seen in the previous section under similar setups. Moreover, the addition of an interim analysis for accelerated approval could substantially shorten the time to drug approval. Last but not least, this basket trial has the potential to get an experimental therapy approved in up to six tumor indications based on a comparable sample size to a conventional Phase 3 trial for one tumor indication.

For simplicity, we have only considered one interim analysis in the above hypothetical example. In practice, multiple interim analyses may be conducted. For example, an OS analysis for overwhelming survival benefit may be added mid-way between the interim analysis and the final analysis. An early futility analysis may be conducted based on response rate.

3. Discussion

We have demonstrated that a basket trial with pruning of indications based on an interim analysis is feasible and, after adjusting for Type I error control and accounting for the risk of inactive indications, will have superior overall performance characteristics when comparing with a basket trial without pruning. The rigor of this design may facilitate evaluation and approval of an experimental therapy in multiple tumor types in patients with a common predictive biomarker signature by health authorities, while the efficiency of the design makes it appealing to patients, physicians and drug developers. We note that the required penalty for using internal data for pruning can be significant. Credible external data, whenever available, should be used to help with the pruning decision to reduce penalty. Further, there is no penalty when tumor indications are pruned solely because of unexpectedly slow accrual, or due to evolution of SOC that renders the study in some of the tumor indications obsolete. Relaxation of the pruning bar can also reduce the penalty.

The ongoing discovery of subgroups of common cancers defined by predictive biomarkers creates small indications which may be difficult to enroll. This has led to the basket study in which the fundamental classification is based on molecular subtypes rather than histologies. Previous basket study designs have either been for exploratory work or for confirmation in the setting of potentially transformational agents and/or extraordinarily strong prior evidence in patients with no other therapy options. The basket design described in this chapter is a rigorous design which is broadly applicable to any effective agent (transformative or not), in patients with or without other therapy options, and also provides opportunities for accelerated approval of indications in the basket. The approach presented here has the potential to improve and accelerate access to therapies for patient populations defined by molecular subtypes. The design may also make development more feasible and cost effective and provide more optimal datasets for health authority evaluation in these molecularly defined indications.

The Type I error control in this chapter is based on a null hypothesis of all indications being inactive. Rejection of the null hypothesis at the pooled analysis doesn't automatically mean that the tumor indications in the pool are equally active. To reduce the chance of highly active indications driving the final result, these indications may be stopped early for efficacy so that they will not be included in the pooled analysis (22). Hierarchical clustering techniques (23) may in principle be employed to identify outlier indications that are either inactive or highly active in the final pool. This is an important topic for future research. Meanwhile, in the current formulation, we demand that any accepted indication show a trend consistent with the overall positive result and be judged as having a positive risk-benefit ratio based on the available data. Graphic tools (e.g., forest plot and Galbraith plot) may be used to assist with the regulatory decision. Possible heterogeneity in treatment effect across remaining tumor indications in the pooled population is an issue similar to conventional Phase 3 trials. For example, treatment effect in these trials may differ by age or gender, and the impact of baseline characteristics on treatment effect is routinely investigated. Regulatory decisions on drug approval or the scope of the label hinges upon the outcome of such ad hoc analyses despite an overall positive outcome from the trial. The issue is also similar to regional effects in a multi-regional study or the trial effect in a meta-analysis, which is well studied and understood. Therefore, concerns about heterogeneity shouldn't deter us from performing pooled analyses of basket trials.

This chapter provides an in-depth discussion of statistical considerations in a confirmatory Phase 3 basket trial design with the goal of achieving approvals in multiple indications simultaneously, emphasizing type I error control which is a high priority for confirmatory studies. Selection unavoidably leads to bias (24). The estimation property of the bias is investigated in (25). In recent years, advances have been achieved in the design of basket trials, primarily focused the application of Bayesian adaptive strategies to Phase 2 studies (26,27,28,29,30). While this chapter focuses on frequentist approaches and attempts to mirror current approval paradigms, incorporation of strategies such as hierarchical clustering, shrinkage and others in the current Phase 3 design requires further investigation. Collaborative research is ongoing to bridge basket trials with umbrella trials, hybrid trial designs that combine multiple targeted agents and molecular subgroups of a specific tumor type in a single study (1,31,32,33,34).

References

1. Barker AD, Sigman CC, Kelloff GJ, Hylton NM, Berry DA, Esserman LJ. I-SPY2: An adaptive breast cancer trial design in the setting of neoadjuvant chemotherapy. *Clinical Pharmacology & Therapeutics* 2009; 86: 97–100.
2. Kopetz S. Right drug for the right patient. In *Hurdles and the path forward in colorectal cancer*. ASCO Educational Book, 2013. http://meetinglibrary.asco.org/content/19-132.

3. Lacombe D, Burocka S, Bogaertsa J, Schoeffskib P, Golfinopoulosa V, Stuppa R. The dream and reality of histology agnostic cancer clinical trials. *Molecular Oncology* 2014; 8: 1057–1063.

4. Meador CB, Micheel CM, Levy MA, Lovly CM, Horn L, Warner JL, et al. Beyond histology: Translating tumor genotypes into clinically effective targeted therapies. *Clinical Cancer Research* 2014; 20: 2264–2275.

5. Sleijfer S, Bogaerts J, Siu LL. Designing transformative clinical trials in the cancer genome era. *Journal of Clinical Oncology* 2013; 31: 1834–1841.

6. Demetri G, Becker R, Woodcock J, Doroshow J, Nisen P, Sommer J. *Alternative trial designs based on tumor genetics/pathway characteristics instead of histology.* Issue Brief: Conference on Clinical Cancer Research 2011. www.focr.org/conference-clinical-cancer-research-2011.

7. Beckman RA, Antonijevic Z, Kalamegham R, Chen C. Design for a basket trial in multiple tumor types based on a putative predictive biomarker. *Clinical Pharmacology & Therapeutics* 2016; 100(6): 617–625. doi: 10.1002/cpt.446.

8. Chen C, Li N, Yuan S, Antonijevic Z, Kalamegham R, Beckman RA. Statistical design and considerations of a phase 3 basket trial for simultaneous investigation of multiple tumor types in one study. *Statistics in Biopharmaceutical Research* 2016; 8(3): 248–257. doi: 10.1080/19466315.2016.1193044.

9. Heinrich MC, Joensuu H, Demetri GD, Corless CL, Apperley J, Fletcher JA, et al. Phase II, open-label study evaluating the activity of imatinib in treating life-threatening malignancies known to be associated with imatinib-sensitive tyrosine kinases. *Clinical Cancer Research* 2008; 14: 2717–2725.

10. Chapman PB, Hauschild A, Robert C, Haanen JB, Ascierto P, Larkin J, et al. Improved survival with vemurafenib in melanoma with V600E mutation. *The New England Journal of Medicine* 2011; 364: 2507–2516.

11. Prahallad A, Sun C, Huang S, Di Nicolantonio F, Salazar R, Zecchin D, et al. Unresponsiveness of colon cancer to BRAF(V600E) inhibition through feedback activation of EGFR. *Nature* 2012; 483: 100–103.

12. Hyman DM, Puzanov I, Subbiah V, Faris JE, Chau I, Blay J-Y, et al. Vemurafenib in multiple nonmelanoma cancers with BRAF V600 mutations. *The New England Journal of Medicine* 2015; 373: 726–736.

13. Magnusson B, Turnbull BW. Group sequential enrichment design incorporating subgroup selection. *Statistics in Medicine* 2013; 32: 2695–2714.

14. Chen C, Beckman RA. Optimal cost-effective Go-No Go decisions in late-stage oncology drug development. *Statistics in Biopharmaceutical Research* 2009; 1(2): 159–169.

15. Simon R. Optimal two-stage designs for phase II clinical trials. *Controlled Clinical Trials* 1989; 10: 1–10.

16. Chen C, Sun L, Chih C. Evaluation of early efficacy endpoints for proof-of-concept trials. *Journal of Biopharmaceutical Statistics* 2013; 23: 413.

17. Li X, Chen C, Li W. Adaptive biomarker population selection in phase III confirmatory trials with time-to-event endpoints. *Statistics in Biosciences* 2016; Early online. doi: 10.1007/s12561-016-9178-4.

18. Sargent D, Wieand S, Haller DG, Gray R, Benedetti JK, Buyse M, et al. Disease-free survival (DFS) vs. overall survival (OS) as a primary endpoint for adjuvant colon cancer studies: Individual patient data from 20, 898 patents on 18 randomized trials. *Journal of Clinical Oncology* 2005; 23: 8664–8670.

19. Tang PA, Bentzen SM, Chen EX, Siu LL. Surrogate end points for median overall survival in metastatic colorectal cancer: Literature-based analysis from 39 randomized controlled trials of first-line chemotherapy. *Journal of Clinical Oncology* 2007; 25: 4562–4568.

20. Whitehead A. *Meta-analysis of controlled clinical trials.* UK: Wiley, 2002.

21. *SAS/STAT® software: Changes and enhancements through release 6.12.* Cary, NC: SAS Institute Inc., 1997.

22. Yuan S, Chen A, He L, Chen C, Gause CK, Beckman RA. On group sequential enrichment design for basket trials. *Statistics in Biopharmaceutical Research* 2016; 8(3): 293–306. doi: 10.1080/19466315.2016.1200999.

23. Thall PF, Wathen JK, Bekele BN, Champlin RE, Baker LH, Benjamin RS. Hierarchical Bayesian approaches to phase II trials in diseases with multiple subtypes. *Statistics in Medicine* 2003; 22(5): 763–780.

24. Bauer P, Koenig F, Brannath W, Posch M. Selection and bias – Two hostile brothers. *Statistics in Medicine* 2010; 29(1): 1–13. doi: 10.1002/sim.3716.

25. Li W, Chen C, Li X, Beckman RA. Estimation of treatment effect in two-stage confirmatory oncology trials of personalized medicines. *Statistics in Medicine* 2017; 36(120): 1843–1861.

26. Berry DA. The brave new world of clinical cancer research: Adaptive biomarker-driven trials integrating clinical practice with clinical research. *Molecular Oncology* 2015; 9(5): 951–959. doi: 10.1016/j.molonc.2015.02.011.

27. Berry SM, Broglio KR, Groshen S, Berry DA. Bayesian hierarchical modeling of patient subpopulations: Efficient designs of phase II oncology clinical trials. *Clinical Trials* 2013; 10(5): 720–734.

28. Neuenschwander B, Wandel S, Roychoudhury S, Bailey S. Robust exchangeability designs for early phase clinical trials with multiple strata. *Pharmaceutical Statistics* 2016; 15(2): 123–134. doi: 10.1002/pst.1730.

29. Simon R, Geyer S, Subramanian J, Roychowdhury S. The Bayesian basket design for genomic variant-driven phase II trials. *Seminars in Oncology* 2016; 43 (1): 13–18. doi: 10.1053/j.seminoncol.2016.01.002.

30. Wathen JK, Thall PF, Cook JD, Estey EH. Accounting for patient heterogeneity in phase II clinical trials. *Statistics in Medicine* 2008; 27: 2802–2815.

31. Herbst RS, Gandara DR, Hirsch FR, Redman MW, LeBlanc M, Mack OC, et al. Lung Master Protocol (lung-MAP)–A biomarker-driven protocol for accelerating development of therapies for squamous cell lung cancer: SWOG S1400. *Clinical Cancer Research* 2015; 21(7): 1514–1524. doi: 10.1158/1078-0432.CCR-13-3473.

32. Kim ES, Herbst RS, Wistuba II, Lee JJ, Blumenschein GR Jr., Tsao A, et al. The BATTLE trial: Personalizing therapy for lung cancer. *Cancer Discovery* 2011; 1: 44–53.

33. McNeil C. NCI-MATCH launch highlights new trial design in precision-medicine era. *JNCI: Journal of the National Cancer Institute* 2015; 107: 7.

34. Trusheim M, Shrier A, Antonijevic Z, Beckman RA, Campbell RK, Chen C, et al. PIPELINEs: Creating comparable clinical knowledge efficiently by linking trial platforms. *Clinical Pharmacology & Therapeutics* 2016; 100(6): 713–729. doi: 10.1002/cpt.514.

16

Benefit-Risk Assessment for Platform Trials

Chunlei Ke and Qi Jiang

1. Introduction

Every drug product is targeted to have some benefits with favorable effects for patients. A drug product also inevitably has certain risks (harms) and it is important to manage the events when they occur. Benefit-risk assessment (BRA) is an evaluation on whether or not the benefits outweigh the risks for a particular product in the context of treatment options available to patients.

Benefit-risk assessment is fundamental and important for drug development and life-cycle management. BRA is critical for all decision-makers such as patients, physicians and health care providers, regulators, payors, and sponsors. For many years, BRA was often an informal process. Many decisions are easy. However, for hard decisions, informal BRA can lead to institutional biases. As a result, companies, regulatory agencies, and other governance bodies are increasingly relying on the use of formal, structured BRA approaches for critical decision points. A structured BRA is the application of a benefit-risk framework that guides the user in presenting the relevant information and accompanying rationale in a systematic and standardized format. Having structured BRA enhances transparency, consistency, efficiency, and communication.

The FDA started to develop a structured BRA framework for drugs and biologics in 2009. In 2013, the FDA issued "Structured Approach to Benefit-Risk Assessment in Drug Regulatory Decision-Making Draft PDUFA V Implementation Plan" (1) and described their benefit-risk assessment framework to guide regulatory decision making. In 2016, FDA issued "Factors to Consider Regarding Benefit-Risk in Medical Device Products."(2) EMA had put similar efforts into BRA as well. BRA in the context of a new drug application is a central element of the scientific evaluation of a marketing authorization application and related variations (3). As a part of the EMA BRA efforts, an Effects Table is now required for the Rapporteur day 80 critical assessment report. Furthermore, ICH M4E elaborated on the inclusion of BR consideration in a Clinical Overview report for the Common Technical Document.

The Pharmaceutical Research and Manufacturers of America (PhRMA) established a benefit-risk assessment working team in 2005, developing their BRAT framework and providing several case studies using the framework (4). In 2013, a benefit-risk working group was formed mainly among US statisticians under the sponsorship of Quantitative Sciences in the Pharmaceutical Industry (QSPI BRWG) with a vision to promote use of structured BRA and understand and improve BRA methods. Some of the efforts from QSPI BRWG are included in the book edited by (5).

As discussed in other chapters of this book, platform design provides an innovative approach to efficiently evaluating multiple compounds and/or multiple indication together in one trial. Various decisions will be made during and after the trial pertaining to the drugs' benefit-risk profile. There isn't a well accepted definition of a platform design yet. In fact, the terminology including platform design, basket design, and umbrella design has been used interchangeably for various types of design in literature. Regardless of the specific type of design, the principle of BRA based on the trial data is similar. For the purpose of the BRA discussion in this chapter, we mainly consider the following types of design (Figure 16.1)

- Design 1: A design to evaluate multiple treatment arms or treatment regimens for the same disease population or indication
- Design 2: A design to evaluate the same treatment for each of the several patient populations or indications
- Design 3: A design to evaluate the same treatment for the combination of related populations with the same biomarker or genetic features.

The distinction between Design 2 and Design 3 lies where the inference on the treatment benefit-riskprofile is evaluated for individual populations (Design 2) and for the pooled (selected) patient populations (Design 3). In the literature, Design 3 is referred to as a basket design. In practice, a design can be a combination of these types, but the BRA evaluation can be adapted accordingly. In addition, although a platform design can be used at all stages of drug life-cycle management, we will mainly focus our discussion on the platform design used in early- and late-phase drug development.

The goal of BRA is to form an integral view of the benefit-risk profile of the treatment under study in the context of the disease state and treatment options available to support decision making on the study and ultimately on the treatment. In the platform design, BRA is important to facilitate decision-makings in the process of drug development including:

- Interim analysis to decide whether any changes need to be made to the current trial. The changes may include early drop of an inferior treatment, early conclusion of an efficacious treatment, and potential

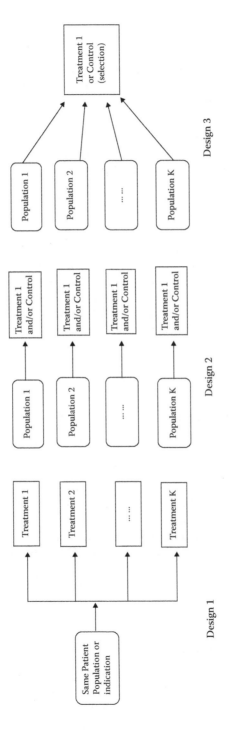

FIGURE 16.1
Three types of platform design considered in this chapter.

increase of sample size. In a basket design, the decision is needed to select a target population to move forward. This applies to both early and late phase platform trials.

- Go or no-go decision after the end of phase 2 trials. The BRA can be used to assess whether a given treatment should be moved to the confirmation stage. It could also be used to evaluate any biomarker or subgroup effect to determine the study population for the phase 3 study.
- At conclusion of phase 3 trials, BRA can be used to evaluate whether any of the treatments studied provides a favorable benefit-risk profile to inform regulatory decision and patient use.

In this chapter, we will discuss use of the BRA in the platform trial. In Section 2, we will introduce the general BRA methods for platform trials, and discuss some quantitative methods to support the BRA. We will also develop methods for benefit-risk interim analysis and subgroup analysis. A few examples will be used to illustrate the methods. As a platform trial usually involves large number of treatment arms and is performed in early stages of drug development, the information available may be very limited, which leads to many uncertainties in the BRA. These and other uncertainties will be discussed in Section 3. Some discussions and conclusions will be provided in Section 4.

2. BRA Approaches for the Platform Trials

BRA approaches refer to any qualitative or quantitative methods to integrate or balance evidence on benefits and risks to carry out a comprehensive benefit-risk assessment. Many approaches have been proposed in the literature for BRA for different considerations with various scopes. For example, (6) reviewed 18 methods, and the IMI-PROTECT working group reviewed and evaluated 47 methods (3). Several efforts were attempted to categorize and appraise various methods and provide recommendations for their use (7)). For example, QSPI BRWG recommends a structured BRA approach which includes a descriptive B-R framework complemented with some general quantitative methods (8). We will consider this structured BRA approach for the platform trials.

2.1. BRA Framework for Platform Trials

The BRA is a very complicated process. A descriptive BRA framework is recommended to be used to select, organize, summarize the relevant facts, uncertainties, and key areas of judgment, and communicate data relevant to any benefit-risk decision. Due to the complex nature of the BRA, it is necessary to have a systematic framework to structure and guide the process of benefit-risk assessment and to articulate reasoning behind BRA decisions.

Several frameworks have been proposed in the literature including FDA B-R framework (2016), EMA framework, the Pharmaceutical Research and Manufacturers of America (PhRMA) BRAT framework (4), and the Centre for Innovation in Regulatory Science (CIRS) Unified Methodologies for Benefit-Risk (UMBRA). All these frameworks share some common features. QSPI BRWG summarizes these features and recommends the following 4-step B-R framework (Figure 16.2) (8).

Step 1: Define decision context. At this step, a summary and analysis of the disease condition that the drug is targeted to treat and other therapeutic options available to treat the disease population will be provided. The perspective of the stakeholders including patients on the disease and treatment outcome (e.g., weighting) can also be included. The decision context should be developed separately for each population or indication. In Design 3 (Figure 16.1), biological, clinical, and non-clinical evidence needs to be provided to justify pooling selected populations or cohorts, for example, the biomarker evidence underlying the identification of the intended patients.

Step 2: Identify benefit and risk endpoints. The benefit endpoints typically include the primary and secondary efficacy endpoints of the clinical trials, the clinical meaning of primary and secondary endpoints, and appropriate analyses of subpopulations. The risk endpoints include the identified and emerging adverse events, the severity and reversibility of adverse events, inadequacy of the safety database, and the potential for sub-optimal management in the post-market setting that may be of concern. Other considerations include non-clinical pharmacology and toxicology data; clinical pharmacology, and dosing route convenience, etc. There are

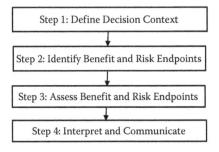

FIGURE 16.2
Benefit-Risk Assessment Framework

usually multiple benefits or risks relevant to BRA and the value tree is an effective graphic tool to visually display and summarize the endpoints identified. Figure 16.3 shows an example of decision tree for an oncology indication. The benefits include objective tumor response, progression free survival (PFS), and a quality of life (QoL) score. The potential risks include cardiovascular (CV) and gastrointestinal (GI) adverse events.

For the platform trials, one decision tree can be built for each population/indication. While multiple decision trees will be developed for Design 2, some overlapping is expected among the decision trees.

Step 3: Assess Benefit and Risk Endpoints. Relevant data sources will be identified, which usually include all phases of clinical studies. Non-clinical study data should also be included and described. The benefits and risks identified will be evaluated against the data sources. If applicable, meta-analysis techniques may be used to integrate evidences from multiple studies. The benefit and risk results are summarized and presented together in a tabulate or figure format. While the BRA still relies on expert judgment, quantitative approaches can provide valuable insight and instrumental information to support the benefit-risk decision, in particular for cases where the benefit-risk decision is not obvious or involves a large number of benefits and risks with various sources of evidence. Several quantitative methods will be discussed in Section 2.2.

Step 4: Interpret and communicate. To interpret the B-R analysis results, relative importance of the benefits and risks should be taken into account. Weighting, assigning weights to each of benefit and risk endpoints, is a common way to represent the relative importance. There are various

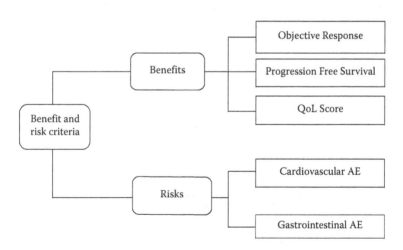

FIGURE 16.3
An Example of Decision Tree.

approaches to deriving the weights, such as ranking and swing weights (5,9). However, it is acknowledged that weighting is highly subjective, and that different stakeholders likely have different preferences. It is also not clear whose weighting should be considered in the benefit-risk assessment and what to do if different B-R decisions arrive as a function of the weights. Recently, there has been a focus on the patients' perspective in drug development (8,10). It is natural to consider weighting from patients on the benefits and risks in BRA. Some standards need to be established on how to elicit and use patients' preferences in BRA.

The BRA framework should be developed separately for each indication. For Design 1, as there is only one indication involved, all treatment arms will be evaluated under the same framework. For Design 2, a framework needs to be established for each indication. However, some data from the different arms (e.g., safety data) may be useful to be pooled to support B-R evaluation for different indications. For Design 3, one B-R framework is needed and there should be strong evidence supporting such a design, for example biomarker data.

Example 1. Consider a platform phase 2 trial for an oncology indication where 400 advanced cancer patients are randomized to three experimental arms and a control arm in 1:1:1:1 ratio. The objective is to select promising treatment arms to further test in phase 3 trials. The efficacy and safety endpoints identified to be relevant to BRA are shown in Figure 16.3. The CV risk is relatively rare and the GI risk is more common for some treatment arms. A QoL endpoint is included, for which a responder analysis (>2 point) is used. The treatment effect is based on hazard ratio (HR) for PFS and odds ratio (OR) for the other endpoints.

Table 16.1 summarizes the benefit and risk results based on the simulated data. Treatment 1 did not show any notable difference from the control arm for both benefits and risks. Treatment 2 improved the objective response rate, but did not show evidence for improvement in PFS. On the other hand, the risk for CV and GI events was higher in Treatment 2 compared to the control. Treatment 3 improved both PFS and ORR, but also observed increased risk for CV and GI events. In order to form an overall view of the B-R profile, the relative importance of these endpoints should be considered. As mentioned previously, there are a number of ways to derive the weighting, For simplicity, we weight these endpoints by ranking with PFS and CV AE being more important endpoints to consider for BRA. Based on the evidence observed and the ranking, Treatment 1 did not show a favorable B-R profile; the benefit of ORR in Treatment 2 may not outweigh the increased risk; and Treatment 3 showed some promise for a favorable B-R profile and may be worthwhile to move to next stage of drug development. Graphic display is a useful tool to assist interpretation and communication of the BRA results (11). Figure 16.4 is a forest plot of comparison of treatment arms against the control arm.

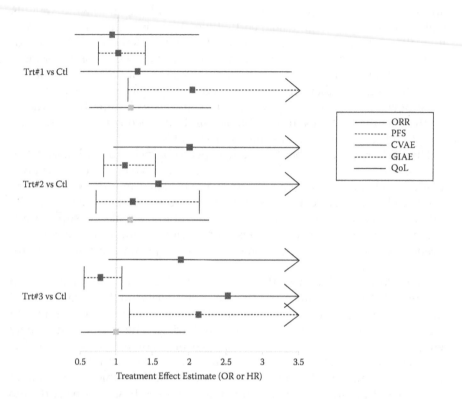

FIGURE 16.4
Benefit-risk endpoint comparison with the control arm

2.2. Quantitative Benefit-Risk Assessment Methods

Although decision making on the B-R profile of a treatment requires judgement and preference and is qualitative in nature, some quantitative methods can be instrumental to facilitate the BRA. Quantitative methods can be used to process, integrate, and synthesize large amounts of evidence and data from various sources to provide insights and inform decision-making. There are many methods in the literature that may be used for BRA [e.g., (6)]; some of them are very similar and others may be limited in their use or have a different level of scientific rigor. With an aim to standardize the BRA process, QSPI BRWG evaluated many available approaches and recommended several quantitative methods that should be considered in the BRA (5). In this section, we will describe the methods and considerations relevant to BRA for platform trials.

TABLE 16.1

Summary of benefit and risk endpoints based on the simulated platform trial.

	Control	Treatment 1		Treatment 2		Treatment 3		Ranking (Weight)
		Incidence	Relative Effect [95%CI]	Incidence	Relative Effect [95%CI]	Incidence	Relative Effect [95%CI]	
PFS	75%	74%	1.00 (0.73, 1.38)	78%	1.11 (0.81, 1.53)	63%	0.77 (0.55, 1.08)	1
CV AE	8%	10%	1.28 (0.48, 3.38)	12%	1.57 (0.61, 4.02)	18%	2.52 (1.04, 6.11)	2
ORR	13%	12%	0.91 (0.39, 2.11)	23%	2.00 (0.95, 4.22)	22%	1.89 (0.89, 4.00)	3
GI AE	50%	67%	2.03 (1.15, 3.60)	55%	1.22 (0.70, 2.13)	68%	2.13 (120, 3.77)	4
QoL	22%	25%	1.18 (0.61, 2.27)	25%	1.18 (0.61, 2.27)	22%	1.00 (0.51, 1.95)	5

2.2.1. Methods for Single Benefit and Risk

This is the simplest situation where single benefit and risk endpoints are considered for evaluating the B-R profile. Arguably, many B-R decisions can be narrowed down to one key benefit and one key risk. In this case, 'number needed to treat' (NNT) is a useful and simple approach for BRA. NNT is defined for a binary endpoint as the reciprocal of an absolute risk reduction between a treatment and a control (12). NNT is explained as, on average, the number of patients needed to be treated by the experimental treatment to prevent exactly one patient from experiencing the endpoint event compared to the control treatment. It provides a measure that can translate the treatment effect to the clinical practice and "tells physicians and patients in more concrete terms how much effort they must expend to prevent one event" (12), therefore it is very popular in interpreting clinical trial results. NNT is initially used to describe a benefit outcome. When used for the safety or risk outcome, it is also named as 'number needed to harm' (NNH). NNH is interpreted as the number of patients needed to treat to cause one patient to experience the risk event compared to the control treatment.

To contrast the benefit and risk for BRA, the ratio $r = NNH/NNT$ is proposed to combine the benefit and risk to form an integral view. The ratio is interpreted as number of patients who have efficacy events prevented by Treatment 3 for each additional patient with the risk event compared to the control. A threshold c (>1) can be defined so that a ratio larger than the threshold represents a favorable B-R profile. Determination of the threshold is challenging and should reflect relative importance of the benefit and risk endpoints or weighting. The discussion above on weighting applies to determination of the threshold. It should be noted that there is some criticism on the statistical properties of NNT and its use [e.g., (13)]. Particularly, one issue is concerned with some difficulty in constructing and interpreting confidence intervals for NNT if two arms do not show a significant difference (14,15). However, we consider NNT as a useful measure to interpret the results, not as an inferential statistic, and thus having some merits in evaluating B-R profile. Ke and Jiang extend the concept of NNH/NNT to the case of the time-to-event endpoint (15).

For Design 1, NNT and NNH can be presented as in Table 16.2. The benefit and risk endpoints are typically the same for all arms and then the threshold for the ratio will be the same. It is possible that the risk could be different for a different treatment arm. Then c_i's could be different, too. When it is of interest to compare among the active arms, the different thresholds should be taken into consideration. One way could be based on calculating the normalized ratio $\tilde{r}_i = r_i/c_i$. For Design 2, a similar table can be constructed where each arm corresponds to different indications. In general, one may not want to compare the B-R profile across indications. However, if a portfolio-level decision is needed to prioritize the development programs, it is possible to also compare the normalized ratio across

TABLE 16.2

NNH and NNT for Platform Trials

	Arm 1	Arm 2	...	Arm K
Benefit: NNT	x_1	x_2		x_k
Risk: NNH	y_1	y_2	...	y_k
Ratio: NNH/NNT	$r_1 = y_1/x_1$	$r_2 = y_2/x_2$	...	$r_k = y_k/x_k$
(threshold)	(c_1)	(c_2)		(c_k)

indications to support such portfolio decision. However, such a comparison has several statistical challenges, for example multiplicity control and a low power. For Design 3, one NNH and NNT ratio can be calculated once the population is selected. The ratio could also be used to select which subpopulations should be included for further development (see Section 2.2.3).

Example 1. In the simulated example, we assume that PFS and CV risk are two important endpoints to the BRA. We only consider Treatment 3 vs control. NNT is 8.3 for PFS and NNH is 10 for CV AE. Then the NNH and NNT ratio is 1.2, which means that on average 1.2 patients had a disease progression or death event prevented by Ttreatment 3 for each additional patient with a CV event. Whether this ratio represents a favorable profile depends upon how important one disease progression or death event is relative to a CV adverse event.

2.2.2. Methods for Multiple Benefits and Risks

It is common that data are collected on multiple benefits and risks in clinical trials. The stakeholders need to assess all evidence to determine whether the experimental treatment possesses a favorable B-R profile. Quantitative methods can be helpful to synthesize the evidence and to explore uncertainties to facilitate decision-making. Several methods have been proposed in literature to combine multiple benefits or risks [e.g., (16, 17)]. However, these methods share some common components as in multiple criteria decision analysis (MCDA) (18). In this section, we will describe the MCDA approach in detail.

Denote E_i as measurement for the i-th endpoint including benefits and risks, $v_i(x)$ as a value function to standardize E_i, and w_i the weight assigned to E_i with $\sum_{i=1}^{K} w_i = 1$. Then define a B-R score for each treatment arm as

$$S = \sum_{i=1}^{K} w_i v_i(E_i).$$

The B-R score combines all benefits and risks together in a meaningful way, and comparison of the B-R profile between treatment arms can be based on the score. For example, we can use the absolute or relevant difference in the B-R score

$$\Delta S = S_1 - S_2, \; r_s = S_1/S_2$$

The difference of the benefit-risk scores can be rewritten as

$$\Delta S = \sum_{i=1}^{K} w_i v_i(E_{1i}) - \sum_{i=1}^{K} w_i v_i(E_{2i}) = \sum_{i=1}^{K} w_i[v_i(E_{1i}) - v_i(E_{2i})],$$

and $w_i[v_i(E_{1i}) - v_i(E_{2i})]$ represents the contribution from the i-th criterion to the overall benefit-risk balancing. Given the weight w_i, the B-R score can be estimated by plugging in the estimate of E_i

$$\hat{s} = \sum_{i=1}^{K} w_i v_i(\widehat{E}_i)$$

$$v(\hat{s}) = w^T Cov(v_i(\widehat{E}_i), i = 1, \dots, K)w,$$

where $w = (w_1, \dots, w_K)$ and $Cov(v_i(\widehat{E}_i), i = 1, \dots, K)$ is the covariance matrix of the transformed endpoints. The correlation matrix needs to be estimated. Then confidence intervals can be constructed for $\hat{S}$ to account for the sampling variation and the Wald-type test statistic can be used to compare $\hat{S}$ between the treatment arms. A resampling-based method can also be employed.

Some notes on the MCDA-type analysis are as follows:

- Selection of E_i. The benefits and risks should be selected to be meaningful for the BRA. For example, the clinical endpoints would be preferred for benefits to a pharmacodynamic or lab endpoint. This selection should be justified in the BRA framework and presented in the value tree.
- Value function v_i. As the endpoint E_i can be of different variable type (e.g., continuous, binary) or of different scales, the value function is employed to transform the endpoints to the same scale to be comparable. A simple example of a value function is a linear interpolation when the minimum (L) and maximum (U) levels of a criterion can be identified and their values are set as 0 and 1 respectively

$$v(x) = \begin{cases} 1, & x=U \\ \dfrac{x - L}{U - L}, & L < x < U. \\ 0, & x=L \end{cases}$$

The minimum and maximum levels could be specified based on expert judgment or based on the percentile of the distribution of the criterion.

- Weight w_i. The weight represents the relative importance of endpoints. But there is no objective measure of the weight and the view of importance can be highly subjective.

- Several important assumptions are made in the MCDA approach, and thus sensitivity analyses should be used to demonstrate the impact any assumption has on the final weighted BR score and the BR conclusion. The sensitivity analysis should take into account, among other things, endpoint selection, value functions, and weights.

For Design 1 and Design 2, a similar summary table of B-R scores can be provided to Table 16.2. For Design 3, the B-R score can also be used to select subpopulations.

Example 1. We apply the MCDA analysis to Example 1. For the purpose of illustration, we analyze PFS based on incidence of progressive disease or death instead of a time-to-event endpoint. Since all endpoints are binary, we take the value function as $v(x) = x$ for response endpoints and $v(x) = 1 - x$ for AE and PFS. In practice, one could pick a narrow range to define the value function instead of 0 to 1. Table 16.3 shows the MCDA results assuming the weight $w = c$ (0.5, 0.2, 0.1, 0.1, 0.1). As shown, BR scores for Treatment 1 and 2 are comparable to the control arm, confirming no favorable B-R profile in Treatment 1 or 2 relative to the control. Treatment 3 has an improvement of 8% in BR score compared with the control. Treatment 3 may be promising for further study, particularly with some measures taken to mitigate the CV risk. Sensitivity analyses should also be conducted to evaluate the robust of the B-R conclusion against endpoints, value function, and weight selection.

TABLE 16.3

MCDA analysis for Example 1

	Weight	Control	Treatment 1	Treatment 2	Treatment 3
PD or Death	0.5	75%	74%	78%	63%
CV AE	0.2	8%	10%	12%	18%
ORR	0.1	13%	12%	23%	22%
GI AE	0.1	50%	67%	55%	68%
PRO	0.1	22%	25%	25%	22%
BR Score		0.394	0.38	0.379	0.425
(SE)	–	(0.023)	(0.024)	(0.023)	(0.026)

In addition, QSPI BRWP also recommends methods for eliciting patient preference. It has come to consensus that patients, as the consumer of the drug treatment, should play a key role in the BRA decision-making process. For example, FDA CDRH (2)

> would consider evidence relating to patients' perspective of what constitutes a meaningful benefit when determining if the device is effective, as some set of patients may value a benefit more than others. It should also be noted that if, for a certain device, the probable risks outweigh the probable benefits for all reasonable patients, FDA would consider use of such a device to be inherently unreasonable.

Since the patient preference data is not collected in clinical studies, some survey-based approaches such as conjoint analysis are useful to collect patients' data on weighting benefits and risks. Refer to (8) and (10) for more discussions.

2.2.3. B-R Interim Analysis

The platform designs are mostly useful in the exploratory early stage studies, e.g., phase 2 studies. Early decision based on interim analysis (IA) is important to drop non-promising arms and to advance promising arms as soon as possible to achieve efficiency. In this section, we will discuss considerations of using B-R methods to support decision making at IA.

In the case of one benefit and one risk, we use NNH/NNT ratio to formulate the BR decision criteria. In the platform design, early decision criteria are commonly defined based on efficacy. For example, the decision criteria were based on the pathologic complete response rate in I-SPY2 study (19). We propose to formulate the decision criteria based on B-R considerations, for example

- Potentially stop the study or a treatment arm for a positive B-R profile if the $a\%$ confidence lower limit of the ratio NNH/NNT > Cp
- Stop the study or a treatment arm for a futile B-R profile if Pr ($a\%$ confidence lower limit of the ratio at the final > Cp | interim data) < b
- Otherwise continue the study.

C_p is the threshold selected in consideration of the relative importance of the benefit and risk. Because clinical studies are usually only powered for efficacy, not B-R balancing, appropriate thresholds for a and b should be selected, for example through simulations to achieve certain design characteristics. While it is possible to implement the B-R based decision criteria, it may be more reasonable to supplement the efficacy criteria with the B-R criteria to support the decision-making. Below is an example combining efficacy and B-R criteria for interim analysis.

- If the efficacy boundary is crossed and if the $a\%$ confidence lower limit of the ratio NNH/NNT > Cp, stop the study or the treatment arm for a positive B-R profile
- If the futility efficacy boundary is crossed or if Pr ($a\%$ confidence lower limit of the ratio at the final > Cp | interim data) < b then stop the study or treatment arm for futility
- Otherwise continue the study.

The above criteria can also be stated under the Bayesian framework using posterior and predictive probabilities. Denote $Y_i \sim$ Bernoulli (p_i) and $X_i \sim$ Bernoulli (r_i), as the benefit and risk endpoint respectively, $i = 1, 2$ for treatment and control. Then NNT=$1/(\hat{p}_2 - \hat{p}_1)$, NNH = $/(\hat{r}_1 - \hat{r}_2)$,, assuming that more events indicate worse outcome for both benefit and risk endpoints. Further assume a total of N_i patients will be enrolled into treatment arm i and there is one interim analysis when endpoint data is available for n_i patients. Assume S_{1i} and T_{1i}, $i = 1, 2$, are the number of events for benefit and risk endpoints observed in treatment arm i by the IA. The predictive probability can be expressed as

$$\Pr\left(\frac{\text{NNH}}{\text{NNT}} > C_p | S_{1i}, T_{1i}\right) = \Pr(\text{NNH} > C_p * \text{NNT} | S_{1i}, T_{1i})$$

$$= \text{pr}((\hat{p}_2 - \hat{p}_1) + C_p * (\hat{r}_2 - \hat{r}_1) > 0 | S_{1i}, T_{1i})$$

Assume Beta(A_{pi}, B_{pi}) and Beta(A_{ri}, B_{ri}) as the prior distributions for p_i and r_i, where Beta(A, B) represents a Beta distribution with parameters A and B. Then the posterior distribution of p_i and r_i are: Beta($A_{pi} + S_{pi}$, $B_{pi} + n_i - S_{pi}$) and Beta($A_{ri} + S_{ri}$, $B_{ri} + n_i - S_{ri}$). And the posterior predictive distribution of ΔS_i, the number of new events after IA is a beta-binomial distribution:

$$p(\Delta S_i | S_{1i}) = \binom{N_i - n_i}{\Delta S_i} \frac{B(\Delta S_i + \alpha, N_i - n_i - \Delta S_i + \beta)}{B(\alpha, \beta)}$$

where $\alpha = A_{pi} + S_{1i}$, $\beta = B_{pi} + n_i - S_{1i}$. Define the estimate of the subject incidence as $\hat{p}_i = \frac{S_{2i}}{N_i} = \frac{S_{1i} + \Delta S_i}{N_i}$, where S_{21} is the number of benefit events observed for treatment arm i by the end of study. The posterior predictive distribution for the estimate $\hat{p}_i$ can be derived accordingly. So do the risk differences $\hat{p}_2 - \hat{p}_1$ and $(\hat{r}_2 - \hat{r}_1)$. Note that if the support of the predictive distribution covers zero, the distribution for NNH, NNT, and the NNH/HHT may be problematic. The posterior predictive probability can be obtained by using Markov-Chain Monte Carlo simulations.

For multiple benefits and risks, similar decision criteria can be set up using the MCDA analysis.

2.2.4. B-R Subgroup Analysis

In practice, patients may respond to a treatment differently for many reasons, therefore possessing a different benefit-risk profile. B-R subgroup analysis is proposed to evaluate whether the B-R profile of a treatment changes according to some baseline covariates, i.e., whether there is an interaction effect on B-R balancing. If such interaction exists, subgroup analysis can be used to identify patients who benefit from the treatment with a favorable B-R profile, which falls into the framework of precision medicine. In Design 3, the primary goal is to identify such responder patient populations (baskets) for further evaluation. The decision should take into consideration both efficacy and safety, and thus utilizes the benefit-risk assessment techniques. Of note, the B-R subgroup analysis is similar to the patient-level BRA approach recommended by QSPI BRWG (8).

Assume that we have patient-level data available. Define a B-R score or index for patient i

$$Y_i = f(E_{i1}, \ldots, E_{iK}; w),$$

where f is a known function and w is the weight vector. An example is the B-R score in the MCDA approach. Subgroup analysis can then be conducted based on Y_i. For example, treatment-by-covariate interaction can be evaluated based on the following model:

$$h(\mu_{Yi}) = \beta_1 X_i + \beta_2 T_i + \beta_{12} X_i T_i$$

where β_{12} β_{12} represents the interaction effect, $h(x)$ is a known link function, and T_i is treatment arm indicator.

B-R profile heterogeneity may come from interplay of benefits, risks, and judgement or weight.

To investigate the source of heterogeneity, we consider the MCDA method for one benefit and one risk. Denote $X = 0$, or 1 as a baseline variable, and Y as the B-R score in MCDA-type analysis. Then we have

$$\mu(x, w) = E(Y; x, w) = w_x \mu_B(x) + (1 - w_x)\mu_R(x), \text{ and}$$
$$\Delta\mu = \mu(1, w) - \mu(0, w) = [w_1 \mu_B(1) + (1 - w_1)\mu_R(1)] - [w_0 \mu_B(0)$$
$$+ (1 - w_0)\mu_R(0)].$$

There are three simple scenarios of heterogeneity and a general situation can be a combination of these three scenarios.

1. Heterogeneity due to benefit. If $\mu_R(1) = \mu_R(0)$ and $w_1 = w_0 = w$, then $\Delta_\mu = w(\mu_B(1) - \mu_B(0))$. In this case, the difference in the benefit with respect to X will leads to a different B-R profile.
2. Heterogeneity due to risk. If $\mu_B(1) = \mu_B(0)$ and $w_1 = w_0 = w$, then $\Delta\mu = (1-w)(\mu_R(1) - \mu_R(0))$. In this case, the difference in the risk with respect to X will leads to a different B-R profile.
3. Heterogeneity due to weight. If $\mu_B(1) = \mu_B(0) = \mu_B$ and $\mu_R(1) = \mu_R(0)$, then $\Delta\mu = (w_1 - w_0)(\mu_B - \mu_R)$. In this case, when the weight assigned to the benefit and risk varies with the covariate X, the B-R profile will be different.

Example 2. Vorapaxar for secondary prevention of CV events. The phase 3 study of Thrombin Receptor Antagonist in Secondary Prevention of Atherothrombotic Ischemic Events (TRA 2P)–Thrombolysis in Myocardial Infarction (TIMI) 50 trial, was designed to evaluate the efficacy and safety of vorapaxar in reducing atherothrombotic events in patients with established atherosclerosis who were receiving standard therapy. At an interim analysis, after completion of enrollment and a median of 24 months of follow-up, the data and safety monitoring board (DSMB) reported an excess of intracranial hemorrhage in patients with a history of stroke in the treatment arm. The DSMB recommended discontinuation of the drug in all patients with previous stroke, including those with a new stroke during trial but continuation of the study in patients without a history of stroke (20). There was no significant heterogeneity for the benefit of vorapaxar on the primary efficacy endpoint across most of the major subgroups examined. Vorapaxar was eventually approved with an indication of reduction of thrombotic cardiovascular events in patients with a MI or PAD history. The heterogenous B-R profile seems driven by the difference in safety in this case.

Example 3. Talimogene Laherparepvec (T-VEC) for melanoma. The primary evidence is based on a randomized phase 3 study designed to evaluate whether treatment with T-VEC resulted in an improved durable response rate (DRR) compared with GM-CSF in patients with unresected stage IIIB to IV melanoma (21). The study data showed the drug had a consistently well tolerated safety profile. As of the efficacy results, some variation was observed in the treatment effect on overall survival in relation to the disease stage: HR = 0.57 (95%CI: 0.40, 0.80) in patients of Stage IIIB/IIIC/IVM1a and HR = 1.07 (95%CI: 0.75, 1.53) in patients of stage IVM1B/IVM1C (Table 5 in T-VEC SPC). T-VEC was deemed to have a favorable B-R profile and was subsequently approved for use in a subset of patient population of unresectable melanoma that is regionally or distantly metastatic (Stage IIIB, IIIC, and IVM1a) with no bone, brain, lung or other visceral disease by EMA and for the local treatment of unresectable cutaneous, subcutaneous, and nodal lesions in patients with melanoma recurrent after initial surgery by FDA. This example demonstrates heterogeneity in the B-R profile due to the variation of the benefit.

Finally, in Design 3, the basket selection can be based on the B-R index defined above. For example, in a phase 2 oncology basket trial, many small cohorts, such as primary tumor types, are studied to evaluate the drug activity and potentially screen the subset of tumor types for confirmatory studies. Response rate is a typical benefit measurement, and some specific adverse event can be considered as the risk. We can define the B-R index for each basket or cohort as:

$$Y = \frac{q}{1-p}\frac{w_B}{w_R}$$

where q is the rate of some adverse event, p is the objective response rate, and w_B and w_R are weights assigned to the response and AE. Please refer to other chapters in this book for methods to select baskets.

---

3. Uncertainties

Uncertainty has been recognized as a key issue in B-R assessment, due to the challenges it adds to the decision-making process. There are clear imbalances in the sources, timing, and nature of information available throughout a drug's lifecycle (22), which could cause uncertainties in B-R assessment.

While some uncertainties are known and can sometimes be quantified and addressed, others may not be known. One obvious source of uncertainty is the confidence interval around the effect, but there are several other important sources of uncertainty. For example, results from pre-specified hypotheses are more credible than unexpected findings. Incomplete follow-up and resulting missing data add uncertainty. Relative importance of benefits vs risks could bring uncertainty as well. Different stakeholders may have different understandings about this. Another uncertainty source is about benefit-risk assessment in post-marketing. In post-marketing, we often put more emphasis on assessing safety than efficacy, which brings uncertainties related to BR assessment. There are other sources of uncertainties in addition to these. Some could relate to endpoint definitions which result in double counting. One option in this case is to conduct sensitivity analysis using endpoints that do not overlap. Note that it is important to address uncertainty considering the complexity of the decision-making process. There have been many efforts to date devoted to improving the biopharmaceutical community's understanding of uncertainty and approaches to addressing different sources of uncertainty in benefit-risk assessment.

How to minimize and assess BR uncertainty? Uncertainty present throughout benefit-risk assessment and associated with study design and conduct such as missing data could be addressed by proactive planning and prevention of issues. For example, patients could be encouraged to stay in follow-up even if they stop taking the study therapy. Estimates of BR could be provided with measures of uncertainty such as confidence interval and sensitivity analysis. Well designed and conducted meta-analyses for safety endpoints can be used to synthesize information from different sources. Statistical tools such as graphical tools are helpful to understand the impact of uncertainty.

4. Conclusions and Discussion

Structured benefit-risk assessment has recently gained much attention in drug development and life-cycle management. Many decisions regarding development, regulation, and use of a drug treatment are concerned with both benefits and risks, and therefore are B-R decisions. While the B-R evaluation was mostly informal and qualitative in the past, many efforts from regulatory, academia, and industry have been put forth to improve the B-R assessment process and to increase clarity and transparency in the B-R decision making. The platform designs are a group of innovative alternatives to traditional study designs to address the emerging issues in drug development to achieve efficiency and precision. In this chapter, we discussed benefit-risk assessment methods and challenges as well as their application in platform trials. We recommended a structured benefit-risk assessment approach including the use of a descriptive framework complemented with some quantitative BRA approaches to inform decision making in the course of clinical development and life-cycle drug management in general.

The platform designs are primarily used in early stage clinical trials, for example, phase 2 trials, and have some special features that should be considered when implementing BRA. For example, most of the decisions in the platform trials are concerned with the sponsor's go or no-go decision based on early data. Other stakeholders including patients may not be involved in these assessments. However, a robust BRA should take into account considerations from the perspective of different stakeholders. Another feature is that studies using the platform design may have small amount of data available for decision making, surrogate efficacy endpoints are typically used, and some data, such as long-term safety, may be missing, which makes the early benefit-risk evaluation very challenging.

It is critical that BRA should incorporate all available data cumulatively, including non-clinical and clinical data, using meta-analysis, and modeling and simulation techniques.

Since BRA is very complicated and qualitative in nature, there are many uncertainties when implementing the BRA. For example, weighting the benefit and risk endpoints is largely subjective, and it may not be realistic to reach a consensus on the relative importance of one endpoint relative to another endpoint. To account for the uncertainties in the BRA, e.g., through sensitivity analyses, is critical to a robust B-R decision. Some standard processes to elicit and use the weight should be established to further achieve consistency and transparency.

Quantitative methods are critical in complicated decision making such as BRA. Some quantitative B-R evaluation methods were proposed for the platform trials. We also developed the methods for B-R interim analysis and B-R subgroup analysis for the platform trials. We will look to implement the methods to some real trial data as further work. More research is needed in this area.

References

1. FDA. Enhancing benefit-risk assessment in regulatory decision-making. Draft PDUFA V implementation plan: Structured approach to benefit-risk assessment in drug regulatory decision-making. February 2013. www.fda.gov/down loads/ForIndustry/UserFees/PrescriptionDrugUserFee/UCM329758.pdf
2. FDA CDRH. Guidance for Industry and Food and Drug Administration Staff – Factors to Consider When Making Benefit-Risk Determinations in Medical Device Premarket Approvals and De Novo Classifications. Silver Spring, MD: FDA CDRH, 2012.
3. EMA benefit-risk methodology project. www.ema.europa.eu/ema/index. jsp?curl=pages/special_topics/document_listing/document_listing_ 000314.jsp&murl=menus/special_topics/special_topics.jsp&mid= WC0b01ac0580223ed6&jsenabled=false
4. Coplan PM, Noel RA, Levitan BS, Ferguson J, Mussen F. Development of a framework for enhancing the transparency, reproducibility and communication of the benefit-risk balance of medicines. *Clinical Pharmacology and Therapeutics* 2011; 89(2): 312–315.
5. Jiang Q, He W. *Benefit-risk Assessment Methods in Medical Product Development: Bridging Qualitative and Quantitative Assessments*. Boca Raton, FL: Taylor and Francis, 2016.
6. Guo JJ et al. A review of quantitative risk-benefit methodologies for assessing drug safety and efficacy-report of the ISPOR risk-benefit management working group. *Value in Health* 2010; 13(5): 657–666.
7. IMI Pharmacoepidemiological Research on Outcomes of Therapeutics by European Consortium (PROTECT). WP5: Benefit-risk integration and representation. www.imi-protect.eu/wp5.html

8. Quartey G et al. Overview of benefit-risk evaluation methods: A spectrum from qualitative to quantitative. In *Benefit-risk Assessment Methods in Medical Product Development: Bridging Qualitative and Quantitative Assessments*. Edited by Jiang Q, He W. Boca Raton, FL: Taylor and Francis, 2016.

9. Ke C, Jiang Q, Snapinn S. Benefit-risk assessment approach. In *Quantitative Evaluation of Safety in Drug Development: Design, Analysis and Reporting*. Edited by Jiang Q, Amy Xia H. Boca Raton, FL: Taylor and Francis, 2014.

10. Johnson F, Zhou M. Quantifying patient preferences for regulatory benefit-risk assessment. In *Benefit-risk Assessment Methods in Medical Product Development: Bridging Qualitative and Quantitative Assessments*. Edited by Jiang Q, He W. Boca Raton, FL: Taylor and Francis, 2016.

11. Shi W et al. Visualization of benefit-risk assessment in medical products with real example. In *Benefit-Risk Assessment Methods in Medical Product Development: Bridging Qualitative and Quantitative Assessments*. Edited by Jiang Q, He W. Boca Raton, FL: Taylor and Francis, 2016.

12. Laupacis A, Sackett DL, Roberts RS. An assessment of clinically useful measures of the consequences of treatment. *New England Journal of Medicine* 1988; 318(26): 1728–1733.

13. Hutton JA. Number needed to treat: Properties and problems. (with discussion). *Journal of the Royal Statistical Society* 2000; 163: 403–419.

14. Altman DG. Confidence intervals for the number needed to treat. *British Medical Journal* 1998; 317: 1309–1312.

15. Ke C, Jiang Q. Benefit–risk assessment using number needed to treat and number needed to harm for time-to-event endpoints. *Statistics in Biopharmaceutical Research* 2016; 8: 379–385.

16. Chuang-Stein C. A new proposal for benefit-less-risk analysis in clinical trials. *Controlled Clinical Trial* 1994; 15: 30–43.

17. Ouellet D. Benefit-risk assessment: The use of clinical utility index. *Expert Opinion on Drug Safety* 2010; 9(2): 289–300.

18. Mussen F, Salek S, Walker S. A quantitative approach to benefit-risk assessment of medicines – Part 1: The development of a new model using multi-criteria decision analysis. *Pharmacoepidemiology and Drug Safety* 2007; 16(Suppl 1): S2–S15.

19. Park JW et al. Adaptive randomization of neratinib in early breast cancer. *New England Journal of Medicine* 2016; 375: 11–22.

20. Marrow DA et al. Vorapaxar in the secondary prevention of atherothrombotic events. *New England Journal of Medicine* 2012; 366: 1404–1412.

21. Robert HI et al. Talimogene Laherparepvec improves durable response rate in patients with advanced melanoma. *Journal of Clinical Oncology* 2015; 33: 2780–2788.

22. Hammad TA, Neyarapally GA, Iyasu S, Staffa JA, Dal Pan G. The future of population-based postmarket drug risk assessment: A regulator's perspective. *Clinical Pharmacology & Therapeutics* 2013; 94(3): 349–358.

17

Effect of Randomization Schemes in Umbrella Trials When There Are Unknown Interactions between Biomarkers

Janet J. Li, Shuai Sammy Yuan, and Robert A. Beckman

Background

Umbrella Trials

The past decade has brought about progress in tumor biology and cancer research that has had many implications in translational and clinical cancer research. The classical design of oncology clinical trials targets one tumor type with one specific biomarker. This "one trial for one drug" strategy requires large resources and can make the evaluation of target agents inefficient when multiple agents are each potentially effective for many different tumor types, and collectively for multiple biomarkers. Recent advances in targeted therapy have made it possible to treat cancer patients in a more precise and more personalized way. The underlying rationale of targeted therapy may require dividing the patient population into many small subpopulations, each of which has a specific target biomarker. In trying to find treatments for patients with different tumor types or different mutations, it becomes difficult for patients to get the right treatment in a timely manner due to the resources and time needed to investigate and get regulatory approval for each potential agent. To shorten the investigational period and streamline the regulatory approval process, more innovative study designs that can utilize limited resource more efficiently and be flexible and rigorous enough to meet the needs and objectives of the sponsor, regulatory agents and patients at the same time are needed. One design that addresses this need is the master protocol framework. A master protocol consists of one overarching protocol that includes multiple diseases, multiple treatments, and/or multiple markers. Types of master protocols include umbrella trials, cloud trials, and basket trials (LaVange and Sridhara, 2014).

Umbrella trials are designed to test the impact of different drugs on different mutations in a single tumor type in one overarching protocol. For certain diseases that have very small patient pools to test investigational therapies, umbrella trials can borrow information from different parts of the integrated trial, share resources among sub-studies, and thus speed up the regulatory approval process (Menis, Hasan, and Besse, 2014).

In general, a central screening component exists in the umbrella trial infrastructure to screen patients for a specific set of biomarkers, and the trial design involves strata (also can be referred to as substudies or subtrials) that are defined on the basis of biomarker profile and/or other baseline factors. Patients are assigned to a specific stratum if they have one of the target biomarkers. If they are negative on all markers, they may be assigned to a non-match stratum. Strata can have different investigational therapies or share the same therapy or control, follow different randomization schemes, and be conducted according to different timelines. There is the flexibility to add, drop, or modify the strata while other strata are ongoing. See Figure 17.1 for a generalized schematic representation of the umbrella trial framework.

The LUNG-MAP trial is an example of a phase II/III umbrella trial for patients with advanced lung squamous cell carcinoma (SCCA) (Herbst et al., 2015). In this study, a drug that is found to be effective in phase II will move directly into the phase III registration setting. Other ongoing umbrella trials include the ALCHEMIST trial and FOCUS4 master protocol. The ALCHEMIST trial uses the umbrella design to identify and screen patients with the EGFR and ALK mutations in early-stage resected nonsquamous non-small cell lung cancer (NSCLC). The FOCUS4 Master Protocol is a multi-arm, multi-stage umbrella trial for patients with colorectal cancer that opened in the UK in 2014 and is similar in design to the LUNG-MAP trial.

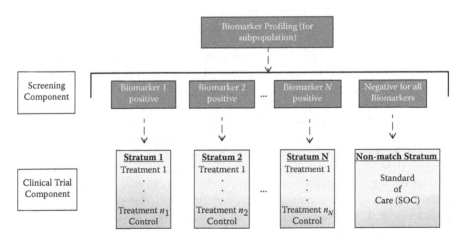

FIGURE 17.1
A generalized schematic representation of the umbrella trial design.

NCI-MATCH (National Cancer Institute-Molecular Analysis for Therapy Choice), which has been referred to as an umbrella/basket or hybrid trial, was initiated in August 2015 as a master protocol for molecular screening with many phase II subprotocols aimed to determine whether a drug or drug combination targeted to a specific molecular abnormality could produce responses (Conley, 2016).

Prioritization and Randomization Schemes in Patients Positive for Multiple Markers

Since the strata are usually created according to the status of target biomarkers in the umbrella trial framework, it is important to note that patients may have more than one of the positive target biomarkers that they are being screened for. It needs to be decided which biomarker-driven stratum these patients are assigned to. Patients may be assigned to one of the targeted strata they qualify for by either random assignment or a set of pre-determined, fixed rules. If prevalence of the biomarker or mutation group is not rare, random assignment is preferred. However, in the case where one of the mutations is truly rare, patients who qualify for more than one stratum may be assigned to the stratum with the lower accrual rate. In the LUNG-MAP study, patients who qualify for more than one stratum are assigned to strata using an algorithm that combines these two assignment strategies in that the probability of being assigned to a given stratum is inversely proportional to biomarker prevalence (Woodcock and LaVange, 2017).

NCI-MATCH uses a fixed-rule algorithm for assignment. If the cancer carries more than one mutation or copy number variant, the mutation with the highest allele frequency and at least 15% higher than the next frequent mutation is considered the most actionable. Mutations that are within 15% frequency of each other will be considered "equal." If there is a tie for the most "actionable" mutation, the patient will be assigned to the corresponding arm with the least enrollment. In this trial, patients are also re-assessed for mutations or markers upon initial disease progression and then assigned to second matched cohorts within the same trial on the basis of those results (Conley and Doroshow, 2014).

Objective

We investigated the impact that prioritization versus random assignment of patients to a biomarker-defined stratum (when patients meet criteria for multiple strata) has on treatment evaluation and trial performance including estimation bias by conducting simulations with different assignment schemes under different settings. In considering the impact of assignment schemes other than balanced randomization, it is important to note that multiple biomarkers cannot necessarily be assumed to be independent of each other in their effects on drug response. In fact, some authors have attributed the apparent tissue dependence of marker effects to interaction between markers (Tabchy et al., 2013). The research is part of an overall effort to simulate and understand master protocols by the Master Protocol Subteam of the Small Populations Workstream of the Drug Information Association (DIA) Adaptive Design Scientific Working Group.

Master Protocol Simulation Study Design

To investigate if the stratum assignment scheme will result in any bias on the treatment effect estimation of the drug on cancer patients with a specific biomarker, we considered a master protocol design with two biomarkers, Biomarker A and Biomarker B, where the prevalence of Biomarker A is 0.6 and prevalence of Biomarker B is 0.4, and the prevalences are independent (i.e., the prevalence of Biomarker B is independent of whether Biomarker A is present or absent) (Figure 17.2). We considered a subject who is positive for Biomarker A to be defined as A+ regardless of the status of other biomarkers, and a

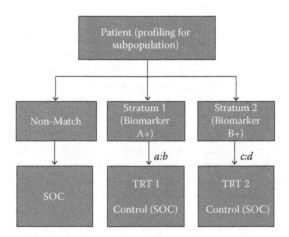

FIGURE 17.2
Master protocol simulation study design. The treatment assignment randomization ratio within Stratum 1 is denoted as *a:b* and the treatment assignment randomization ratio within Stratum a 2 is denoted as *c:d* when there are only two treatment arms in each stratum.

subject who is positive for Biomarker B is defined as B+. Similarly, a subject who is negative for Biomarker A is denoted as A– and a subject who is negative for Biomarker B is denoted as B–.

In this setup, we have four sub-populations:

1. A+B–
2. A–B+
3. A+B+
4. A–B–

We assume, without loss of generality, two active drugs, Treatment 1 (TRT1) and Treatment 2 (TRT2) for investigation, and one common control (standard of care, SOC) for this tumor type. We consider cases where neither biomarker affects the therapeutic significance of the other (independence) and cases where one biomarker affects the therapeutic response to the other (dependence).

Master Protocol Simulation Tool Development

Input Parameters

The simulation tool was created using R software (3.3.1) to allow users to be able to input parameters to generate a master protocol data set. There are two types of data considered: binary response and survival response (i. e., time to event or TTE). Each type of data can be generated under each of the above mentioned trial settings.

The parameters in the R functions include:

1. Number of patients in the trial and number of patients within each stratum
2. Prevalence of target biomarkers
3. Treatment assignment randomization ratios within each stratum
4. Number of treatment arms within each stratum
5. True response probabilities (to generate binary response data)
6. Hazard ratios (to generate time-to-event, TTE, data)
7. Median TTE value for either progression free survival or overall survival
8. Accrual Time (for TTE data)
9. Censoring Time (for TTE data)

10. Control options—the user can specify whether controls will be common or separate across different strata

Output of the Simulation Tool

The output of the simulation tool is a master protocol data set with the following variables:

1. Patient ID
2. Biomarker Screening Results (whether a patient tested positive or negative for each target biomarker)
3. Stratum Assignment
4. Treatment Assignment (within each stratum)
5. Binary response data (0 = No response, 1 = Response)
6. Time-to-event data
7. Censoring Status
8. Enrollment time (time at which patient enrolls into the trial)

Simulation Study

Stratum Assignment Strategies

In the case where a subject is positive for both biomarkers (A+B+), the subject will be assigned to a stratum (Stratum 1 or 2 in Figure 17.2) based on the following assignment strategies:

1. Random assignment with equal probability
2. Assignment to the stratum corresponding to the biomarker with the lowest prevalence
3. Assignment to the highest level of actionability based on allele frequency or other fixed prioritization scheme (we consider both the case where the priority is greater for Biomarker A and the case where the priority is greater for Biomarker B)
4. Inverse weighted assignment based on biomarker prevalence

Sample Size and Power Calculations

The sample size per group per stratum (powered on expected effect size of 30% response rate (P_1) on treatment and 5% response rate (P_2) on control at 80% power ($1 - \beta = 0.8$) and a one-sided alpha of 10%

$(\alpha = 0.1)$) can be approximated (based on the normal approximation to the binomial) by:

$$n = \frac{(Z_\alpha + Z_\beta)^2 (p_1(1-p_1) + p_2(1-p_2))}{(p_1 - p_2)^2} \approx 19$$

Since there are two groups per stratum, we will require 38 subjects per stratum. In total, 95 subjects (38 × 2 biomarker strata + 19 × 1 non-match stratum) were accrued for the simulation study. EAST 6.3 was used for the calculation.

Analysis

The true treatment effect is defined as the difference of the true response rates (as defined in Table 17.1) between treatment and control for each drug on each subpopulation (A+, B+) respectively. The patients with both biomarkers positive (A+B+) are not viewed as a separate subpopulation to mimic the practice in the LUNG-MAP or other study where the interaction between biomarker A and B is neither known nor suspected, and the assignment of the patients to a stratum is based on the status of a single relevant biomarker for that stratum.

Three different scenarios for response rates to Treatment 1 and Treatment 2 in the A+B+ population were considered:

1. Treatment 1 and Treatment 2 response rates of 30% (i.e., assuming independence; no interaction of Biomarkers A and B)
2. Treatment 1 response rate of 40% and Treatment 2 response rate of 20% (presence of Biomarker B increases the response rate to Treatment 1 in the A+ population; presence of Biomarker A decreases the response rate to Treatment 2 in the B+ population)
3. Treatment 1 response rate of 20% and Treatment 2 response rate of 40% (presence of Biomarker A increases the response rate to Treatment 2 in

TABLE 17.1

True response rates (RR) assumed in the three simulation scenarios.

Population		TRT1 True Response Rate	TRT2 True Response Rate	SOC True Response Rate
A+B−		30%	10%	5%
A−B+		10%	30%	5%
A+B+	*Scenario 1*	30%	30%	5%
	Scenario 2	40%	20%	5%
	Scenario 3	20%	40%	5%
A−B−		5%	5%	5%

the B+ population; presence of Biomarker B decreases the response rate
to Treatment 1 in the A+ population)

Since we were interested in the effect of Treatment 1 on the A+ population
regardless of the subject's status of Biomarker B and also interested in the
effect of Treatment 2 on the B+ population regardless of the subject's status
of Biomarker A, the true treatment response rates were calculated using
weighted averages of response rates from Table 17.1. For instance, the true
treatment response rate (TRT RR) of Treatment 1 in the A+ population was
calculated by the following (Equation 1):

$$True\ TRT\ RR = Prevalence_{B+} \times RR_{A+B+} + (1 - Prevalence_{B+}) \times RR_{A+B-} \quad (1)$$

where $Prevalence_{B+}$ is the prevalence of Biomarker B+, RR_{A+B+} is the
response rate of Treatment 1 in the A+B+ population, and RR_{A+B-} is the
response rate of Treatment 1 in the A+B− population. In our simulations, we
are considering the prevalence of one marker is independent of the prevalence of the other marker. However, for cases where the prevalence may
not be independent, the true treatment response rate of Treatment 1 in the A
+ population can be calculated by a more general formula (Equation 2):

$$True\ TRT\ RR = \frac{Prevalence_{A+B+}}{Prevalence_{A+}} \times RR_{A+B+} + \frac{Prevalence_{A+B-}}{Prevalence_{A+}} \times RR_{A+B-} \quad (2)$$

The estimated treatment effects, or the difference of estimated response
rates between Treatment 1 and Control on the A+ population (Stratum 1)
and the difference of estimated response rates between Treatment 2 and
Control on the B+ population (Stratum 2), were compared to the true
treatment effects. We investigated the bias, or systematic difference
between the true treatment effect and the estimated treatment effect.

Since five different assignment strategies (including the two different sub-
methods for stratum assignment method 3, where we consider both the case
where priority is greater for Biomarker A and the case where the priority is
greater for Biomarker B) and three different A+B+ treatment response rate
scenarios were considered, fifteen scenarios were investigated. The estimated
treatment effects were calculated 1,000 simulations for each scenario.

Results

The estimated average treatment response rates (for 1,000 simulations for
each scenario) and true treatment effects are summarized below in
Table 17.2.

TABLE 17.2

Summary of treatment (TRT) response rates (RR) and treatment effects

	SOC RR	True SOC RR	TRT RR*	True TRT RR	TRT Effect (95%)CI	True TRT Effect
Stratum Assignment Method 1 (random assignment)						
Scenario 1						
Stratum 1 (A+,TRT 1)	4.99%	5%	30.34%	30%	25.35% (2.47,48.22)	25%
Stratum 2 (B+,TRT 2)	5.10%	5%	29.57%	30%	24.47% (1.69,47.25)	25%
Scenario 2						
Stratum 1 (A+,TRT 1)	4.99%	5%	32.66%	34%	27.66% (4.41,50.91)	29%
Stratum 2 (B+,TRT 2)	5.12%	5%	25.58%	24%	20.46% (−1.52,42.44)	19%
Scenario 3						
Stratum 1 (A+,TRT 1)	5.12%	5%	27.75%	26%	22.63% (0.19,45.07)	21%
Stratum 2 (B+,TRT 2)	5.25%	5%	34.26%	36%	29.01% (5.43,52.58)	31%
Stratum Assignment Method 2 (lowest prevalence)						
Scenario 1						
Stratum 1 (A+,TRT 1)	5.08%	5%	29.56%	30%	24.47% (1.70,47.25)	25%
Stratum 2 (B+,TRT 2)	5.03%	5%	30.55%	30%	25.52% (2.60,48.45)	25%
Scenario 2						
Stratum 1 (A+,TRT 1)	5.13%	5%	30.10%	34%	24.97% (2.09,47.86)	29%
Stratum 2 (B+,TRT 2)	5.04%	5%	24.41%	24%	19.37% (−2.30,41.04)	19%
Scenario 3						
Stratum 1 (A+,TRT 1)	5.08%	5%	30.01%	26%	24.92% (2.07,47.77)	21%
Stratum 2 (B+,TRT 2)	5.08%	5%	36.03%	36%	30.95% (7.21,54.68)	31%
Stratum Assignment Method 3 (when priority A>B)						
Scenario 1						
Stratum 1 (A+,TRT 1)	4.78%	5%	30.35%	30%	25.57% (2.78,48.36)	25%
Stratum 2 (B+,TRT 2)	4.98%	5%	29.73%	30%	24.75% (1.99,47.51)	25%
Scenario 2						
Stratum 1 (A+,TRT 1)	5.11%	5%	34.16%	34%	29.05% (5.54,52.56)	29%
Stratum 2 (B+,TRT 2)	5.02%	5%	30.01%	24%	24.99% (2.17,47.82)	19%
Scenario 3						
Stratum 1 (A+,TRT 1)	4.97%	5%	26.59%	26%	21.62% (−0.52,43.76)	21%
Stratum 2 (B+,TRT 2)	4.86%	5%	29.67%	36%	24.81% (2.11,47.51)	31%
Stratum Assignment Method 3 (when priority A<B)						
Scenario 1						
Stratum 1 (A+,TRT 1)	4.82%	5%	29.83%	30%	25.01% (2.30,47.42)	25%
Stratum 2 (B+,TRT 2)	4.78%	5%	29.42%	30%	24.64% (2.01,47.26)	25%

(Continued)

TABLE 17.2 (Cont.)

	SOC RR	True SOC RR	TRT RR*	True TRT RR	TRT Effect (95%)CI	True TRT Effect
Scenario 2						
Stratum 1 (A+,TRT 1)	4.97%	5%	30.15%	34%	25.18% (2.35,48.02)	29%
Stratum 2 (B+,TRT 2)	5.34%	5%	24.26%	24%	18.92% (−2.85,40.68)	19%
Scenario 3						
Stratum 1 (A+,TRT 1)	4.96%	5%	29.81%	26%	24.85% (2.08,47.61)	21%
Stratum 2 (B+,TRT 2)	4.70%	5%	35.83%	36%	31.13% (7.56,54.70)	31%
Stratum Assignment Method 4 (weighted assignment based on prevalence)						
Scenario 1						
Stratum 1 (A+,TRT 1)	5.09%	5%	30.38%	30%	25.29% (2.37,48.21)	25%
Stratum 2 (B+,TRT 2)	5.11%	5%	29.72%	30%	24.62% (1.81,47.43)	25%
Scenario 2						
Stratum 1 (A+,TRT 1)	5.11%	5%	33.04%	34%	27.93% (4.58,51.28)	29%
Stratum 2 (B+,TRT 2)	4.68%	5%	26.63%	24%	21.94% (−0.09,43.97)	19%
Scenario 3						
Stratum 1 (A+,TRT 1)	4.98%	5%	27.11%	26%	22.13% (−0.13,44.38)	21%
Stratum 2 (B+,TRT 2)	5.07%	5%	33.41%	36%	28.34% (4.94,51.73)	31%

* True TRT RR was calculated using weighted averages of RR from Table 1. For example, in the A+ arm: $True\ TRT\ RR = Prevalence_{B+} \times RR_{A+B+} + (1 - Prevalence_{B+}) \times RR_{A+B-}$

Some of the stratum assignment strategies led to overestimation or underestimation of the treatment effect. For instance, when using the lowest prevalence method in Scenario 2, the estimated treatment effect is for Treatment 1 in the A+ population is 24.97% whereas the true treatment effect is 29%. This is due to the fact that A+B+ patients were assigned to Stratum 2 (B+) only since the prevalence of Biomarker B (0.4) was less than the prevalence for Biomarker A (0.6), and those A+B+ patients would have raised the overall Treatment 1 response rate according to Scenario 2. In general, errors in estimates of the true response rate were greater for the lowest prevalence method and other fixed prioritization methods than for the randomization of inverse-prevalence weighted randomization.

Discussion/Implications

Advantages of the Master Protocol Simulation Tool

We created a master protocol simulation tool with a high-level approach that allows users to select choices (by logical or index variables) for different scenarios. The flexible and branching logic structure of the tool will enable investigators to explore different statistical considerations for the master protocol platform.

Impact of Different Patient Assignment-to-Stratum Strategies Is a New Problem under the Master Protocol Framework

The impact of the different patient assignment-to-stratum strategies is a new problem under the Master Protocol framework. In our simulation study, we found that some of the stratum assignment strategies led to overestimation or underestimation of the treatment effect. This was due to the fact that the A+B+ patients were sometimes assigned only to one stratum and not the other depending on which assignment strategy was used. The bias is due to the fact that the estimand and the estimator are not fully matching. For instance, when using the lowest prevalence method, A+B+ patients were assigned to Stratum 2 (B+) since the prevalence of Biomarker B (0.4) was less than the prevalence for Biomarker A (0.6). This is a problem only when there is therapeutic interaction between the biomarkers, i.e., the presence of one biomarker affects the therapeutic response to an agent targeted at the other one.

It is likely that there are multiple unknown interactions between individual biomarkers given that individual markers represent single nodes in complex signaling and/or regulatory networks. Similarly, while many therapies primarily affect a single node, some affect several. The underlying networks have a high degree of redundancy and robustness, as well as feedback loops. These features would tend to make the independence assumption for therapeutic response unlikely although it is a useful default assumption. Investigators who wish to conduct umbrella trials in which they assume that the target biomarkers do not interact may be misled by their findings. The magnitude of the resulting bias in umbrella trial results depends on the frequency of double positives and the strength of the interaction. We note that this study assumed that the prevalence of the two biomarkers was independent, a simplifying assumption that also is not likely to always be true. Equation 2 is written to be general, but the simulation was performed assuming that the prevalence of the two biomarkers was independent.

Most umbrella trials are studying a limited number of biomarkers, and it may be possible to estimate or detect any relevant pairwise interactions from the trial data itself and adjust for it in the subsequent analysis or interpretation. At a minimum, the trial data should be used to test the independence assumptions to the degree feasible. Given the great utility of master protocols, we merely counsel awareness of these issues if anything other than strict randomization is contemplated.

The problem will also need more investigation requiring simulation studies of more complex situations, such as more than two biomarkers, time to event data, and adaptive randomization.

References

Conley B, Doroshow J. (2014). Molecular analysis for therapy choice: NCI MATCH. *Seminars in Oncology*, 41(3), 297–299.

Conley B. (2016). Molecular analysis for therapy choice (NCI-MATCH): A precision medicine signal-seeking trial in oncology. *Personalized Medicine in Oncology*, 5(8).

Herbst RS, Gandara DR, Hirsch FR, Redman MW, LeBlanc M, Mack PC, Yelensky R. (2015). Lung master protocol (Lung-MAP)—A biomarker-driven protocol for accelerating development of therapies for squamous cell lung cancer: SWOG S1400. *Clinical Cancer Research*, 21(7), 1514–1524.

LaVange LM, Sridhara R. (2014, October 21). *Statistical Considerations in Designing. Innovations in Breast Cancer Drug Development – Next Generation Oncology Trials Workshop*. Bethesda, MD: FDA.

Menis J, Hasan B, Besse B. (2014). New clinical research strategies in thoracic oncology: Clinical trial design, adaptive, basket and umbrella trials, new end-points and new evaluations of response. *European Respiratory Review*, 23(133), 367–378.

Tabchy A, Eltonsy N, Housman D, Mills G. (2013). Systematic identification of combinatorial drivers and targets in cancer cell lines. *PLoS ONE*, 8(4), e60339.

Woodcock J, LaVange LM. (2017). Master protocols to study multiple therapies, multiple diseases, or both. *The New England Journal of Medicine*, 377, 62–70.

18

Combinatorial and Model-Based Methods in Structuring and Optimizing Cluster Trials

Valerii V. Fedorov and Sergei L. Leonov

1 Introduction

Basket, umbrella, and platform clinical studies have become increasingly popular in early phases of drug development; for examples, see Redig and Jänne (2015), Beckman et al. (2016), Chen et al. (2016), Woodcock and LaVange (2017). Studies of these types aim at screening and selection of the best treatment or a group of nearly "optimal" treatments out of many candidates and/or identifying the most sensitive sub-populations. We introduce a concept of "cluster" trials, which by definition comprises a number of sub-trials with common features. This commonality makes it scientifically sound to share information across all cluster members. Usually such an exchange of information is based on the use of statistical modeling.

In oncology, various treatments are currently tested for different cancer types among patients with various biomarkers, genetic mutations, phenotypes, or genotypes. From a classification point of view, both basket and umbrella trials can be put into a single hierarchical framework. The order of "layers" (biomarkers, cancers, treatments, etc., which one goes first, which one second, etc.) defines the type of a particular trial. In umbrella trials, multiple therapies are compared in the context of a single disease; see Figure 18.1, right panel, where the disease can be viewed as a cluster stem. In basket trials, the commonality is manifested through the application of the same therapy to various biomarkers and cancer subtypes (Figure 18.1, left panel). In both cases clusters have a rather simple structure associated with a single stem, either a disease type or a treatment of interest.

In more complex cases, clusters may be defined by a combination of several categories (genotypes, phenotypes, mutational signatures, etc.) that can be determined with various statistical methods like cluster analysis, principal component and factor analysis, or other machine learning or statistical techniques which are beyond the scope of this chapter; cf. De Souto et al. (2008), Alexandrov et al. (2013), Prat et al. (2013), Iorio et al. (2016). It is worth noting that the term "cluster" may

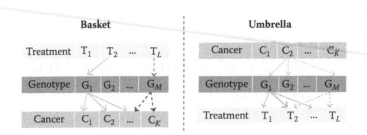

FIGURE 18.1
Schematic presentation of basket and umbrella trials

be overloaded: recall "cluster randomization," as in Donner and Klar (2000), or "cluster cancer," as in Thun and Sinks (2004). "Meta trial" or "compound trial" are competitive alternatives, but they are overloaded even more, so that we decided to stay with "cluster trials" for the needs of this chapter. We stay within the framework of oncology trials but the approach can be applied in other areas, for instance, for the comparison of different antibiotics for the same disease; cf. CODA, https://clinical trials.gov/ct2/show/NCT02800785.

We start Section 2 with a "thought" cluster trial (a medical version of Albert Einstein's *Gedanken-Experiment*), then proceed with related ANOVA models and set up respective trial design problems. Various traditional combinatorial and factorial designs are presented in Section 3. These types of designs are useful for understanding of many features of optimal or near-optimal designs. However, their practical appeal quickly vanishes when various operational, ethical and budget constraints are taken into account. Such constraints are typical for clinical trials, which explains the necessity of developing numerical methods discussed in Section 4. The iterative exchange algorithms of the first and second order (Fedorov, 1972) work well but become increasingly computationally intensive in the presence of multiple drug combinations, various cancer subtypes, etc. This, in turn, was one of the motivations for the start of a "proof-of-concept" project on the use of quantum computing in numerical construction of optimal designs. Related results are discussed in Section 5.

2 Motivating Example: Cluster Trials

2.1 Models and Notations

In a rather general setting, it is assumed that the observed response to a combination treatment is a random vector

$$\mathbf{Y}_{ijk\ell\ell'} \sim \mathcal{F}(\boldsymbol{\mu}_{jk\ell\ell'}). \tag{1}$$

Index i stands for an observation number (subject), j—for a sub-trial (block), k for a cancer type, ℓ and ℓ' stand for two distinct drugs. In the case of multiple drugs we may use more indices; in addition, the number of indices may be extended to cover cases with additional classifiers. In general, $\mathcal{F}$ is a multivariate distribution, e.g., normal or multinomial, or even a distribution that includes variables of different types to cover cases when several responses/endpoints are observed; see Fedorov et al. (2012). Distribution parameters $\boldsymbol{\mu}_{jkll'}$ are unknown and should be either estimated or ranked when the best drug combinations are to be determined.

While model (1) is rather general, it does not provide enough practical guidance on how to structure and perform a cluster trial without additional assumptions. Indeed, let K be the number of cancer types, L be the number of principal drugs/treatments and L' be the number of adjuvant drugs (therapies). Even assuming block homogeneity, we end up with $K \times L \times L'$ parameters to be estimated or compared. Consider a modest case with $K = 2$, $L = 3$, $L' = 5$, i.e., a trial with 30 arms, with normally distributed observations. Let the expected signal-to-noise ratio ("treatment effect-to-standard error") be $1/3$. Then one needs ~ 70 observations (subjects) for each of 30 arms, to assure 75% probability of the correct selection of the best combination and ~ 135 subjects per arm for 95% probability of the correct selection; for details, see Bechhofer et al. (1995), formula (2.2.1) and Table B.2. In practice, the required study sizes may be substantially larger. Moreover, in screening studies we often search for the best set of indices (k, ℓ, ℓ') under the assumption that parameters $\boldsymbol{\mu}_{jk\ell\ell'}$ correspond to "optimal" doses of drugs ℓ and ℓ'. To find these doses, one needs several cohorts assigned to corresponding combinations of the two drugs and, consequently, the resulting study size may become prohibitively large for an early stage screening study. While a sample size reduction can be achieved by applying multistage/adaptive screening (e.g., Bechhofer et al. (1995), Chapters 2 and 6), these types of designs are beyond the scope of this chapter. Complementing model (1) with further assumptions that are based on prior knowledge (previously conducted trials, medical hypotheses, etc.) may also lead to substantial study size reduction.

Let us narrow the scope of model (1) and assume that observations are univariate, $\mathbf{Y}_{ijk\ell\ell'} \rightarrow Y_{ijk\ell\ell'}$, and

$$Y_{ijk\ell\ell'} = \mu_{jk\ell\ell'} + \varepsilon_{ijk\ell\ell'}, i = 1, \ldots, n_{jk\ell\ell'}, \tag{2}$$

where $\varepsilon_{ijk\ell\ell'}$ are normally distributed with zero mean and the constant variance σ^2. The transition from model (1) to model (2) simplifies notations, while preserving the key elements of the methodology. Model (2) naturally leads us towards the well established ANOVA methodology of design and analysis of experiments for statistical selection, screening and multiple comparisons, see Bechhofer et al. (1995), Wu and Hamada (2000), Box et al. (2005). Thus, one has a set of tools for structuring cluster trials statistically and operationally. However, additional assumptions or constraints have to be imposed on the model in order to generate results of practical value. In the case of principal and adjuvant drugs, one may consider the following decomposition:

$$\mu_{jk\ell\ell'} = a + b_j + c_k + d_\ell + d'_{\ell'}, \tag{3}$$

where a is the global mean, b_j stands for block j (sub-trial, medical center, biomarker, etc.), c_k for cancer k, d_l for principal drug l, $d_{l'}$ for adjuvant drug l'. It is often assumed that

$$\sum_{j=1}^{J} b_j = \sum_{k=1}^{K} c_k = \sum_{\ell=1}^{L} d_\ell = \sum_{\ell'=1}^{L'} d'_{\ell'} = 0, \tag{4}$$

to assure identifiability of all unknown parameters.

The construction of optimal or nearly optimal designs for models of type (3) is a well developed area, with numerous elegant mathematical results; see, for example, Box et al. (2005). Unlike classical design applications, of which agriculture and chemistry are popular examples, in clinical trial practice investigators face so many constraints driven by ethical, operational, and budget considerations that it is impossible to cover the existing needs within the framework of classical combinatorial designs. Therefore, while the latter provide a general methodological guidance, one has to resort to numerical methods for optimal design construction.

With the introduction of combination therapies and precision medicine, the number of possible treatments increases dramatically and the standard paradigm (one treatment, one disease, one study at a time) becomes practically infeasible; e.g., see Aanur et al. (2017) or a description of FRACTION-Lung study (2016). In what follows we assume that doses of individual drugs have been selected, which is the standard practice in drug development because mono-therapies are studied prior to using individual drugs in combination settings. Therefore, the presence of a given drug can be coded as 1 and 0 otherwise. For methods of designing dose-finding/ranging studies, including studies with multiple responses and drug combinations, see Chevret (2006), Fedorov et al. (2012), Fedorov and Leonov (2013), Chapters 6 and 8, O'Quigley et al. (2017).

2.2 Motivating Example

In our example, we discuss designs which allow in each sub-trial to treat only a limited number of cancer types with only a limited number of drugs, allowing for two-drug combinations. The statement of this problem was motivated by the discussions with Rosemary Bailey at the workshop "Design and Analysis of Experiments in Healthcare" held at the Isaac Newton Institute for Mathematical Sciences (Cambridge, UK) in July 2015.

Let J be the number of sub-trials, let K be the number of cancer types and L be the number of drugs. The following properties are desirable:

1) All sub-trials involve the same number n_1 of cancer types.
2) All sub-trials use the same number n_2 of drugs.
3) Each pair of distinct cancer types are involved together at the same non-zero number n_3 of sub-trials.
4) Each pair of distinct drugs are used together at the same non-zero number n_4 of sub-trials.
5) Each drug is used on each type of cancer at the same number n_5 of sub-trials.

In the sequel, "sub-trials" will be referred to as "blocks." The non-zero condition in items 3) and 4) is necessary to prevent the confounding of either cancer types or drugs with blocks. Conditions 1) and 3) specify that the design for cancer types is a balanced incomplete-block design (BIBD). Conditions 2) and 4) specify that the design for drugs is a BIBD. Methods of construction of BIBD designs for the above problem were developed by Bailey and Cameron (2018) under the assumption of *equal patient allocation in all arms of the trial*. Numbers $n_1, n_2, ..., n_5$ are defined by operational and time constraints/needs. The cited publication provides tables of designs and methods of their construction for various combinations of $\{n_i\}$.

Table 18.1 shows such a design for $K = 6$ cancer types and $L = 5$ drugs using $J = 10$ blocks; it has $n_1 = 3$, $n_2 = 2$, $n_3 = 2$, $n_4 = 1$, and $n_5 = 2$. For example, in block 1 we use the combination of drugs 1 and 5 and apply this combination to cancers 1, 2, and 3. Block 2 utilizes combination (D1, D2) and cancers C1, C5, C6, etc.

The above design has the following properties:

- With $L = 5$, there exist $C_5^2 = 10$ distinct drug pairs.
- In each block patients with $n_1 = 3$ different cancers are enrolled. There exist $C_6^3 = 20$ different combinations of three cancers out of six. Therefore, the proposed design covers only half of possible drug pairs and, consequently, it is a fraction of the full design.
- Each cancer is treated by five distinct drug pairs (not all 10).

TABLE 18.1

An example of BIBD: $J = 10$ blocks, $K = 6$ cancers, $L = 5$ drugs

(a)	Cancer	Drugs
Block	(subpopulation)	
1	C123	D15
2	C156	D12
3	C134	D23
4	C126	D34
5	C145	D45
6	C245	D13
7	C235	D24
8	C356	D35
9	C346	D14
10	C246	D25

(b)	Cancers					
Block	C1	C2	C3	C4	C5	C6
1	D15	D15	D15			
2	D12				D12	D12
3	D23		D23	D23		
4	D34	D34				D34
5	D45			D45	D45	
6		D13		D13	D13	
7		D24	D24		D24	
8			D35		D35	D35
9			D14	D14		D14
10		D25		D25		D25

During our initial analysis we are not introducing costs. However, when costs are introduced, such as various operational costs, then blocking of cancers within sub-trials may lead to the substantial cost savings.

The design presented in Table 18.1 has good characteristics with respect to several optimality criteria for the traditional ANOVA model

$$\mu_{jk\ell\ell'} = a + b_j + c_k + \left\{ d_\ell \vee d_{\ell'} \right\}, \tag{5}$$

under an assumption that every non-empty cell corresponds to a two-arm sub-trial: one for drug d_ℓ and another for drug $d_{\ell'}$. For this model the design has a D-efficiency of 90% and χ^2 —efficiency of 80%, see SAS-JMP (2017), Chapter 4. For more details on D-efficiency, see Section 4 and Appendix A1.

Interestingly, this design has very reasonable characteristics for other, more complicated models. For instance, if one is interested in drug combinations formed from the same set of five drugs and every non-empty cell is interpreted as a single arm sub-trial with two drugs d_ℓ and $d_{\ell'}$, $\ell < \ell'$, administered to enrolled subjects, then the design's D-efficiency is $\sim 80\%$ for model

$$\mu_{jk\ell\ell'} = a + b_j + c_k + \tau_{\ell\ell'}, \ \ell < \ell', \tag{6}$$

where the pair (ℓ, ℓ') enumerates all 10 distinct combinations.

If non-empty cells contain three arms, two with a single drug and the third with a drug combination, then for model

$$\mu_{jk\ell\ell'} = a + b_j + c_k + \left\{ d_\ell \bigvee d_{\ell'} \right\}, \tag{7}$$

$$\mu_{jk\ell\ell'} = a + b_j + c_k + d_\ell + d_{\ell'} + \zeta_{\ell\ell'}, \ell < \ell'$$

the design's D-efficiency is $\sim 70\%$. Note that models (5), (6), and (7) should be complemented by constraints similar to (4), which are skipped here for brevity.

To summarize, combinatorial methods provide useful designs for many occasions. However, they are not very robust with respect to assumptions. For instance, once the design becomes unbalanced, e.g., the numbers of subjects in non-empty cells of Table 18.1(b) and respective arms are different, or specific combinations of drugs/cancers are infeasible, then the nice statistical properties of BIBD designs, such as orthogonality of parameter estimators, are gone. For these reasons, in the next section we resort to model-based designs, aka designs for response surface models. The model-based designs are less elegant but more flexible in addressing various practical needs, in particular ethical and budget constraints, stochasticity of enrollment process, drop outs, incomplete data.

3 Model-Based Designs

3.1 From Combinatorial Models to Regression Models

Combinatorial models do not include placebo arm explicitly. In the case when all compared drugs are principal, one can add an additional category that corresponds to a "placebo pill." To avoid the introduction of numerous linear constraints in the regression model, we may interpret all five drugs as adjuvant and introduce a model which incorporates the placebo arm:

$$\mu_{jk\ell\ell'} = a + b_j + c_k, \tag{8}$$

$$\mu_{jk\ell\ell'} = a + b_j + c_k + \left\{ d_\ell \vee d_{\ell'} \right\},$$

$$\mu_{jk\ell\ell'} = a + b_j + c_k + d_\ell + d_{\ell'} + d_{\ell\ell'}, \quad \ell < \ell'.$$

Model (8) assumes that there are four distinct arms for each pair of indices (ℓ, ℓ'): placebo, two single drug arms, and a drug combination arm. We remind the reader that doses of individual drugs are assumed selected; see a comment at the end of Section 2.1.

Our immediate aim is to map the model (8) to the standard linear regression model

$$y(\mathbf{x}) = \mathbf{f}^T(\mathbf{x})\, \boldsymbol{\beta} + \varepsilon, \tag{9}$$

where $\mathbf{x}$ is a vector of zeros and ones which indicates experimental conditions, such as block, cancer type, presence or absence of a particular drug, etc.; $f(\mathbf{x})$ is a vector of basis functions; $\boldsymbol{\beta}$ is a vector of unknown parameters to be estimated; ε is a random normally distributed observational error with zero mean and constant variance σ^2.

For each design problem we need to define the set $\mathscr{X}$ of all possible choices of $\mathbf{x}$ which are often called candidate, or support points. In clinical trials, $\mathscr{X}$ is defined by operational and clinical needs. In the example of Section 2.2, a support point can be defined as an arm which is associated with a given cancer, includes no more than two drugs (placebo, drug ℓ, drug ℓ' and their combination), and is allocated to one of ten available blocks. The collection of arms to which subjects can be allocated forms a set of support points. The latter, complemented with the specific number or relative weight of subjects constitutes a "design"; see Appendix A1 for a formal introduction of discrete and continuous designs. Support points for the design from Table 18.1(b) and the regression model (8) are presented in Table 18.2. This design contains 120 arms uniformly allocated to 10 blocks. Non-zero components of x_i define a block, a cancer type and a treatment that can be administered to a subject.

The allocation of subjects to design support points that provide maximum information with respect to the selected optimality criterion is addressed by *model-based optimal experimental design theory*; see Fedorov (1972), Atkinson et al. (2007), Berger and Wong (2009), Goos and Jones (2011), Fedorov and Leonov (2013). In what follows we focus on D-criterion.

The simplest linear regression model has the following form:

$$\boldsymbol{\beta} = (\beta_0; \beta_{b1}, \ldots, \beta_{b10}; \beta_1 \ldots, \beta_6; \beta_7, \ldots, \beta_{11})^T, \tag{10}$$

TABLE 18.2

Set of candidate points $\mathscr{X}$

No	Block effects b_j				Cancer effects c_k						Drug effects d_ℓ			
	b_1	b_2	...	b_{10}	c_1	c_2	c_3	c_4	c_5	c_6	d_1	d_2	...	d_5
1	1	0	0	0	1	0	0	0	0	0	0	0	0	0
2	1	0	0	0	1	0	0	0	0	0	0	0	0	1
3	1	0	0	0	1	0	0	0	0	0	1	0	0	0
4	1	0	0	0	1	0	0	0	0	0	1	0	0	1
5	1	0	0	0	0	1	0	0	0	0	0	0	0	0
6	1	0	0	0	0	1	0	0	0	0	0	0	0	1
7	1	0	0	0	0	1	0	0	0	0	0	1	0	0
8	1	0	0	0	0	1	0	0	0	0	0	1	0	1
9	1	0	0	0	0	0	1	0	0	0	0	0	0	0
10	1	0	0	0	0	0	1	0	0	0	0	0	0	1
11	1	0	0	0	0	0	1	0	0	0	0	1	0	0
12	1	0	0	0	0	0	1	0	0	0	0	1	0	1
...	...	...	...	...	...	...	...	...	...	...	...	...	...	...
109	0	0	0	1	0	1	0	0	0	0	0	0	0	0
110	0	0	0	1	0	1	0	0	0	0	0	0	0	1
111	0	0	0	1	0	1	0	0	0	0	1	0	0	0
112	0	0	0	1	0	1	0	0	0	0	1	0	0	1
113	0	0	0	1	0	0	0	1	0	0	0	0	0	0
114	0	0	0	1	0	0	0	1	0	0	0	0	0	1
115	0	0	0	1	0	0	0	1	0	0	1	0	0	0
116	0	0	0	1	0	0	0	1	0	0	1	0	0	1
117	0	0	0	1	0	0	0	0	0	1	0	0	0	0
118	0	0	0	1	0	0	0	0	0	1	0	0	0	1
119	0	0	0	1	0	0	0	0	0	1	0	1	0	0
120	0	0	0	1	0	0	0	0	0	1	0	1	0	1
	x_{b1}	x_{b2}	...	x_{b10}	x_1	x_2	x_3	x_4	x_5	x_6	x_7	x_8	...	x_{11}

with $\beta_0 = a$, $\beta_{b1 \to b10} = b_{1 \to 10}$, $\beta_{1 \to 6} = c_{1 \to 6}$, $\beta_{7 \to 11} = d_{1 \to 5}$, and

$$\mathbf{f}(x) = (1; x_{b1}, \ldots, x_{b10}; x_1, \ldots x_6; x_7, \ldots, x_{11})^T. \qquad (11)$$

Note that all 22 parameters $\boldsymbol{\beta}$ cannot be estimated with the support points from Table 18.2, which is typical when moving from combinatorial setting to the regression models, cf. Box et al. (2005). This problem can be resolved by adding some parameter constraints, as in

$$\sum_{j=1}^{10} \beta_{bj} = 0; \tag{12}$$

see Wu and Hamada (2000), Chapter 1.6. Incorporating the above constraint in the model defined by (10) and (11) leads to the following model:

$$\boldsymbol{\beta} = (\beta_0; \beta_{b2}, \ldots, \beta_{b10}; \beta_1, \ldots, \beta_6; \beta_7, \ldots, \beta_{11})^T, \tag{13}$$

and

$$\mathbf{f}(\boldsymbol{x}) = (1; x_{b2} - x_{b1}, \ldots, x_{b10} - x_{b1}; x_1, \ldots x_6; x_7, \ldots, x_{11})^T. \tag{14}$$

One can verify that if drug interaction terms are added to (13), (14) and a constraint similar to (12) is added to cancer parameters, then all regression parameters can still be estimated.

To simplify the narrative, we exclude the terms associated with parameters $\beta_0; \beta_{b1}, \ldots, \beta_{b10}$ from further consideration. Instead, we add interaction terms, i.e., we continue with the model (9) where

$$\boldsymbol{\beta} = (\beta_1 \ldots, \beta_6; \beta_7, \ldots, \beta_{11}, \beta_{12}, \ldots, \beta_{21})^T \tag{15}$$

and

$$\mathbf{f}(\boldsymbol{x}) = (x_1, \ldots x_6; x_7, \ldots, x_{11}, x_7 x_8,\ x_7 x_9,\ \ldots\ x_{10} x_{11})^T. \tag{16}$$

Now, after removing block effects the design set consists of 96 distinct candidate points, see Table 18.3.

---

4 Design Comparison

All comparisons in this section are done for the regression model defined in (15), (16), and are performed with respect to:

- D-efficiency, which is defined as $[|\mathbf{D}(\xi^*)|/|\mathbf{D}(\xi)|]^{1/m} \times 100\%$, where design ξ^* is D-optimal, $\mathbf{D}$ is the normalized variance-covariance matrix; see details in Appendix A1.
- $tr\mathbf{D}(\xi)/m$ (trace of $\mathbf{D}$ normalized by the number of estimated parameters) and diagonal elements of $\mathbf{D}$.

TABLE 18.3

Set of candidate points $\mathscr{X}_2$

Points	Cancers						Drugs					Comments
No	c1	c2	c3	c4	c5	c6	d1	d2	d3	d4	d5	
1	1	0	0	0	0	0	0	0	0	0	0	Placebo
2	1	0	0	0	0	0	1	0	0	0	0	Single drugs
3	1	0	0	0	0	0	0	1	0	0	0	**Cancer 1**
4	1	0	0	0	0	0	0	0	1	0	0	
5	1	0	0	0	0	0	0	0	0	1	0	
6	1	0	0	0	0	0	0	0	0	0	1	
7	1	0	0	0	0	0	1	1	0	0	0	Pairs with D1
8	1	0	0	0	0	0	1	0	1	0	0	
9	1	0	0	0	0	0	1	0	0	1	0	
10	1	0	0	0	0	0	1	0	0	0	1	
11	1	0	0	0	0	0	0	1	1	0	0	Pairs with D2
12	1	0	0	0	0	0	0	1	0	1	0	
13	1	0	0	0	0	0	0	1	0	0	1	
14	1	0	0	0	0	0	0	0	1	1	0	Pairs with D3
15	1	0	0	0	0	0	0	0	1	0	1	
16	1	0	0	0	0	0	0	0	0	1	1	Pairs with D4
17	0	1	0	0	0	0	0	0	0	0	0	Placebo
18	0	1	0	0	0	0	1	0	0	0	0	Single drugs,
19	0	1	0	0	0	0	0	1	0	0	0	**Cancer 2**
...					...	...						
22	0	1	0	0	0	0	0	0	0	0	1	
23	0	1	0	0	0	0	1	1	0	0	0	Pairs with D1
...					...	...						
26	0	1	0	0	0	0	1	0	0	1	0	
...					...	...						
32	0	1	0	0	0	0	0	0	0	1	1	Pairs with D4
...					...	...						
81	0	0	0	0	0	1	0	0	0	0	0	**Cancer 6**
...					...	...						
96	0	0	0	0	0	1	0	0	0	1	1	Pairs with D4
	x_1	x_2	x_3	x_4	x_5	x_6	x_7	x_8	x_9	x_{10}	x_{11}	

- Normalized variance of prediction $d(\mathbf{x}, \xi)$, which for D-criterion coincides with the sensitivity function:

$$d(\mathbf{x}, \xi) = \mathbf{f}^T(\mathbf{x})\mathbf{D}(\xi)\mathbf{f}(\mathbf{x}); \qquad (17)$$

for details, see Appendix A1 or Fedorov and Leonov (2013), Chapter 2.5.

- Average normalized variance of prediction $d_{uv}(\mathbf{x}, \xi)$ averaged over all 96 candidate points from Table 18.3.
- Number of support points of the design.

We confine ourselves to designs with the uniform allocation, i.e., to designs with the same number of subjects on all arms. The results are summarized in Table 18.4 and Figures 18.2 and 18.3.

Design ξ_{96}^* has all 96 support points from the set $\mathscr{X}_2$. Designs ξ_n^* have n support points that are selected by backward elimination from ξ_{96}^*, i.e., by using (26), with the weight

$$p = 1/(N_0 - s) \tag{18}$$

on step s, with $N_0 = 96$. Design ξ_{66} has 66 support points, obtained from the BIBD design (120 points) by removing replications from the set $\mathscr{X}$:

(a) Placebo arm is included for each of the three cancers in each of the 10 blocks, i.e., 30 times, while in the set $\mathscr{X}_2$ it is included only six times, once for each cancer.

(b) Each drug (5 total) is used for each cancer (6 total) in two different combination arms, which results in 30 replications.

(c) In total, there are 54 replications in the set $\mathscr{X}$ and, consequently, 66 distinct support points.

Design ξ_{48} with 48 support points is obtained from ξ_{66} by backward elimination, i.e., using (26) and (18) with $N_0 = 66$.

It turns out that design ξ_{96}^* is D-optimal, which can be verified by plotting the normalized variance of prediction $d(\mathbf{x}, \xi)$, see (17), and

TABLE 18.4

Comparison of designs

Design	$\|D\|^{1/21}$	Efficiency (%)	Variances trD/21	$d_{av}(x_i, \xi)$	c_j	d_k	d_{k_1, k_2}
ξ_{96}^*	13.80	100	44.1	21	21	32	64
ξ_{48}^*	14.56	94.8	48.3	23.6	21–26	33–36	67–73
ξ_{32}^*	15.6	88.4	54.8	27.8	21–31	37–43	73–90
ξ_{30}^*	16.2	85.4	64.3	30.8	20–34	36–64	65–127
ξ_{66}	14.76	93.5	36.7	24.06	16.5	22	56.1
ξ_{48}	14.56	94.8	48.4	22.96	21–26	33–36	65–73

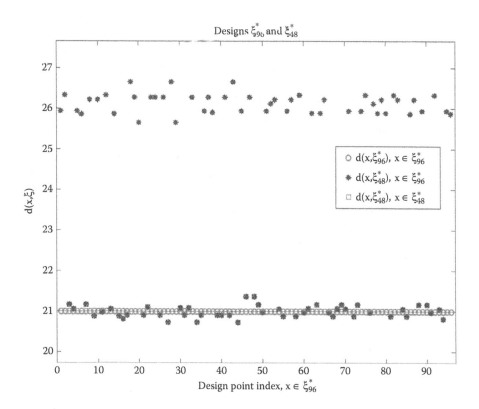

FIGURE 18.2

Normalized variance of prediction, designs ζ_{96}^* and ζ_{48}^*

utilizing the Equivalence Theorem. The Equivalence Theorem states that for the D-optimal design the maximum of this function over all candidate points should be equal to the number ($m = 21$) of estimated parameters; cf. Fedorov and Leonov (2013, Chapter 2.5). See Figure 18.2 (circles).

While design ζ_{96}^* is D-optimal, it utilizes all 96 admissible design points. If costs are taken into account, then one may be interested in reducing the number of distinct points. Such a reduction may still keep the statistical efficiency almost intact while reducing costs of originating additional arms.

Deleting 48 points leads to design ζ_{48}^*. The loss of efficiency of this design is only 5.2% compared to D-optimal; the variance $d(x, \xi)$ of prediction is marked by stars in Figure 18.2. The x-axis corresponds to indices of 96 candidate design points from $\mathscr{X}_2$. The loss of D-efficiency can be compensated by $\sim 5\%$ increase of the total sample size (total number of enrolled subjects), but elimination of 48 arms may lead to the dramatic reduction of the total cost of the respective cluster trial.

The loss of D efficiency of design ξ_{66} is 6.5%; see Figure 18.3 for the plot of the sensitivity function (crosses). The points at the level 16.5 correspond to all placebo and single arms; the points at the level 26.4 correspond to those combination arms (30 total) which belong to $\mathcal{X}_2$; the points at the level 30.8 correspond to those combination arms (30 total) which do not belong to $\mathcal{X}_2$. This plot immediately suggests how to improve the quality of the design: the enrollment to placebo and single arms has to be reduced, while all combination arms should be included.

One can further reduce the number of support points starting from design ξ_{66} by using backward elimination procedure. Removing 18 points from ξ_{66} leads to design ξ_{48}. Its sensitivity function is shown in Figure 18.3 (pluses). Again, one has to perform a cost analysis to decide which option is preferable, either a minor increment in the total sample size or the substantial reduction in the number of active arms.

Our simple example illustrates the comparative analysis of various designs which is the integral part of the quantitative support of decision

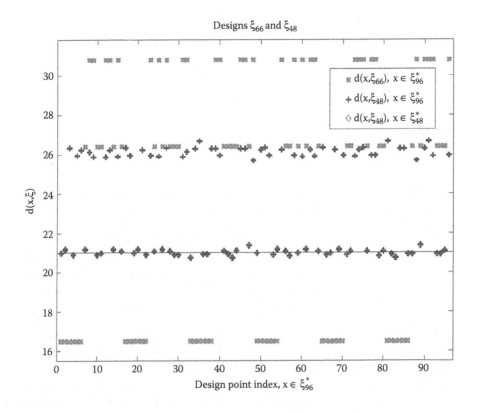

FIGURE 18.3
Normalized variance of prediction, designs ξ_{66} and ξ_{48}

making and should be used more often in pharmaceutical studies. For real-life problems, such analysis often requires substantial computational efforts which can be enhanced by the development of more efficient algorithms and/or moving to more advanced computational platforms. To a large extent, this was the motivation for starting a joint project between ICON's Innovation Center and Lockheed Martin on implementation of quantum computing in statistics and machine learning. In 2017, Lockheed Martin and ICON, together with the Department of Statistics at George Washington University, co-organized a workshop on the application of quantum computing in drug development; see *https://statistics.columbian.gwu.edu/workshop-quantum-comput ing-and-its-application*. The work stream on the application of quantum computing to the design of cluster trials is briefly discussed in the next Section.

5 Quantum Computing in Optimal Design

Quantum computing has drawn extensive attention in recent years in a number of diverse areas, from financial engineering to cryptography to artificial intelligence. New quantum computing algorithms, including quantum Monte Carlo, are developed in parallel with building first functioning quantum computers. While the theory of quantum information and various theoretical aspects of quantum computing have attracted statisticians and probabilists for decades, the examples of practical applications are still rather rare.

Quantum computers provide a computational power many times the order of existing computers, which is critical for training machine learning algorithms to predict clinical trial outcomes from genomic and phenotypic information. Other optimization problems that arise in statistical applications may benefit from developments in quantum computing, e.g., simulated annealing algorithms in optimal model-based experimental design; see Bohachevsky et al. (1986), Haines (1987). Rather than store information using bits represented by 0s or 1s as conventional digital computers do, quantum computers use quantum bits, or qubits, to encode information as 0s, 1s, or both at the same time. This superposition of states, along with the other quantum mechanical phenomena of entanglement and tunneling, enables quantum computers to manipulate enormous combinations of states at once; see D-Wave Systems (2017, 2018).

In the spring of 2017, ICON was granted access to D-Wave quantum computer of Lockheed Martin through its affiliates program. D-Wave computer (*www.dwavesys.com*) is a quantum annealer which is designed to solve quadratic unconstrained optimization problems (QUBO):

$$x^* = \text{Arg} \min_{x} \left[x^T Q x + h^T x \right], \tag{19}$$

where elements of $n \times 1$ vector x are either 0 or 1, Q is an $n \times n$ symmetric matrix, and h is an $n \times 1$ vector. A popular Ising problem, with elements $x_i' = \pm 1$ can be put into the framework of (19) by a transformation $x_i = (1 + x_i')/2$; see Lewis and Glover (2017) for details on the use of quantum annealing for solving QUBO problems. In (19), vector h represents weights of qubits, while elements of matrix Q_{ij} define the "coupling" strengths of the interaction between qubits.

We noticed similarities of the optimization problems arising in iterative algorithms for the construction of model-based designs with the QUBO problem (19) and realized that various popular optimal design settings can be put into the QUBO framework in a straightforward fashion. One of such examples is the construction of designs with the fixed number of support points, including saturated designs (i.e., the number of support points coinciding with the number of unknown parameters) for linear regression models on a hypercube:

$$y_i = \beta_0 + x_i^T \beta + \varepsilon_i, x_i \in \mathcal{X}, \tag{20}$$

with $\mathcal{X}$ containing all vertices of an $(m - 1)$-dimensional hypercube, i.e., $x \in \{0, 1\}^{m-1}$. To solve this problem, one may use the second-order exchange algorithm (27) — (29) described in Appendix A2, where $f(x) = (1, x_1, \ldots, x_{m-1})^T$. However, even for moderate m a "brute-force" implementation of this algorithm on existing classical computers might be very challenging. For example, for the construction of the saturated optimal design for $m = 7$, the total number of all possible combinations is $C_{26}^7 \sim 0.6 * 10^9$, in which case one needs to apply various tricks to avoid running out of memory/acceptable computer time.

As a "proof-of-concept," we implemented the second-order exchange algorithm with $m = 5, 6$ on D-Wave computer (1152 qubits) and validated the results by running the same algorithm on a standard computer, for which the maximization in (28) was performed by the enumeration of the finite number of candidate points on each iteration.

To obtain the solution of QUBO on D-Wave computer, several preliminary steps have to be performed in order to map the original optimization procedure to the QUBO problem wired at D-Wave computer. The D-Wave system has a web API (Application Programming Interface) with client libraries available for various programming languages, including MATLAB. This allows us to perform all preliminary calculations on a standard computer, in particular, the calculation of the matrix Q in (29) on each step of the iterative procedure, and running embedding algorithms to match "logical" and "physical" cubits.

Because a quantum computer is probabilistic rather than deterministic, the computer returns multiple solutions—not only the best solution found but also other "good" alternatives. For details on the conversion of "physical" solutions to "logical" solutions, see Pudenz (2016).

Note, however, that in the settings of cluster trials, as in Sections 2–4, additional steps are needed to reduce the encountered optimization problems to QUBO. Unlike the search on a hypercube, where any possible combinations of 0s and 1s is admissible, in cluster trials vectors $\mathbf{x}$ must satisfy additional constraints. For example, the following constraints must be satisfied for model (15) − (16):

$$\mathbf{1}_1^T\mathbf{x} = 1, l_{1i} = 1, \ i = 1,\ldots,6; \ l_{1i} = 0, \ i = 7,\ldots,11; \tag{21}$$

$$0 \leq \mathbf{1}_2^T\mathbf{x} \leq 2, \ \mathbf{1}_2 = 1 - \mathbf{1}_1, \tag{22}$$

where $\mathbf{1}$ is an 11×1 vector of ones. To reduce the optimization problem (27) − (29) to QUBO under constraints (21) and (22), one has to do the following:

(a) Introduce auxiliary variables $u_1, u_2 \in \{0,1\}$ to reduce the inequalities in (22) to the equality

$$\mathbf{1}_2^T\mathbf{x} + u_1 + u_2 = 2. \tag{23}$$

(b) Introduce penalty functions

$$\Psi_1(\mathbf{x}) = w_1\left[\mathbf{1}_1^T\mathbf{x} - 1\right]^2, \Psi_2(\mathbf{x}, u_1, u_2) = w_2\left[\mathbf{1}_2^T\mathbf{x} + u_1 + u_2 - 2\right]^2. \tag{24}$$

(c) Identify "reasonable" values of weights w_1, w_2 in (24) to solve the optimization problem

$$\{\mathbf{x}_s^+, \mathbf{x}_s^-\} = \arg\min_{\mathbf{x}\in\mathscr{X}, \mathbf{x}'\in\mathscr{X}_{N,s}; u_1, u_2} [\Psi_1(\mathbf{x}) + \Psi_2(\mathbf{x}, u_1, u_2) - \Delta_s(\mathbf{x}, \mathbf{x}')]; \tag{25}$$

see (28) in Appendix A2.

---

6 Concluding Remarks

While generalizing the ideas of various modern clinical studies (basket, umbrella, etc.) and embedding them into the framework of cluster trials, we show that bringing together combinatorial techniques and model-based optimal design of experiments may lead to useful recommendations on structuring large early phase projects which include multiple studies with similar diseases, various population signatures, and competing treatments. The next natural step is fusing the proposed approach with optimal design of dose finding studies, which will lead to the more efficient information sharing between different sub-trials. Bayesian techniques and random parameters (population) models may provide an important tool in expanding the approach. Complementing the above mentioned techniques with modeling of operational processes and with cost analysis will make the problem even more computationally challenging. Foreseeing this, we realized the need for the exploration of various modern computing platforms which naturally led us in the direction of quantum computing. Iterative algorithms for the construction of optimal model-based experimental designs are well suited for using quantum annealing at each iteration. The implementation of these algorithms on a quantum computer became possible within a "proof-of-concept" collaborative project with the group of researchers from Lockheed Martin corporation.

Acknowledgement

The authors are grateful to Rosemary Bailey for the discussions that led to the motivating example and to Greg Tallant and Kristen Pudenz for their help with the implementation of iterative algorithms on D-Wave computer.

Appendix: Model-Based Optimal Design of Experiments

A1. Optimization Problem for Linear Regression Models

- Model:

$$y_{ij} = \mathbf{f}^T(\mathbf{x}_i)\,\boldsymbol{\beta} + \varepsilon_{ij},$$

where ε_{ij} has zero mean and constant variance σ^2.

- The set of candidate (support) points: $\mathcal{X}$.
- Design: $\xi_N = \{n_j,\ \mathbf{x}_j\}_1^n$, $\sum_{j=1}^n n_j = N$, $\mathbf{x}_j \in \mathcal{X}$, where n_j is the number of observations at support point $\mathbf{x}_j$.
- Normalized design: $\xi = \{p_j,\ \mathbf{x}_j\}_1^n$, $\sum_{j=1}^n p_j = 1$, $p_j = n_j/\mathbf{n}$.
- Best linear unbiased estimators or least square estimators (coincide with the maximum likelihood estimators in the normal case):

$$\hat{\beta} = \mathbf{M}^{-1}(\xi) \sum_{j=1}^{u} p_j \mathbf{f}(\mathbf{x}_j) \sum_{i}^{n_i} y_{ij}, \mathbf{M}^{-1}(\xi) = \mathbf{D}(\xi) = \sum_{j=1}^{n} p_j \mathbf{f}(\mathbf{x}_j) \mathbf{f}^T(\mathbf{x}_j),$$

where $\mathbf{M}(\xi)$ and $\mathbf{D}(\xi)$ are normalized information and variance-covariance matrices, respectively.

- Variance-covariance matrix of β:

$$Var[\hat{\beta} \mid \xi] = N^{-1} M^{-1}(\xi)$$

- Popular optimality criteria $\Psi[\mathbf{M}^{-1}(\xi)]$:

$$\det \mathbf{M}^{-1}(\xi) = |\mathbf{M}^{-1}(\xi)| (\mathrm{D-criterion}), tr\mathbf{M}^{-1}(\xi)(\mathrm{A-criterion}),$$

$$\max_{x \in \mathscr{X}} \mathbf{f}^T(x)\mathbf{M}^{-1}(\xi)\mathbf{f}(x) \ , \ \int_{\mathscr{X}} \mathbf{f}^T(x)\mathbf{M}^{-1}(\xi)\mathbf{f}(x),$$

where $d(\mathbf{x}, \xi) = \mathbf{f}^T(x)\mathbf{M}^{-1}(\xi)\mathbf{f}(x)$ is the variance of predicted response $\mathbf{f}^T(\mathbf{x}_i)\hat{\beta}$ [see (17)], and $\mathscr{X}$ is a zone of interest.

- Design problem for continuous designs:

$$\xi^* = \mathrm{Arg} \min_{\xi} \Psi[M^{-1}(\xi)].$$

- Design problem for discrete designs:

$$\xi_N^* = \mathrm{Arg} \min_{\xi_N} \Psi[M^{-1}(\xi_N)],$$

A2. Iterative Algorithms for Discrete Design Problem

Exchange Algorithm of the First Order

In what follows, all results are reported for D-criterion (minimization of determinant). The results for other criteria are very similar. Only algorithms for discrete case are used in this chapter and, consequently, only these algorithms are presented. Details on numerical algorithms can be found in Fedorov and Leonov (2013), Chapter 3.

The following algorithm can be used to construct "improved" designs for a given N. To find optimal design, one should repeat procedure multiple times with different initial designs $\xi_{N,0}$. For finite N, the convergence to the global minimum is not guaranteed. However, when $N \to \infty$, then the limiting design ξ^* will be close to the optimal continuous design.

1. *Forward step*: given $\xi_{N,s}$, with the support set $\mathscr{X}_{N,s}$, and $\mathbf{M}^{-1}(\xi_{N,s})$ find

$$x_s^+ = \arg\max_{x \in \mathscr{X}} \mathbf{f}^T(x)\mathbf{M}^{-1}(\xi_{N,s})\mathbf{f}(x),$$

and add weight $p = 1/N$ to point x_s^+.

2. *Backward step*: find

$$x_s^- = \arg\min_{x \in \mathscr{X}_{N,s}} \mathbf{f}^T(x)\mathbf{M}^{-1}(\xi_{N,s})\mathbf{f}(x),$$

and subtract weight $1/N$ from point x_s^-, i.e., create design $\xi_{N,s+1}$ by "swapping" of two points.

3. Compute $\mathbf{M}^{-1}(\xi_{N,s+1})$ and return to step 1.

4. Stop when either there is no substantial improvement seen after step 2, or when s exceeds a given upper bound s^*.

There exist numerous modifications of this algorithm. For instance, a forward step may be replaced by a forward excursion which consists of several forward steps. A forward excursion should be followed by the backward excursion of the same length if one wants to preserve the sample size N. The information matrix can be recomputed after both forward and backward steps, not only after the backward step as above.

Exchange Algorithm of the Second Order

1. Given design $\xi_{N,s}$, find points $x_s^+ \in \mathscr{X}$ and $x_s^- \in \mathscr{X}_{N,s}$ such that their swapping maximizes the increment of the ratio of determinants; see Fedorov (1972), Chapter 3.2, pp. 160–164:

$$\frac{|\mathbf{M}(\xi_{N,s+1})|}{|\mathbf{M}(\xi_{N,s})|} = 1 + \Delta_s(x_s^+, x_s^-), \tag{27}$$

and

$$\{x_s^+, x_s^-\} = \arg\max_{x \in \mathscr{X}, x' \in \mathscr{X}_{N,s}} \Delta_s(x, x'), \tag{28}$$

where

$$\Delta_\sigma(x, x') = f^T(x)M_s^{-1}f(x) - f^T(x')M_s^{-1}f(x')$$
$$+ f^T(x)M_s^{-1}f(x')f^T(x')M_s^{-1}f(x) - f^T(x)M_s^{-1}f(x)f^T(x')M_s^{-1}f(x') \quad (29)$$
$$= f^T(x)Qf(x) - q,$$

$$M_s = M^{-1}(\xi_{N,s}), \quad q = f^T(x')M_s^{-1}f(x'), \quad Q = \left[(1-q)M_s^{-1} + M_s^{-1}f(x')f^T(x')M_s^{-1}\right].$$

Note that the maximization of the increment $\Delta_s(x, x')$ with respect to x is equivalent to the maximization of a quadratic form $f^T(x)Qf(x)$ in (29).

2. Update the design together with the information matrix and return to step 1.

3. Stop when no substantial improvement is seen, or when s exceeds a given upper bound s^*.

References

1. Aanur P et al. (2017). FRACTION (Fast Real-time Assessment of Combination Therapies in Immuno-Oncology)-gastric cancer (GC): A randomized, open-label, adaptive, phase 2 study of nivolumab in combination with other immuno-oncology (IO) agents in patients with advanced GC. *J. Clin. Oncol.*, 35 (15_suppl.), TPS4137.

2. Alexandrov LB et al. (2013). Signature of mutational processes in human cancer. *Nature*, 500, 415–421.

3. Atkinson AC, Tobias R, Donev A. (2007). *Optimum Experimental Designs, with SAS*. Oxford University Press, Oxford.

4. Bailey RA, Cameron PJ. (2018). Designs which allow each medical centre to treat only a limited number of cancer types with only a limited number of drugs. Available at: https://arxiv.org/pdf/1803.00006.pdf.

5. Bechhofer RE, Santner TJ, Goldsman DM. (1995). *The Design and Analysis of Experiments for Statistical Selection, Screening, and Multiple Comparisons*. Wiley, New York.

6. Beckman RA, Antonijevic Z, Kalamegham R, Chen C. (2016). Adaptive design for a confirmatory basket trial in multiple tumor types based on a putative predictive biomarker. *Clin. Pharmacol. Ther.*, 100(6), 617–625.

7. Berger MPF, Wong WK. (2009). *An Introduction to Optimal Designs for Social and Biomedical Research (Statistics in Practice)*. Wiley, Chichester.

8. Bohachevsky I, Johnson ME, Stein ML. (1986). Generalized simulated annealing for function optimization. *Technometrics*, 28(3), 209–217.

9. Box GEP, Hunter S, Hunter WG. (2005). *Statistics for Experimenters: Design, Innovation, and Discovery*. 2nd Edition. Wiley, New York.

10. Chen C, Li N, Yuan S, Antonijevic Z, Kalamegham R, Beckman RA. (2016). Statistical design and considerations of a phase 3 basket trial for simultaneous

investigation of multiple tumor types in one study. *Stat. Biopharm. Res.*, 8(3), 248–257.

11. Chevret. S (ed). (2006). *Statistical Methods for Dose-Finding Experiments.* Wiley, Chichester.

12. De Souto MCP et al. (2008). Clustering cancer gene expression data: A comparative study. *BMC Bioinformatics*, 9, 497.

13. Donner A, Klar N. (2000). *Design and Analysis of Cluster Randomization Trials in Health Research.* Arnold, London.

14. D-Wave Systems. (2017). *Quantum Performance Evaluation: A Short Reading List.* Available at: www.dwavesys.com/sites/default/files/14-1019A-A_Quantum_Performance_Evaluation_Short_Reading_List.pdf.

15. D-Wave Systems. (2018). *Quantum Computing: How D-Wave Systems Work.* Available at: www.dwavesys.com/quantum-computing.

16. Fedorov VV. (1972). *Theory of Optimal Experiment.* Academic Press, New York.

17. Fedorov VV, Leonov SL. (2013). *Optimal Design for Nonlinear Response Models.* Chapman & Hall/CRC Biostatistics Series, Boca Raton, FL.

18. Fedorov V, Wu Y, Zhang R. (2012). Optimal dose-finding designs with correlated continuous and discrete responses. *Stat. Med.*, 31(3), 217–234.

19. FRACTION-Lung. (2016). *An Investigational Immuno-Therapy Study to Test Combination Treatments in Patients with Advanced Non-Small Cell Lung Cancer.* Available at: http://clinicaltrials.gov/ct2 (accessed February 27, 2018) (ClinicalTrials.gov Identifier: NCT02750514).

20. Goos P, Jones B. (2011). *Optimal Design of Experiments: A Case Study Approach.* Wiley, New York.

21. Haines LM. (1987). The application of the annealing algorithm to the construction of exact optimal designs for linear regression models. *Technometrics*, 29(4), 439–447.

22. Iorio F et al. (2016). A landscape of pharmacogenomic interactions in cancer. *Cell*, 166(3), 740–754.

23. Lewis M, Glover F. (2017). Quadratic unconstrained binary optimization problem preprocessing: Theory and empirical analysis. *Networks*, 70(2), 79–97. Available at: https://arxiv.org/ftp/arxiv/papers/1705/1705.09844.pdf.

24. O'Quigley J, Iasonos A, Bornkamp B (eds). (2017). *Handbook of Methods for Designing, Monitoring, and Analyzing Dose-Finding Trials.* Boca Raton, FL, Chapman & Hall/CRC Handbooks of Modern Statistical Methods.

25. Prat A et al. (2013). Genomic analyses across six cancer types identify basal-like breast cancer as a unique molecular entity. *Sci. Rep.*, 3, 3544.

26. Pudenz KL. (2016). Parameter setting for quantum annealers. Available at: https://arxiv.org/pdf/1611.07552.pdf.

27. Redig AJ, Jänne PA. (2015). Basket trials and the evolution of clinical trial design in an era of genomic medicine. *J. Clin. Oncol.*, 33(9), 975–977.

28. SAS-JMP. (2017). *JMP 13 Design of Experiments Guide.* 2nd Edition. SAS Institute Inc, Cary, NC.

29. Thun MJ, Sinks T. (2004). Understanding cancer clusters. *CA Cancer J. Clin.*, 54 (5), 273–280.

30. Woodcock J, LaVange L. (2017). Master protocols to study multiple therapies, multiple diseases, or both. *N. Engl. J. Med.*, 377, 62–70.

31. Wu CFJ, Hamada M. (2000). *Experiments. Planning, Analysis, and Parameter Design Optimization.* Wiley, New York.

Part IV

Conclusions

19

An Executive's View of Value of Platform Trials

David Reese and Phuong Khanh Morrow

A Spark Begun from a Confluence of Events

One of the core responsibilities of a research and development executive is management of a portfolio of assets, a task that requires integrating a blend of technical and non-technical sets of data, often hedged by considerable uncertainty. From one point of view, the spark igniting the explosion of interest in platform trials in the pharmaceutical industry has been created by the confluence of the urgent need for molecules to treat life-threatening diseases and the escalating resources required to develop innovative medicines in an increasingly cost-constrained environment. One way to address this predicament is through novel clinical study designs, which in some cases may supplant traditional, staged development programs and avoid evaluation of a hypothesis only with the conduct of a large, randomized, phase III trial. Such trials are typically conducted to compare an experimental agent to a standard regimen, either directly in a head-to-head design or as an add-on therapy, approaches that usually necessitate a large sample size in order to demonstrate clinical benefit. The current revolution in drug development is founded upon innovative mechanisms such as platform trials, designed to advance the most promising molecules and novel combinations with the greatest effect sizes, in order to provide value to patients, caregivers, physicians, and society as a whole. Development of platform trials is supported by early collaboration between industry partners and regulatory agencies in order to advance the mutual goal of efficient approval of drugs with transformational potential.

The Job Is Harder than Ever

The complex road to approval is costly and inefficient, often with multiple trials competing for trial subjects, all of whom are volunteers for a study without a known outcome. We are now on the threshold of an era in which much deeper insights into human genetics, disease biology, and the ability to engineer new classes of medicines that precisely modulate molecular pathways will enhance our ability to improve the cycle time of drug development (time from laboratory to commercialization) as well as the success rate. One of the challenges of the new approach is that the target population for many new drugs may shrink, as we are able to identify patients most likely to benefit. Practically, then, the increasing precision of medicine thus leads to screening many potential subjects in order to treat the few whose genetic subtype corresponds to a particular targeted agent [1]. For example, the recently conducted RATIFY trial, a phase III, placebo-controlled study that led to the approval of midostaurin, screened more than 3,200 patients with acute myelogenous leukemia in order to enroll 717 patients with fms-like tyrosine kinase 3 (FLT3) mutations [2]. The approach seeks not only to identify the right patient for the right target, but it also reduces the risk of unnecessary toxicities for patients who may never benefit from a drug. An even greater denominator would be required for a rarer disease, leading to a need for increasingly robust screening infrastructure. The question for the R&D executive then becomes how to most efficiently prosecute development programs in the age of molecular medicine.

The Potential Value of Platform Trials

If designed robustly, a platform trial creates the development engine that can nimbly test a hypothesis with the same urgency that a disease encroaches upon a patient. Importantly, from the vantage point of a decision-making executive, the trials themselves are not a "one size fits all" category. For instance, I-SPY2 (Investigation of Serial Studies to Predict Your Therapeutic Response With Imaging And molecular Analysis 2) employs adaptive randomization to assign no more than 120 patients to each experimental arm, based upon biomarker assessment. By applying a Bayesian predictive probability of success in a simulated phase III trial, I-SPY2 is able to identify promising agents for breast-cancer subgroups and replace less effective agents with new molecules in its trial, reducing time, cost, and risk of exposing more patients to ineffective therapies [3]. The Lung-Master Protocol (Lung-MAP) tests potential subjects once according to a master protocol; it then assigns each subject to a sub-study. Each sub-study evaluates a different drug from a distinct developer, with the ultimate goal to enable a rapid registrational path for active agents that are identified in the initial phase II study [4]. In each case, the unifying tenet of these trials is the need to generate a robust set of data that may inform developers on where to differentially invest resources across their pipeline—the question with which executives grapple daily.

Limitations of Platform Trials

As an executive contemplates resource allocation across a portfolio, one of the key variables is the probability of technical success of any given program. As with any experimental approach, a significant concern in evaluating the outcomes of platform trials involves the potential for both Type I and Type II errors. For example, a basket trial, which employs several independent two-stage designs (one per basket), has a much higher false-positive rate than a standard phase II study [5]. To illustrate, if the trial contains five baskets, each having a 5% false-positive rate, there is a 23% chance that one or more of the baskets will demonstrate an effect in the absence of true benefit. To address this error, investigators may adjust the sample size or decision rules in order to reduce the false-positive rate per basket. In addition, blinding can be affected in platform trials, as the use of agents with diverse modes of administration and frequency can reduce the ability to blind the investigator and/or subject [6]. Beyond those effects, the development and execution of a platform trial is a complex process, requiring negotiation of study endpoints and inclusion criteria between sponsors, frequent and transparent communication among developers to maintain an accelerated pace, shared costs, and a reduction in autonomy in order to deliver a mutually-agreed upon trial. Ultimately, without sufficient commitment among the sponsors to effectively operationalize such a study, a platform trial may be less attractive due to increased lead times and lack of perceived value to the sponsor. Nevertheless, the inherent advantages to platform trials should in many instances outweigh these potential challenges, especially as they become more commonly used and routine methodologies are established.

The Future of Platform Trials

The biopharmaceutical industry is at a critical inflection point of drug development. Almost everyone agrees that, to increase the return on investment, innovation in the form of novel trial design and data sharing must occur, in order to leverage collective knowledge across the industry and stakeholders. Recently, the Food and Drug Administration (FDA) approved tocilizumab for the treatment of CAR (chimeric antigen receptor) T cell-induced cytokine release syndrome, based upon retrospective analysis of pooled outcome data from clinical trials by independent pharmaceutical companies [7]. Such an event occurred as a result of a shared understandiing among industry partners, regulators, physicians, and patients, of the importance of approving an agent that significantly impacts the treatment course of leukemia patients undergoing CAR-T therapy. This desire to collaborate is a necessary component of the future of platform trials, enabling pathways to approval that are founded upon disease biology and a large treatment effect.

Beyond registrational intent, timely engagement with payers is crucial in order to establish mutual agreement upon the value of the trial outcomes to patients and to society. Greater incentives in support of transformational medications, rather than "me too" drugs, help to lay the foundation for such engagement. Finally, appropriate risk taking by developers is essential to the success of platform trials, enabled by early and frequent dialogue with academia, regulatory agencies, patients, payers, and organizations. This enables key stakeholders to regularly review current and future unmet needs, as well as address logistical barriers to effective drug development. These regular interactions may also enable the building and continued refinement of registrational pathways, in order to support drug development through such mechanisms as platform trials. For example, discussions among FDA, Friends of Cancer Research, and key stakeholders led to the development of initiatives such as the Breakthrough Therapy Designation, which established that, for drugs that have the potential to produce a substantial improvement over existing therapies, the FDA and the drug developer must work closely together to determine the most efficient path forward [8]. Such valuable additions to the current infrastructure enable efficient development of molecules with transformative capacity. Ultimately, these platform trials have the capacity to play an increasingly critical role in the development pathway, serving as engines for discovery and development of critical medicines. At any moment in time, an executive has to make difficult choices regarding resource allocation, while laboring under significant uncertainty. It is clear that platform trials can increase efficiency and help to reduce uncertainty, and in our view their use will undoubtedly increase—and rapidly.

References

1. Woodcock J, LaVangeLM. Master Protocols to Study Multiple Therapies, Multiple Diseases, or Both. *N Engl J Med*, 2017. 377(1): p. 62–70.
2. Stone RM, et al. Midostaurin Plus Chemotherapy for Acute Myeloid Leukemia with a FLT3 Mutation. *N Engl J Med*, 2017. 377(5): p. 454–464.
3. Bartsch R, de Azambuja E, I-SPY2: Optimising Cancer Drug Development in the 21st Century. *ESMO Open*, 2016. 1(5): p. e000113.
4. Herbst RS, et al. Lung Master Protocol (Lung-MAP)-A Biomarker-Driven Protocol for Accelerating Development of Therapies for Squamous Cell Lung Cancer: SWOG S1400. *Clin Cancer Res*, 2015. 21(7): p. 1514–1524.

5. Cunanan KM, et al. Basket Trials in Oncology: A Trade Off between Complexity and Efficiency. *J Clin Oncol*, 2017. 35(3): p. 271–273.
6. Saville BR BerrySM. Efficiencies of Platform Clinical Trials: A Vision of the Future. *Clin Trials*, 2016. 13(3): p. 358–366.
7. Genentech. *FDA Approves Genentech's Actemra (Tocilizumab) for the Treatment of CAR T Cell-Induced Cytokine Release Syndrome* 2017 [cited 2017 December 1]; www.gene.com/media/press-releases/14679/2017-08-30/fda-approves-genen techs-actemra-tocilizu.
8. Friends of Cancer Research. *About Breakthrough Therapies*. 2017 [cited2017 December 1]; www.focr.org/about-breakthrough-therapies.

Index

A

Accelerated Approval (AA), 105, **106**, 107
acute coronary syndrome (ACS), 100
adaptive alpha allocation, 146
Adaptive Design Scientific Working
    Group, xiii, xv, 51, 256
adaptive designs in RCTs, 100–2
adaptive patient allocation, 182
adaptive-randomization algorithm, 6,
    290
ADAPT platform trial, 190, 199
adjuvant therapy trials, 5, 6, *8*, 13, 16,
    109–10
administrative claims data, 55, *56*
African trypanosomiasis, 128
agent *vs.* control randomized clinical
    trial, 10
AIDS *see* HIV/AIDS
ALCHEMIST trial, 254
ALK mutation, 254
Alzheimer's Disease
    Dominantly Inherited Alzheimer
        Network, 184
    Dominantly Inherited Alzheimer's
        Disease (DIAN-TU), 189–90, 194
    European Prevention of Alzheimer's
        Dementia Consortium (EPAD),
        189–90
    platform trials, 184–5, 189–90
American Society of Clinical Oncology
    (ASCO), 31, 59, 111, 169
American trypanosomiasis, 128
ANOVA methodology, 266, 268
anthracycline-based chemotherapy, 6
antibiotics platform trials, 190
anti-EGFR antibody Cetuximab, 179
anti-HER2 tyrosine kinase inhibitor, 13
antiretroviral therapy (ART), 125

B

balanced incomplete-block design
    (BIBD), 269

basket trials
    with accelerated approval, 159–62,
        160, *161*
    application examples, 45–7
    Bayesian basket designs, 171–4, 228
    biomarker hypothesis, 50
    companion diagnostic assay, 49
    confirmatory basket trial, *61*, 61–7, *65*
    decision analysis, 148
    discussion, 227–8
    high screen failure rate, 50
    interim and final endpoints, 50–1
    hypothetical example of special
        interest, 226–7
    introduction to, 37–40, *38*, 211–13
    operating characteristic comparisons,
        218–20, *219*, **220**, **221**
    overview of design, 40–3, *41*
    in pharmaceutical frameworks, 79, *79*
    Phase II basket trials, 167–9, *169*,
        174–7, *175*
    Phase III basket trials, 174–7, *175*,
        213–27
    pooling risks, 47–9
    power and sample size calculations,
        216–18, *217*
    pruning, 40–2, 43–5
    pruning and pooling with different
        endpoints, 222–7
    pruning and pooling with same
        endpoint, 214–22
    randomized basket trials, 177–8, 226
    regulatory approval, 114
    single-arm basket trial example,
        221–2
    statistical designs for, 170–1
    statistical designs of Phase III basket
        trials, 213–27
    summary of, 51
    tissue acquisition and processing,
        49–50
Bayesian basket designs, 171–4, 228
Bayesian hierarchical modeling, 39, 183

Bayesian probabilities, 7, 9–10, 183
Bayesian updating, 74
BCR/ABL fusion protein, 23
benefit/cost ration (BCR), 142
benefit-risk assessment (BRA)
    approaches of, 234
    discussion, 249–50
    frameworks of, 234–7, *235, 236, 238*
    graphic tool use, 228, 237
    interim analysis, 244–6
    introduction to, 231–4, *233*
    multiple benefits and risks, 241–4, **243**
    quantitative methods, 238–48, **239**
    single benefit and risk, 240–1, **241**
    subgroup analysis, 246–8
    uncertainties in, 248–9
between trial heterogeneity parameter, 204
bias model, 203
Bill & Melinda Gates Foundation, 126, 127
binding futility, 44
biomarkers
    absence of, 23
    dependent efficacy *in vitro/in vivo*, 48
    development impact, 181
    hypothesis, 50
    hypothesis-testing biomarkers, 10, **12**
    interventions within multiple groups,
        189
    introduction to, 6, 7
    negative patients, 49, 50
    negative study impact on, 144–5, *145,
        147, 148*
    positive patients, 49
    study designs involving, 146
biopsies, 10, 28, 32, 89
blood mutations, 28–9
BRAF gene, 25–6, 48, 168, 170, 212
BRAFV600 mutant malignancies, 29, 31–2
brain cancer platform trial, 190
breast cancer, 6, 12, 186–8, **187**
B2225 study, 60
bucket trial *see* basket trials
Buruli ulcer, 127

C

cancer
    breast cancer, 6, 12, 186–8, **187**
    endometrial cancer, 30

gastric cancer, 30
    as heterogeneous, 6
    lung cancer, 23, 37, 85
    pancreatic cancer platform trial, 191
    public impact of, 104
    therapeutics increase in, 3
CancerLinQ, 59
cancer trial system, 85–6, 103
cardiovascular (CV) adverse events, 236,
    237, 241, 247
cardiovascular outcome trials (CVOTs),
    102
CAR-T therapy, 291–2
central screening component, 254
chaperone role, 16
chemotherapy
    anthracycline-based chemotherapy, 6
    cytotoxic chemotherapies, 23
    platinum-based chemotherapy, 94
    sorafenib in combination with, 25
chronic myelogenous leukemia (CML), 23
circulating tumor DNA (ctDNA), 28
Clinical Research Associate (CRA)
        certifications, 131
clinical trials
    cancer trial system, 85–6
    challenges to, 91–2
    collaborative clinical trial design,
        88–94
    community sites, 90–1
    costs of, 87
    efficiency of, 66–7
    efficient initiation, 89
    emerging data and, 93–4
    management of patient information,
        92–3
    origins of, 98–9
    patient access, 91
    patient accrual problems, 87–8, 89–90
    perpetual clinical trial, *80*, 80–1
    role of, 97
    shortcomings of, 86
    summary of, 94–5
    translatability to clinical practice, 88;
        see also Highly Efficient Clinical
        Trials
cluster trials
    design comparison, 274–9, **275, 276,**
        277, 278

exchange algorithms, 284–5
introduction to, 265–6, *266*
iterative algorithms, 283–4
model-based designs, 271–4, **273**
models and notations, 266–8
motivating example, 269–71, **270**
quantum computing, 279–81
summary of, 281–2
Cochrane Collaboration, 128
co-data setting, 203
collaborative clinical trial design, 88–94
colorectal cancer, 29–30, 48
combination therapies, 32, 97, 113, 268
combinatorial models, 271–4, **273**
commensurate prior, 203
common control protocol, 6, 111, 114,
    149, 184, 192, 200, 257
community acquired pneumonia (CAP),
    188
community sites for clinical trials, 90–1
companion diagnostic assay, 49
concurrent comparisons in platform
    trials, 193
concurrent control, 51, 78, 99, 201, *202*,
    203–5, 207
Conditional Marketing Authorization
    (CMA), 107
control data leveraging, 184–5
cysticercosis, 128
cystic fibrosis platform trial, 190–1
cytotoxic chemotherapies, 23

D

data and safety monitoring board
    (DSMB), 247
data management, 114–15
Data Monitoring Committee (DMC),
    101–2
decision analysis, 141–50, *143*, *145*, *147*, *148*
Operating Characteristics, 74
discrete design problems, 283–4
disease-free survival (DFS), 5
disease population of interest, 57
DNA alterations of tumors, 167, 168
Docetaxel experimental treatments, 206,
    206
driver DNA alterations, 167
drug development

benefit-risk assessment, 231
decision analysis and, 141
parallel approach, 153–4, 155–6, *161*
sequential approach, 153, 154–5, *155*,
    160; *see also* multiple stake-
    holders' requirements in drug
    development
drug-diagnostic development, 112
Drug Efficacy Study Implementation
    (DESI), 98
Drug Information Association (DIA)
    xiii, xv, 51, 256
durable response rate (DRR), 247

E

Ebola virus disease (EVD), 127, 182,
    188–9
echinococcosis, 128
effective sample size (ESS), 204
efficiencies in platform trials
    application of, 206, **206**
    discussion, 208–9, **209**
    hypothetic trial scenarios, 207
    incorporating historical control data,
        201–3, *202*
    introduction to, 197
    operating characteristics, 207–8, **208**,
        209
    operational efficiencies, 197–8
    statistical efficiencies, 198–201, *199*
electronic health records (EHR), 55, 58–9,
    63
encorafenib/binimetinib (enco/bini)
    treatment, 32
endometrial cancer, 30
engaging investigators, 16
epidermal growth factor receptor
    (EGFR), 23, 24–5, 254
Erdheim–Chester disease, 212
European Medicines Agency (EMA),
    111, 119–20
European network for health technology
    assessment (EUnetHTA),
    119–20
evidence generation, *57*, 57–60, 75
evidentiary requirements, 99–100
exchangeability, 201, 203–4, 207, 209
exchange algorithms, 284–5

expected Net Present Value (eNPV), 74, 76–7
experimental treatments, 200–1, 206, **206**, 211
extended phase II trials, 174–7, *175*

F

false positive rate control, 43–5
FDA Amendments Act, 58
FDA Modernization Act (FDAMA), 99
final endpoints in basket trials, 50–1
fit-for-purpose RWD sources, 67
fms-like tyrosine kinase 3 (FLT3) mutations, 290
FOCUS4 master protocol, 254
Fogarty International Center, 126
Food, Drug, and Cosmetic Act, 86
Food and Drug Administration (FDA)
    BRA framework, 231, 244
    breakthrough therapy designation (BTD), 105, 107–8
    Center for Biologics (CBER), 108
    Center for Devices and Radiologic Health (CDRH), 108
    Center for Drug Evaluation and Research (CDER), 90, 108
    drug-diagnostic development, 112
    Fast Track Designation (FTD), 105, 106–7
    Lung-MAP trial, 85
    New Drug Application (NDA), 107, 108
    off-label use of drugs, 170
    Priority Review Designation, 105
    regulatory approval by, 212, 228, 291
    response-adaptive randomization procedure, 127
    review of medical effectiveness, 98
    support for platform trials, 110–11, 115
    U.S. Food Drug & Cosmetic Act (FD&CA), 98, 99
Food and Drug Administration Reauthorization Act (FDARA), 102
Food and Drug Administration Safety and Innovation Act (FDASIA), 107–8
formalin fixed paraffin embedded (FFPE) block, 27

Foundation for the National Institutes of Health (FNIH), 14, 85
Foundation Medicine, 28
FRACTION-Lung study, 268
French SHIVA clinical trial, 177
Friends of Cancer Research, 85–6
functional research environment, 128–30

G

gastric cancer, 30
gastrointestinal (GI) adverse events, 236
Gaucher Disease, 115
GBM-AGILE trial, 199
good clinical practice (GCP), 99, 103, 130
graduated agent combination, 13

H

hazard ratio (HR), 13, 67, 175–6, 213, 218, 220, 226, 237, 257
health authority views on platform trials, 108–9
health technology agencies (HTA), 119–22
hematological malignancies, 60
heterogeneity, 45, 48, 247
hierarchical modeling of platform trials, 183
Highly Efficient Clinical Trials (HECT)
    functional research environment, 128–30
    introduction to, 125–6
    lessons learned before, 126–8
    role of, 131–6, *134*, *136*
    summary of, 137
high screen failure rate, 50
histology independent Phase III basket trials, 174–7, *175*
historical control, 58, 201–3, *202*
HIV/AIDS, 104, 107, 125, 126–8
hormone receptor (HR), 6, 16
hypothesis-testing biomarkers, 10, **12**
hypothetic trial scenarios, 207

I

immune system, 5–6
immunotherapy, 13, 18, 28–32, 85, 89
influenza platform trials, 191

institutional review board (IRB), 93
Intel, 4
Intention to Treat (ITT), 102–3
interactive response systems (IRS), 192–3
interactive voice response system
(IVRS), 188
inter-company platform trials, 198
interim analysis (IA), 244–6
interim endpoints in basket trials, 50–1
International Conference on
Harmonization (ICH), 103
In Vitro Diagnostic (IVD) test, 111
IRB review, 14
I-SPY trials
breast cancer, 186–8, **187**
design of, 6–10, **7**, *8*, *9*, *10*
engaging investigators, 16
faster knowledge turns, 4
introduction to, 3–4
lessons from, 13–14
precompetitive model, 14–15
predicting therapeutic response, 109,
110
progress of, 10–13, *11*, **12**
protocol approvals, 4–5
regulatory pathway, 15–16
shared control arm in, 199
smarter approach, 5–6
smarter outcomes, 5
standardization, 16–17
summary of, 18–19
iterative algorithms, 283–4

K

Kefauver-Harris Drug Amendments, 86
KEYNOTE-158 studies, 110–11
knowledge turns, 4–6, 10, 13, 16, 19
KRAS mutations, 25, 31, 179

L

Langerhans histiocytosis, 29, 212
life-cycle management, 231
LOGIC-2 study, 32
longitudinal models, 183
low prevalent histologies in Phase III
basket trials, 177
lung cancer, 23, 37, 85

Lung Master Protocol (Lung-MAP),
85–6, 89–90, 92–4, 199, 254, 290
lymphatic filariasis, 128

M

Markov-Chain Monte Carlo simulations,
246
MassARRAY (Sequenom), 27
master protocols
in clinical trials, 88–94
decision analysis, 141, 147
introduction to, 6, 10, 14
simulation study design, *256*, 256–7
simulation tool development, 257–8,
262–3
Subteam of the Small Populations
Workstream, 256
unlocking potential of, 17–18
Medical Research Council (MRC), 126
melanoma, 25–6, 247
meta-analytic combined (MAC)
approach, 203–5, 207–8, **208**
meta-analytic predictive (MAP)
approach, 203, 205
metastatic melanoma, 25–6
metastatic solid tumors, 28
microsatelliteinstability high (MSI-H),
110, 111
mis-match-repair-deficient (dMMR),
110, 111
mitogen activated protein kinase
(MAPK) pathway, 26
model-based optimal experimental
design theory, 271–4, **273**
Molecular Analysis for Therapy Choice
(MATCH) clinical trial, 93,
168–70
Molecular Profiling-Based Assignment of
Cancer Therapy (MPACT), 177
Moore's Law, 4
MRI volume change, 16
multi-arm, multi-drug trials, 119–23
multi-armed targeted therapy trials
blood mutations, 28–9
BRAF inhibitors in melanoma, 25–6
design of, 30–1
development of, 29–30

EGFR Inhibitors in non-small cell
        lung cancer, 24–5
    introduction to, 23–4
    multiplexed assays, 26–7
    summary of, 32–3
    tissue mutations, 27–8
multiple criteria decision analysis
        (MCDA), 241–4, **243**, 246
multiple stakeholders' requirements
    basket designs with accelerated
            approval, 159–62, *160, 161*
    case study, 156–7
    development options, 154–6
    introduction to, 153–4
    portfolio-level optimization, *157,*
            157–9
    summary of, 162–3
multiplexed assays, 26–7
mutations
    ALK mutation, 254
    blood mutations, 28–9
    fms-like tyrosine kinase 3 (FLT3)
            mutations, 290
    hematological malignancies with, 60
    KRAS mutations, 25, 31, 179
    tissue mutations, 27–8
    V600E mutations, 29, 168, 170

N

National Cancer Institute (NCI), 85
National Cancer Institute-Molecular
        Analysis for Therapy Choice
        (NCI-MATCH), 30–1, 255
needed to treat (NNT), 240–1, **241**, 244–5
neoadjuvant therapy, 5, 6, *8,* 13, 16,
        109–10
neratinib, 13
New Drug Application (NDA), 107, 108
New World cutaneous leishmaniasis, 128
next generation sequencing (NGS), 27–8,
        91, 92–3, 112
non-mutated cell lines, 26
non-oncology trials, 103
non-randomized basket trial, 48
non-small cell lung cancer (NSCLC)
    blood mutations, 28
    efficiencies in platform trials, 203–5,
            206, **206**

epidermal growth factor receptor,
        24–5
    multiple molecularly-defined
            categories in, 30
    mutations in, 254
    Vemurafenib therapy, 212
normal-normal hierarchical model
        (NNHM), 205
null hypothesis, 176, 178, 200, 214–15,
        223, 227–8
number needed to harm (NNH), 240–1,
        241, 244–5

O

objective decision criteria, 74–5
objective response rate (ORR), 107, 212,
        221–2, 225
O'Brien- Fleming group sequential
        stopping boundaries, 133–4,
        134
odds ratio (OR), 171, 237
off-label prescribing, 62–3, 66
oncogenic DNA alterations, 167
oncology trials
    Bayesian basket designs, 171–4
    cancer trial system, 85–6, 103
    discussion over, 178–9
    introduction to, 167
    Phase II basket trials, 167–9, *169*
    Phase III basket trials, 174–7, *175*
    platform trials in, 115
    randomized basket trials, 177–8
    statistical designs for basket trials,
            170–1; *see also* basket trials with
            Type I errors
operating characteristics, 74, 218–20,
        219, **220, 221**
operational bias in platform trials, 193–4
operational efficiencies, 197–8, 207–8, **208**
optimality in pharmaceutical
        frameworks, 75
orphan drug programs, 104–5, **105**
overall survival (OS), 40, 45–7

P

paclitaxel, 6, 24–5
pancreatic cancer platform trial, 191

parallel approach to drug development, 153–4, 155–6, *161*
partial exchangeability, 203
pathological complete response (pCR), 9, 13, 15, 109–10, 186
patient access to clinical trials, 91
patient accrual problems, 87–8, 89–90
patient assignment-to-stratum strategies, 263
PCORNET ADAPTABLE (Aspirin Dosing
A Patient-centric Trial Assessing Benefits and Long-term Effectiveness) trial, 59
PD-L1 staining, 30
PD-1/PD-L1 immune checkpoint inhibitors, 212
pediatrics and platform trials, 113–14
pembrolizumab immunotherapy, 13
perpetual clinical trial, *80*, 80–1
perpetual research trials, 131–6, *134, 136,* 184
pertuzumab, 12, 31, 110
pharmaceutical frameworks (PF)
    basket trials in, 79, *79*
    Bayesian updating, 74
    including platform trials, 78–80
    introduction to, 73
    objective decision criteria, 74–5
    optimality in, 75
    options and operating characteristics, 74
    perceived *vs.* objective risk, 73–4
    perpetual clinical trial, *80*, 80–1
    portfolio level quantitative work, 77–8, *78*
    Program-Level Quantitative Framework, 75–7, *76*
    summary, 81
    umbrella trials in, 80, *80*
Pharmaceutical Research and Manufacturers of America (PhRMA), 232
pharmacokinetic/pharmacodynamic (PK/PD) modelling, 100
Phase II basket trials, 167–9, *169*, 174–7, *175*
Phase III basket trials, 174–7, *175*, 213–27
PIPELINE of platform trials, 51

platform trials
    adaptive patient allocation, 182
    Alzheimer's Disease, 184–5, 189–90
    antibiotics, 190
    applications of, 186–91
    brain cancer, 190
    breast cancer, 186–8, **187**
    case studies, **109**, 109–11
    combination therapies, 113
    community acquired pneumonia, 188
    concurrent comparisons, 193
    control data leveraging, 184–5
    cystic fibrosis, 190–1
    drug-diagnostic development, 112
    Ebola virus, 127, 182, 188–9
    embedding within healthcare systems, 192–3
    future trends, 114–16, 291–2
    health authority views, 108–9
    hierarchical modeling, 183
    influenza, 191
    introduction to, 97, 181–2
    key statistical tools, 182–5
    limitations of, 291
    operational bias, 193–4
    other considerations, 191–4
    pancreatic cancer, 191
    pediatrics and, 113–14
    perpetual trial design, 184
    pharmaceutical frameworks including, 78–80
    population drift modeling, 185
    potential value of, 290–1
    predictive modeling, 183
    regulatory pathways, 103–8, **105, 106,** 194
    role of, 103–11
    simulation studies, 185
    special considerations, 112–14
    statistical efficiencies of, 191–2, 198–201, *199*
    summary of, 289–90; *see also* efficiencies in platform trials; I-SPY trials
platinum-based chemotherapy, 94
polymerase chain reactions (PCR) assays, 26
pooling of samples, 114
pooling risks in basket trials, 47–9

population drift modeling, 185
portfolio-level optimization, *157*, 157–9
power prior, 203
precompetitive model, 14–15
predictive modeling, 183
pre-market approved (PMA) test, 112
PREPARE-ALICE platform trial, 191
Prescription Drug User Fee Act
    (PDUFA), 57
President's Emergency Plan for AIDS
    Relief (PEPFAR), 125–6
prevalent histologies in Phase III basket
    trials, 174
Probability of Success (PoS), 74
Probability of Technical and Regulatory
    Success (PTRS), 74, 76–7
Program-Level Quantitative Framework
    (PLF), 75–7, *76*
progression free survival (PFS), 40, 45–6,
    222, 225, 226, 236, 241
proof of concept (POC) trials, 15, 142–4,
    143, 149
protocol approvals, 4–5
pruning and pooling with different
    endpoints, 222–7
pruning and pooling with same
    endpoint, 214–22
pruning external data, 40–2, 43–5
public-private platform trials, 198

Q

quadratic unconstrained optimization
    problems (QUBO), 279–81
quality of life (QoL) data, 120, 122, 236,
    237
Quantitative Sciences in the
    Pharmaceutical Industry (QSPI
    BRWG), 232, 238, 244, 246
quantum computing, 279–81
Quantum Leap Healthcare Collaborative
    (QLHC), 14

R

rabies, 128
randomized basket trials, 177–8, 226
randomized controlled trials (RCTs)
    agent *vs.* control, 10
    efficiency of, 3–4

emergence of adaptive designs, 100–2
evidentiary requirements, 99–100
future innovation in, 102–3
general considerations, 98
historical development of, 98–103
oncology trials, 167
origins of, 98–9
recording of, 9
Random high bias, 43–5
Randomized Embedded, Multifactorial,
    Adaptive Platform (REMAP)
    trial, 188, 190, 191, 192
RATIFY trial, 290
real-world data (RWD)
    confirmatory basket trial, *61*, 61–7, *65*
    for evidence generation, *57*, 57–60
    future considerations, 67–8
    to inform innovative platform trial
        designs, 60–1
    introduction to, 55–6, *56*
real world evidence (RWE), 56, 102, 121
redundancy issues, 4–5
regenerative medicine advanced therapy
    (RMAT), 105, 108
regression models, 271–4, **273**
regulatory pathways in platform trials,
    103–8, **105**, **106**, 194
resampling-based method, 243
Residual Cancer Burden (RCB), 17
resistance to therapy, 5–6
response adaptive randomization
    (RAR), 127, 182, 188
response rates (RR), **259**, 259–62, **261–2**
Return on Investment (RoI), 74
RISE (Rheumatology Informatics System
    for Effectiveness) registry, 59
ROS1 rearrangements, 28

S

Sentinel Initiative, 58–9
sequential approach to drug
    development, 153, 154–5, *155*,
    160
shared control, 199, 201
simulation studies, 185, *256*, 256–7
simulation tool development, 257–8, 262–3
single-arm basket trial, 221–2
small estimation bias, 40

sorafenib, 25
Southwest Oncology Group (SWOG), 85
squamous cell cancer (SCCA), 85
standardization in platform trials, 198
standardization of contracts, 14–15
standard of care (SOC), 212–13, 227
statistical efficiencies, 191–2, 198–201, *199*
stratum assignment strategies, 258
subgroup analysis, 246–8
surrogate endpoint, 41

T

Talimogene Laherparepvec (T-VEC) for
        melanoma, 247
Targeted Agent and Profile Utilization
        Registry (TAPUR), 31–2,
        169–70
targeted agent and profiling utilization
        registry (TAPUR) study, 111
Thrombin Receptor Antagonist in
        Secondary Prevention of
        Atherothrombotic Ischemic
        Events (TRA 2P), 247
Thrombolysis in Myocardial Infarction
        (TIMI) 50 trial, 247
Thrombus Aspiration in ST-Elevation
        Myocardial Infarction in
        Scandinavia (TASTE) trial, 59
tissue acquisition and processing,
        49–50
tissue mutations, 27–8
tocilizumab therapy, 291
tumor DNA, 167, 168
21st Century Cures Act, 102
Type I error, 40, 100, 170
Type II error, 144, 213

Type III error, 149
tyrosine kinase inhibitor (TKI), 25

U

umbrella trials
        analysis of response rates, 259,
                259–62, 261–2
        background on, 253–5, *254*
        decision analysis, 148–9
        discussion and implications, 262–3
        introduction to, 37–8, *38*
        Lung Master Protocol, 85–6, 89–90,
                92–4, 199, 254
        objective, 255–7, *256*
        in pharmaceutical frameworks, 80, *80*
        patient assignment-to-stratum
                strategies, 263
        patients positive for multiple
                markers, 255
        sample size and power calculations,
                258–9
        stratum assignment strategies, 258
up-front investment, 197
utility function, 141–2, *145*, *146*,
        146–9

V

Vemurafenib therapy, 26, 212
V600E mutations, 29, 168, 170
Vorapaxar treatment, 247

W

WASH interventions, 134, 135, *136*
Wellcome Trust, 127

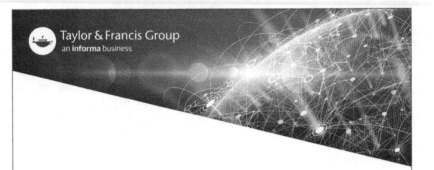